D0960315

Attachment and Psychopathology

ATTACHMENT
AND
PSYCHOPATHOLOGY

Edited by

LESLIE ATKINSON
KENNETH J. ZUCKER

THE GUILFORD PRESS
New York   London

All chapters in this book evolved from presentations made by the authors at a conference entitled "Attachment and Psychopathology," chaired by H. Bruce Ferguson, Ph.D., and held in Toronto, September 29–October 1, 1994. The conference was partially funded by the National Health Research and Development Program, Health and Welfare Canada, and the Ontario Mental Health Foundation.

© 1997 The Guilford Press
A Division of Guilford Publications, Inc.
72 Spring Street, New York, NY 10012

Printed in the United States of America

This book is printed on acid-free paper.

Last digit is print number: 9 8 7 6 5 4 3 2 1

Library of Congress Cataloging-in-Publication Data

Attachment and psychopathology / edited by Leslie Atkinson, Kenneth J. Zucker.
    p.   cm.
  Includes bibliographical references and index.
  ISBN 1-57230-191-0
  1. Attachment behavior. 2. Mental illness—Etiology. 3. Object relations (Psychoanalysis) 4. Attachment behavior in children. I. Atkinson, Leslie, Ph.D. II. Zucker, Kenneth J.
  [DNLM: 1. Object Attachment—in infancy & childhood. 2. Mother–Child Relations. 3. Child Behavior Disorders. WS 105.5.F2 A882 1997]
RC455.4.A84A88 1997
616.89′017—dc21
DNLM/DLC
for Library of Congress   96-49001
                                                                    CIP

Contributors

Leslie Atkinson, Ph.D., Clarke Institute of Psychiatry and University of Toronto, Toronto, Ontario, Canada

Marian J. Bakermans-Kranenburg, Ph.D., Center for Child and Family Studies, Leiden University, Leiden, The Netherlands

Diane Benoit, M.D., Psychiatric Research Unit, Hospital for Sick Children, and Department of Psychiatry, University of Toronto, Toronto, Ontario, Canada

Inge Bretherton, Ph.D., Department of Child and Family Studies, University of Wisconsin–Madison, Madison, Wisconsin

Patricia McKinsey Crittenden, Ph.D., Family Relations Institute, Miami, Florida

Michelle DeKlyen, Ph.D., Department of Psychiatry and Behavioral Sciences, University of Washington, Seattle, Washington

Marya C. Endriga, Ph.D., Department of Psychiatry and Behavioral Sciences, University of Washington, Seattle, Washington

Elizabeth Finley-Belgrad, M.D., Department of Psychiatry, St. Elizabeth's Hospital, Youngstown, Ohio; Northeast Ohio College of Medicine, Rootstown, Ohio

Peter Fonagy, Ph.D., Department of Psychology, University College London, and Anna Freud Centre, London, United Kingdom

Heather Georgeson, B.A., Department of Psychology, University of Wisconsin–Madison, Madison, Wisconsin

Susan Goldberg, Ph.D., Psychiatric Research Unit, Hospital for Sick Children, and Departments of Psychiatry and Psychology, University of Toronto, Toronto, Ontario, Canada

Mark T. Greenberg, Ph.D., Department of Psychology, University of Washington, Seattle, Washington

Roger Kennedy, M.D., Cassel Family Unit, and Charing Cross and Westminster Medical Schools, London, United Kingdom

Tom Leigh, MRc, Adult Department, Tavistock Clinic, London, United Kingdom

Molly Lependorf, B.A., Department of Psychology, University of Wisconsin–Madison, Madison, Wisconsin

Alice Levinson, MRCPsych., Cassel Hospital, London, United Kingdom

Alicia F. Lieberman, Ph.D., Department of Psychiatry, University of California, San Francisco, and San Francisco General Hospital, San Francisco, California

Michael Rutter, M.D., FRS, MRC Child Psychiatry Unit, and Social, Genetic, and Developmental Psychiatry Research Centre, Institute of Psychiatry, London, United Kingdom

Matthew L. Speltz, Ph.D., Department of Psychiatry and Behavioral Sciences, University of Washington, Seattle, Washington

Howard Steele, Ph.D., Department of Psychology, University College London, London, United Kingdom

Miriam Steele, Ph.D., Department of Psychology, University College London, and Anna Freud Centre, London, United Kingdom

Mary Target, Ph.D., Department of Psychology, University College London, and Anna Freud Centre, London, United Kingdom

Marinus H. van IJzendoorn, Ph.D., Center for Child and Family Studies, Leiden University, Leiden, The Netherlands

Reghan Walsh, B.A., Waisman Center, University of Wisconsin–Madison, Madison, Wisconsin

Charles H. Zeanah, M.D., Department of Psychiatry, Louisiana State University School of Medicine, New Orleans, Louisiana

Contents

III. IN THE CLINIC

SECTION I

GENERAL CONSIDERATIONS

1

Attachment and Psychopathology: From Laboratory to Clinic

LESLIE ATKINSON

In this chapter I offer a brief history of attachment theory as it relates to the study of psychopathology. This history serves as a context within which to conceptualize the themes that emerge across the following chapters. As the contributing authors struggled to import attachment theory from laboratory to clinic, they faced a common set of issues. The ways in which they addressed these concerns represent further "growing points of attachment theory and research."

FROM LABORATORY TO CLINIC

The necessity of importing attachment theory into the clinic is ironic. As a physician and psychoanalyst, John Bowlby advanced a model of human behavior which, first and foremost, was intended to explain abnormal development. He believed that psychoanalytic hypotheses were limited in this regard, being "so framed that they are not susceptible to test" (Bowlby, 1979, p. 26). Bowlby also derided the behavioral theories of academic psychologists as "struggling to cram a gallon of obstreperous human nature into a pint pot of prim theory" (p. 26). He won friends in neither camp.

However, it was the academic psychologists who first took up Bowlby's lead. Consistent with his medical training, Bowlby advanced a theory of trauma emphasizing physical separation, whether threatened or actual, and extreme emotional adversity. Whereas Bowlby (1978) also probed the implications of less dramatic attachment processes for the development of the nondisturbed personality, he recognized that supporting evidence was thin. It was Mary Ainsworth, a developmental psychologist, who amplified the conceptual link between attachment and typical development and who provided the empirical means to study it.

Conceptually, Ainsworth defined "separation" as a dimensional, interactive phenomenon reflected in the psychological availability (sensitivity) of the primary caregiver to the infant. Empirically, she provided (1) a set of anchored, context-dependent rating scales of parent–child interaction and (2) a 24-minute laboratory procedure, the Strange Situation, which combines a series of everyday stressors to neatly operationalize many fundamental attachment notions. Ainsworth's scheme for conceptualizing the Strange Situation behavior of infants permits the investigator to draw inferences about the nature of past caregiver–infant interactions and the ways in which they are represented by the infant (Ainsworth, Blehar, Waters, & Wall, 1978; for description of the Strange Situation and classifications derived therefrom, see Goldberg, Chapter 6, and van IJzendoorn & Bakermans-Kranenburg, Chapter 5, this volume; for critical appraisal of the Strange Situation, see Rutter, Chapter 2, this volume). These developments, both conceptual and empirical, permitted the study of attachment in typical, intact families. Theoretically compelling and empirically accessible, the study of attachment was quickly dominated by developmental psychologists (Bowlby, 1988).

Despite their relevance to the study of psychopathology (Bowlby, 1988), early investigations were restricted by the distinct purview of developmental psychology. This scope is limited to the comprehension of universal processes of normal development, including "the age range and sequences generally surrounding the emergence of certain capacities, . . . the changing manifestation of a capacity with development, the changing impact of context on a given capacity, and its changing organization with other capacities" (Sroufe & Rutter, 1984, p. 19). Specifically, investigators studied the predictors and changing organization of attachment, its stability and variation, its manifestations across cultures, and its implications for concurrent and later behavior. Some examples of prediction are offered below so as to map the return of attachment concepts from laboratory to clinic.

Prediction of Attachment Security

The "central" (Sroufe, 1985) or "preeminent" (Belsky & Isabella, 1988) example of the prediction of attachment security involves maternal sensitivity. Researchers, almost invariably studying nonclinical samples (cf.

Capps, Sigman, & Mundy, 1994), "consistently (but not universally)" (Belsky & Isabella, 1988, p. 45) demonstrated that sensitive mothers were more likely to raise securely attached infants than were less sensitive mothers (for meta-analytic review, see Goldsmith & Alansky, 1987; for critical appraisal of the sensitivity literature, see Schneider Rosen & Rothbaum, 1993; for discussion of sensitivity in the context of parental internal working models, see van IJzendoorn & Bakermans-Kranenburg, Chapter 5, this volume). If one accepts that secure attachment increases the probability of integrated personality development, then the implications of the sensitivity–attachment association for the study of psychological disturbance are obvious.

But it was the study of disturbed and maltreating parents that more immediately bridged the chasm between laboratory and clinic. For example, Radke-Yarrow, Cummings, Kuczynski, and Chapman (1985) found a greater incidence of insecure attachment among 2- and 3-year-old children with a parent experiencing a major affective disorder than among (1) children with a parent with minor depression or (2) youngsters whose parents were not depressed. In explaining these findings, Radke-Yarrow et al. invoked traditional developmental concerns, as forwarded by Ainsworth and colleagues. Radke-Yarrow et al. (1985) explained the link between parental depression and infant insecurity in terms of unpredictable and inconsistently sensitive caregiving. However, these authors also emphasized the influences of untoward affective communication and maternal sadness, irritability, hopelessness, helplessness, and confusion, factors not typically addressed by developmental psychologists. Furthermore, the study of depressed parents in the context of attachment theory invited consideration of factors such as increased marital conflict, assortative mating (the tendency of people with depression to choose partners with psychological difficulties), adverse interpersonal environment for both parents and children, comorbid diagnoses, and genetic factors, all associated with maternal depression (Downey & Coyne, 1990) and all potentially related to increased incidence of insecure attachment. Indeed, consideration of such a matrix of transacting factors constitutes the discipline of developmental psychopathology (Cicchetti, 1984, 1987; Cicchetti & Cohen, 1995a, 1995b; Sroufe & Rutter, 1984), a field that owes its resurgence, in large part, to attachment theory and research (Belsky & Isabella, 1988).

Prediction from Attachment Security

An analogous process occurred in which attachment security was used to predict subsequent behavior. For example, Matas, Arend, and Sroufe

(1978) found that infant attachment security was positively related to enthusiasm, persistence, and compliance in toddlerhood. Waters, Wippman, and Sroufe (1979) showed that infant attachment security was associated with later peer competence and ego strength/effectance. Whereas such findings are relevant to the study of psychopathology, a set of studies on attachment security and behavior disorders more explicitly combined attachment theory and clinical concerns.

Lewis, Feiring, McGuffog, and Jaskir (1984) showed that attachment security, as measured at 1 year, predicted degree of psychopathology at age 6. Specifically, insecurely attached boys showed significantly more internalizing behaviors, as reported by their mothers, than did securely attached boys. Lewis et al. found that the strength of the prediction from attachment security to behavior disorder depended not only on the child's sex, but also upon whether or not the child was planned, number of family life stress events, child's birth order, and number of friends the youngster had. Again, such studies make explicit both the link, and the complexity of the link, between attachment and clinical disturbance. Indeed, it was the Lewis et al. study, and a second investigation addressing similar issues (Erickson, Sroufe, & Egeland, 1985), that provided the direct incentive for the first volume dedicated specifically to the "clinical implications of attachment" (Belsky & Nezworski, 1988c).

The route back to the clinic was long and circuitous. Nevertheless, attachment theory was tested and revised (see Rutter, Chapter 2, this volume), such that it now rests on a firm empirical base derived from the study of typical development. This is an advantage that few other theories of abnormality can claim.

IMPLICATIONS AND APPLICATIONS

Perhaps the most basic theme of *Clinical Implications of Attachment* (Belsky & Nezworski, 1988a) involves the assertion that development is continuous; events occurring at any point in the lifespan have implications for subsequent outcomes, both typical and atypical. This notion is not new. Piaget (1957; cited by Flavell, 1963), for instance, bemoaned the artificial chasm separating those who study children and those who work only with adults. Erikson (1971) went so far as to suggest that the " 'oversight' concerning the fateful importance of childhood" (p. 73) is, in fact, intentional. While psychoanalytic thought might be pointed out as an important exception to this state of affairs (cf. Rutter, Chapter 2, this volume), some basic flaws within the theory can be attributed to extrapolation from the behavior of adults to that of children, rather than vice versa. Indeed, Freud (1920/1955) acknowledged:

So long as we trace the development from its final outcome backwards, the chain of events appears continuous, and we feel we have gained an insight which is completely satisfactory or even exhaustive. But if we proceed the reverse way, if we start from the premises inferred from the analysis and try to follow these up to the final results, then we no longer get the impression of an inevitable sequence of events which could not have been otherwise determined. We notice at once that there might have been another result, and that we might just as well have been able to understand and explain the latter. (pp. 167–168; see also Rieff, 1959, and Sroufe & Rutter, 1984; see Lyons-Ruth, Alpern, & Repacholi, 1993, for discussion of "asymmetrical empirical prediction")

Because of difficulties in demonstrating empirically developmental continuities, and despite isolated concerns regarding the spurious dissection of developmental processes, theoreticians constructed finely articulated models of discontinuity; continuous development was considered impossible, or at least unnecessary (see Belsky & Nezworski, 1988b). In this climate, Bowlby (1969) advanced the contention that early, reality-based experience has implications for normal personality development. Bowlby also argued that early experience played an important role in the development of depression and anxiety disorders, with specific reference to school refusal and agoraphobia as psychopathological manifestations of separation anxiety. In so doing, Bowlby restored to the study of typical and atypical populations the "central proposition underlying a developmental perspective" (Sroufe & Rutter, 1984, p. 21): Development is lawful.

Recent Developments

The contributors to *Clinical Implications of Attachment* (Belsky & Nezworski, 1988) exploited these insights. But they did so with three distinct disadvantages. First, they had little access to data on atypical populations. Only one chapter presented data on a bona fide abnormal sample (of maltreating mothers and their infants; Crittenden, 1988), and two chapters presented data on samples at risk (Speiker & Booth, 1988, on a low-socioeconomic-status sample; and Nezworski, Tolan, & Belsky, 1988, on families with insecure infants). By contrast, the passage of time has permitted the current volume contributors to collect data on divorced mothers, chronically ill infants, Romanian adoptees, children of mothers with anxiety disorders, boys with gender identity disorder, preschoolers with oppositional defiant disorder, forensic psychiatric inpatients, and inpatients with borderline personality disorder. In some respects, *Clinical*

Implications of Attachment represented the perspective of attachment theorists looking out from the laboratory. The present volume reports findings now that attachment researchers have stepped inside the clinic.

The second difficulty encountered by investigators at the time *Clinical Implications* was published involved the need to rely on the traditional A (insecure–avoidant), B (secure), C (ambivalent/resistant) attachment coding scheme. Despite the fact that they may represent less than optimal long-term adaptations, A and C are nonpathological strategies. However, work with atypical samples revealed the existence of pathological forms of attachment (see Goldberg, Chapter 6, and Rutter, Chapter 2, this volume). Given the dearth of such research prior to publication of *Clinical Implications,* only one study (Speiker & Booth, 1988) involved the "disorganized" dimension (D; Main & Solomon, 1986, 1990) and Crittenden (1988), having derived criteria for scoring A/C (Crittenden, 1985), was engaged in the first validation study of that classification. In subsequent years, these patterns were developed and validated such that all empirical studies in the current volume include one or another variant of atypical attachment. This is important because the addition of the disorganized dimension may dramatically improve prediction of subsequent disturbed behavior (Lyons-Ruth et al., 1993).

The third liability faced by *Clinical Implications* contributors was the lack of an assessment technology beyond infancy. Such a restriction can have a fourfold impact on the study of psychopathology.

1. Whereas attachment strategy is stable in low-risk samples (see Bretherton, 1985, for review), it is less so in high-risk populations (Vaughn, Egeland, Sroufe, & Waters, 1979; van IJzendoorn & Bakermans-Kranenburg, Chapter 5, this volume), which, ironically, are of particular import to research in attachment and psychopathology. Therefore, effect sizes linking earlier attachment strategy to later psychopathology may be attenuated by changing patterns of attachment. This difficulty can be diminished through use of attachment assessments that are temporally closer to the outcome measure.

2. The disorganized dimension (D), with its comparatively strong link to psychopathology, is relatively unstable (see Lyons-Ruth et al., 1993). This fact again points to the possible need for temporally close assessments of attachment strategy and psychopathology.

3. Different forms of psychopathology emerge at different stages of the lifespan and the same forms of psychopathology manifest themselves differently with maturation. Technologies for the measurement of attachment beyond infancy are crucial to understanding the (possibly changing) role of attachment in psychopathology as individuals age.

4. Many forms of disturbance are transgenerational in nature. If we

are to demonstrate that attachment strategy plays a part in the transmission of psychopathology, then we must measure attachment in both child and parent.

For these reasons, the assessment of attachment quality beyond infancy is crucial to the joint study of attachment and psychopathology. With one exception (Crittenden, 1988, who assessed preschoolers), contributions to *Clinical Implications* were restricted to assessing attachment security in infancy. By contrast, work in the intervening years (see Goldberg, Chapter 6, this volume) enabled all investigators in the present volume to assess attachment beyond infancy, specifically, in the early childhood and adult years.

Dilemmas of Application

Despite these new tools, however, reentry into the clinic presented attachment theorists and researchers with quandaries not evident from the outside. Goldberg (Chapter 6, this volume), for example, points out some difficulties in research design (low yield of individuals manifesting frank psychopathology in longitudinal study and confounded etiology when attachment strategy and psychological disturbance are measured concurrently) and theory (counterintuitive hypothesizing with regard to the outcome of avoidant and ambivalent attachments). Rutter (Chapter 2, this volume) also discusses a myriad of "unresolved questions," including issues pertaining to the behavioral control system, measurement of attachment security, qualities of attachment, the role of temperament, internal working models, manifestations of attachment after infancy, the influence of one relationship on another, differentiation of attachment relationships from other forms of relationship, the role of attachment in later disorder, and the role of parenting in attachment outcome. Fonagy et al. (Chapter 8, this volume) note the dearth of information about ecological and paternal factors as these influence attachment strategy.

Van IJzendoorn and Bakermans-Kranenburg (Chapter 5, this volume) and Rutter (Chapter 2, this volume) identify a mystery of central importance to the study of attachment. Van IJzendoorn and Bakermans-Kranenburg (Chapter 5, this volume) refer to this problem as the "transmission gap" (see also van IJzendoorn, 1995). Treating the matter differently, Rutter (Chapter 2, this volume) inquires about the "transformation of a dyadic quality into a characteristic of the individual." How do parents transmit their attachment strategies to their infants and children? Related to this issue, Lieberman (Chapter 9, this volume), Fonagy et al. (Chapter 8, this volume), and van IJzendoorn and Bakermans-Kranenburg allude to the oft neglected fact that caregiver and child attachment patterns are frequently mismatched.

Given this host of unresolved issues, both methodological and theoretical, it is not surprising, as Fonagy et al., Goldberg, and Rutter note, that investigators often fail to find the associations sought, or demonstrate the expected links in a highly qualified manner. (Goldberg, Chapter 6, this volume, also reminds us that the difficulties do not lie entirely in the domain of attachment theory, but reflect difficulties in the measurement of psychopathology.)

Some Attempted Resolutions

To meet the challenge of unconfirmed or partially confirmed associations, contributors to the current volume adopted three broad strategies. They (1) deleted or deemphasized aspects of the theory in response to empirical or clinical observations, (2) (re)introduced other theoretical frameworks and modifications to augment attachment concepts and increase the scope of their explanatory power, and/or (3) applied nontraditional data analytic procedures.

Streamlining Theory

With reference to streamlining the theory, Rutter (Chapter 2, this volume) records the failure to confirm empirically the concepts of imprinting, sensitive periods, monotropy, and the deterministic nature of early relationships. In addition, Rutter cautions that the effects of inconsistent caregiving and loss must be carefully parsed from the consequences of associated environmental conditions (see also Bretherton, Walsh, Lependorf, & Georgeson, Chapter 4, this volume) so as not to attribute to one the influence of the other (and thereby exaggerate the effects of attachment issues).

As discussed above, a major hypothesis of attachment theory is that maternal sensitivity influences strongly quality of later attachment. So important is the proposition that it has been addressed in approximately 40 studies (see Atkinson, Paglia, Coolbear, Niccols, & Guger, 1996; Goldsmith & Alansky, 1987). However, Goldsmith and Alansky (1987) showed that the sensitivity–attachment link is only a modest one. In the current volume, van IJzendoorn and Bakermans-Kranenburg (Chapter 5; see also van IJzendoorn, 1995) at once demonstrate the *comparative* weakness of the sensitivity variable and the importance of parental internal working models in influencing the child's attachment strategy. This reversal in emphasis will hasten the move away from the study of caregiver behavior toward the "level of representation" (Main, Kaplan, & Cassidy, 1985).

Discarding unsubstantiated aspects of the theory and deemphasizing others helps ensure the validity of premises adopted to guide research in new areas. As mentioned earlier, one great advantage of the attachment paradigm for the investigation of disorder is that it now rests on an empirical foundation derived from the study of typical development.

Empirical work with typical populations invalidates certain aspects of theory; so too, clinical application reveals that other concepts have less practical value than theoretical or research considerations might suggest. While acknowledging the extreme theoretical utility of attachment classifications, Lieberman (Chapter 9, this volume) and Zeanah, Finley-Belgrad, and Benoit (Chapter 10, this volume) imply that reification of behavior patterns may obscure full comprehension of the individual or dyad in clinical situations. These contributors avoid classifying attachment in their presentations of clinical case material. Crittenden (Chapter 3, this volume), too, recognizes the limitations of classifying attachment quality, presenting instead an expanded, dimensional perspective on attachment behavior.

Corollary to deemphasizing attachment classifications, Lieberman (Chapter 9, this volume) and Zeanah et al. (Chapter 10, this volume) question the role of intergenerational similarities in attachment strategy. In their clinical presentations, Lieberman and Zeanah et al. emphasize the differences between parents and children. Indeed, Fonagy et al. (Chapter 8, this volume) suggest that the study of such mismatches may be critical to understanding some forms of psychopathology. Van IJzendoorn and Bakermans-Kranenburg (Chapter 5, this volume) address systematically some of the conditions under which intergenerational transmission can be blocked (see also van IJzendoorn, Juffer, & Duyvesteyn, 1995). The position of these contributors contrasts with the current emphasis on intergenerational continuity in attachment strategy (cf. van IJzendoorn, 1995).

Integration and Theory Expansion

Volume contributors also integrated complementary conceptual frameworks into attachment theory or modified the theory in other ways. Crittenden (Chapter 3, this volume) expands the purview of attachment theory by suggesting that it must explain two principal evolutionary issues: safety, a central Bowlbian concern, and reproduction, more salient in Freudian thought. In service of such an explication, Crittenden extends the traditional attachment classification scheme and presents it as a continuous dimension with "anchor points" (classifications). Each classification is defined in terms of the cognitive/affective balance it reflects. Crittenden also theorizes about lifespan changes, sex differences, and the extreme adaptive advantages of even the most high-risk attachment patterns.

Noting that there is no simple association between psychopathology and insecure attachment, Fonagy et al. (Chapter 8, this volume) advance three interrelated arguments.

1. These authors review the sociological literature and suggest that attachment serves to protect the individual from criminality by reducing vulnerability to high-risk environments.

2. Rooting their conceptions in the work of Anna Freud, Fonagy et al. conceptualize attachment patterns as mechanisms of defense. Psychopathology occurs when the adopted attachment strategy fails to protect the individual from anxiety. The probability of such an outcome increases when an individual develops an attachment strategy that is asymmetrical with those of his or her primary caregivers.

3. Augmenting their theory of criminality with a selective appraisal of borderline personality disorder, Fonagy et al. argue that criminals lack a "reflective self" function. Criminals do not have the sense of agency and empathy that derives from adequate parenting. Lacking a representational basis for interaction, they seek (sometimes violently) concrete solutions to sociopsychological problems.

In contrast to Fonagy et al. (Chapter 8, this volume), Goldberg (Chapter 6, this volume) and Greenberg, DeKlyen, Speltz, and Endriga (Chapter 7, this volume) argue that simple prediction from child attachment security to later psychopathology does have merit, but that predictions must be founded on observation as well as theory. Basing their hypotheses on the behavior of infants in the Strange Situation (Goldberg) and clinical observation (Greenberg et al.), and contrary to accepted theory, these investigators demonstrate that avoidant preschoolers are more likely than ambivalent youngsters to evince both internalizing and externalizing disturbances. Van IJzendoorn and Bakermans-Kranenburg (Chapter 5, this volume) report a similar finding with regard to adults.

Several contributors address the issue of continuity and discontinuity in the intergenerational transmission of attachment strategy. Van IJzendoorn and Bakermans-Kranenburg (Chapter 5, this volume) synthesize past research to propose a model that includes early attachment experiences, later attachment relationships, attachment representations, social context, parenting behavior, characteristics of the baby, and the infant's attachment experiences. Zeanah et al. (Chapter 10, this volume) substantiate the concepts of derogation and identification with the aggressor across three generations. They demonstrate how these concepts both broaden the explanatory scope of attachment theory and deepen the understanding of human lives in the clinical setting. Also using clinical case material, Lieberman (Chapter 9, this volume) offers a synthesis of attachment, attribution, and psychoanalytic theories. Attribution theory augments the current attachment emphasis on information processing. Complementary to her emphasis on attributions, Lieberman recovers and repositions fantasy in reality-based attachment theory (cf. Rutter, Chapter 2, this volume, on attachment theory as the patricidal misericord of psychoanalysis).

Data Analysis

Other investigators met the challenges of clinical material with less traditional data analytical approaches. To understand the discrepancies between three attachment assessments, for example, Greenberg et al. (Chapter 7, this volume) adopted a "person-oriented view of the data, where the unit of analysis was the individual case" (p. 211). The analysis proved of great heuristic value, suggesting a role for state (as opposed to trait) variables, motivational issues, and historical–environmental concerns. As Greenberg et al. point out, these matters are "what a clinician factors into an evaluation and diagnosis . . . [, explaining] why clinical assessment is . . . an ongoing process, rather than . . . a one-time event" (p. 212). Also trying to comprehend clinical data, Bretherton et al. (Chapter 4, this volume) take a phenomenological, qualitative approach to mothers' perspectives on coparenting after divorce. The strategy affords a textural sense of postdivorce mothering that would have been obscured had Bretherton et al. addressed the data in purely quantitative terms. When investigating clinical issues, researchers who have traditionally relied on nomothetic methods adopt a more idiographic approach.

CONCLUSIONS

Despite roots in the study of psychopathology, attachment theory became a mainstay of developmental psychology. This volume reflects the full return of attachment theory to the clinic. It is hoped that the combination of novel theory, new data, and nontraditional data analytic techniques will fuel the growing interest of attachment theorists and researchers in matters clinical while enhancing the explanatory potential of attachment theory for practicing clinicians.

ACKNOWLEDGMENTS

This chapter was supported in part by a research grant from the Social Sciences and Humanities Research Council of Canada.

REFERENCES

Ainsworth, M. D. S., Blehar, M. C., Waters, E., & Wall, S. (1978). *Patterns of attachment: A psychological study of the Strange Situation.* Hillsdale, NJ: Erlbaum.

Atkinson, L., Paglia, A., Coolbear, J., Niccols, A., & Guger, S. (1996). *Infant attachment security: A meta-analysis of maternal predictors.* Manuscript submitted for publication.

Belsky, J., & Isabella, R. A. (1988). Maternal, infant, and socio-contextual determinants of attachment security. In J. Belsky & T. Nezworski (Eds.), *Clinical implications of attachment* (pp. 41–94). Hillsdale, NJ: Erlbaum.

Belsky, J., & Nezworski, T. (Eds.). (1988a). *Clinical implications of attachment.* Hillsdale, NJ: Erlbaum.

Belsky, J., & Nezworski, T. (1988b). Clinical implications of attachment. In J. Belsky & T. Nezworski (Eds.), *Clinical implications of attachment* (pp. 3–17). Hillsdale, NJ: Erlbaum.

Belsky, J., & Nezworski, T. (1988c). Preface. In J. Belsky & T. Nezworski (Eds.), *Clinical implications of attachment* (pp. xv–xvii). Hillsdale, NJ: Erlbaum.

Bowlby, J. (1969). *Attachment and loss: Vol. 1. Attachment.* Harmondsworth, Middlesex: Penguin.

Bowlby, J. (1978). *Attachment and loss: Vol. 2. Separation.* Harmondsworth, Middlesex: Penguin.

Bowlby, J. (1979). *The making and breaking of affectional bonds.* London: Tavistock.

Bowlby, J. (1988). Developmental psychiatry comes of age. *American Journal of Psychiatry, 145,* 1–10.

Bretherton, I. (1985). Attachment theory: Retrospect and prospect. In I. Bretherton & E. Waters (Eds.), Growing points in attachment theory and research. *Monographs of the Society for Research in Child Development, 50*(1–2, Serial No. 209), 3–36.

Capps, L., Sigman, M., & Mundy, P. (1994). Attachment security in children with autism. *Development and Psychopathology, 6,* 249–261.

Cicchetti, D. (1984). The emergence of developmental psychopathology. *Child Development, 55,* 1–7.

Cicchetti, D. (1987). Developmental psychopathology in infancy: Illustration from the study of maltreated youngsters. *Journal of Consulting and Clinical Psychology, 55,* 837–843.

Cicchetti, D., & Cohen, D. (Eds.). (1995a). *Developmental psychopathology: Vol. 1. Theory and methods.* New York: Wiley.

Cicchetti, D., & Cohen, D. (Eds.). (1995b). *Developmental psychopathology: Vol. 2. Theory and methods*. New York: Wiley.

Crittenden, P. (1985). Maltreated infants: Vulnerability and resilience. *Journal of Child Psychology and Psychiatry, 26*, 85–96.

Crittenden, P. (1988). Relationships at risk. In J. Belsky & T. Nezworski (Eds.), *Clinical implications of attachment* (pp. 136–174). Hillsdale, NJ: Erlbaum.

Downey, G., & Coyne, J. C. (1990). Children of depressed parents: An integrative review. *Psychological Bulletin, 108*, 50–76.

Erickson, E. H. (1971). *Identity: Youth and crisis*. London: Faber & Faber.

Erickson, M., Sroufe, L. A., & Egeland, B. (1985). The relationship between quality of attachment and behavior problems in preschool in a high risk sample. In I. Bretherton & E. Waters (Eds.), Growing points in attachment theory and research. *Monographs of the Society for Research in Child Development, 50*(1–2, Serial No. 209), 147–186.

Flavell, J. H. (1963). *The developmental psychology of Jean Piaget*. Toronto: Van Nostrand Reinhold.

Freud, S. (1955). The psychogenesis of a case of homosexuality in a woman. In J. Strachey (Ed. and Trans.), *The standard edition of the complete psychological works of Sigmund Freud* (Vol. 18, pp. 145–172). London: Hogarth Press. (Original work published 1920)

Goldsmith, H. H., & Alansky, J. A. (1987). Maternal and infant temperamental predictors of attachment: A meta-analytic review. *Journal of Consulting and Clinical Psychology, 55*, 805–816.

Lewis, M., Feiring, C., McGuffog, C., & Jaskir, J. (1984). Predicting psychopathology in six-year-olds from early social relations. *Child Development, 55*, 123–136.

Lyons-Ruth, K., Alpern, L., & Repacholi, B. (1993). Disorganized infant attachment classification and maternal psychosocial problems as predictors of hostile–aggressive behavior in the preschool classroom. *Child Development, 64*, 572–585.

Main, M., Kaplan, N., & Cassidy, J. (1985). Security in infancy, childhood, and adulthood: A move to the level of representation. In I. Bretherton & E. Waters (Eds.), Growing points in attachment theory and research. *Monographs of the Society for Research in Child Development, 50*(1–2, Serial No. 209), 66–104.

Main, M., & Solomon, J. (1986). Discovery of a new, insecure-disorganized/disoriented attachment pattern. In M. Yogman & T. B. Brazelton (Eds.), *Affective development in infancy* (pp. 95–124). Norwood, NJ: Ablex.

Main, M., & Solomon, J. (1990). Procedures for identifying infants as disorganized/disoriented during the Ainsworth Strange Situation. In M. T. Greenberg, D. Cicchetti, & E. M. Cummings (Eds.), *Attachment in the preschool years: Theory, research. and intervention* (pp. 121–160). Chicago: University of Chicago Press.

Matas, L., Arend, R., & Sroufe, L. A. (1978). Continuity in adaptation in the second year: The relationship between quality of attachment and later competence. *Child Development, 49*, 547–556.

Nezworski, T., Tolan, W. J., & Belsky, J. (1988). Intervention in insecure infant attachment. In J. Belsky & T. Nezworski (Eds.), *Clinical implications of attachment* (pp. 352–386). Hillsdale, NJ: Erlbaum.

Radke-Yarrow, M., Cummings, E. M., Kuczynski, L., & Chapman, M. (1985). Patterns of attachment in two- and three-year-olds in normal families and families with parental depression. *Child Development, 56,* 884–893.

Rieff, P. (1959). *Freud: The mind of the moralist.* New York: Viking.

Schneider Rosen, K. S., & Rothbaum, F. (1993). Quality of parental caregiving and security of attachment. *Developmental Psychology, 29,* 358–545.

Speiker, S. J., & Booth, C. L. (1988). Maternal antecedents of attachment quality. In J. Belsky & T. Nezworski (Eds.), *Clinical implications of attachment* (pp. 95–135). Hillsdale, NJ: Erlbaum.

Sroufe, L. A. (1985). Attachment classification from the perspective of infant–caregiver relationships and infant temperament. *Child Development, 56,* 1–14.

Sroufe, L. A., & Rutter, M. (1984). The domain of developmental psychopathology. *Child Development, 55,* 17–29.

van IJzendoorn, M. H. (1995). Adult attachment representations, parental responsiveness, and infant attachment: A meta-analysis on the predictive validity of the adult attachment interview. *Psychological Bulletin, 117,* 387–403.

van IJzendoorn, M. H., Juffer, F., & Duyvesteyn, M. G. C. (1995). Breaking the intergenerational cycle of insecure attachment: A review of the effects of attachment-based interventions on maternal sensitivity and infant security. *Journal of Child Psychology and Psychiatry, 36,* 225–248.

Vaughn, B., Egeland, B., Sroufe, L. A., & Waters, E. (1979). Individual differences in infant–mother attachment at twelve and eighteen months: Stability and change in families under stress. *Child Development, 50,* 971–979.

Waters, E., Wippman, J., & Sroufe, L. A. (1979). Attachment, positive affect, and competence in the peer group: Two studies in construct validation. *Child Development, 50,* 821–829.

2

Clinical Implications of Attachment Concepts: Retrospect and Prospect

MICHAEL RUTTER

The year 1994 marked the 25th anniversary of the publication of the first volume of Bowlby's hugely important trilogy on attachment (Bowlby, 1969/1982, 1973, 1980). It had its origins in his 1951 WHO monograph in which he pointed to the likely ill effects on personality development of prolonged institutional care and/or frequent changes of mother figure during the early years of life (Bowlby, 1951). This led to major improvements in the care of young children in hospitals and residential institutions. Nevertheless, his arguments initially had quite a critical reception from academic psychologists (e.g., O'Connor & Franks, 1960) and his suggestions on the importance of attachment relationships were rejected by the psychoanalytic establishment in a manner that often was personally hostile (see Grosskurth, 1986; Holmes, 1993a, 1993b).

Yet, despite its initially negative reception, most of the key components of attachment concepts have received empirical support (Belsky & Cassidy, 1994; Rajecki, Lamb, & Obmascher, 1978; Rutter, 1991). Moreover, attachment ideas have come to dominate writings on relationships and social development in adult life (Hazan & Shaver, 1994; Parkes, Stevenson-Hinde, & Morris, 1991) as well as in childhood (e.g., Bretherton, 1990; Bretherton & Waters, 1985; Campos, Barrett, Lamb, Goldsmith, & Stenberg, 1983; Greenberg, Cicchetti, & Cummings, 1990; Sroufe, 1983). Finally, there has been a growing awareness of the potentially important implications of attachment concepts for clinical practice (Belsky & Nezworski, 1988). The time seems right for a reconsideration of those clinical implications. Necessarily, however, this requires first a reappraisal of the key components of attachment theory and of the extent to which they have been supported by empirical research findings.

ATTACHMENT THEORY

Bowlby's (1951) WHO monograph proposed that the formation of an ongoing relationship with the child is as important a part of parenting as is the provision of experiences, discipline, and child care. Although rejected by some at the time (see Casler, 1968), this view is now generally accepted (Dunn, 1993; Hinde, 1979; Rutter, 1981, 1991; Sameroff & Emde, 1989; Schaffer, 1990). The argument focused attention on the need to consider parenting in terms of consistency of caregivers over time and parental sensitivity to children's individuality.

Bowlby's (1969/1982, 1973, 1980) trilogy on attachment took matters forward in five key ways. First, it differentiated attachment qualities from other aspects of relationships. Thus, it was noted that whereas anxiety increased attachment behavior, it inhibited playful interactions. Second, Bowlby placed the development of attachments within the context of normal developmental processes and proposed specific mechanisms. Most crucially, Bowlby placed emphasis on the role of attachment in promoting security and, thereby, encouraging independence. The importance of this point lay in its differentiation of attachment from dependency (Maccoby & Masters, 1970; Sroufe, Fox & Pancake, 1983) and, in so doing, underlining that the development of attachments was not just an immature phase of dependency to be "got over," but rather a feature that should serve to foster maturity in social functioning. Third, the development of attachments was placed firmly in a biological framework. The process was seen as an intrinsic feature of human development as social beings and not a secondary feature learned as a result of the rewards of feeding. Fourth, Bowlby suggested a mental mechanism, namely internal working models of relationships, as a means for both the carry forward of the effects of early attachment experiences into later relationships and also a mechanism for change. Fifth, Bowlby made various suggestions about the ways in which an insecurity in selective early attachments might play a role in the genesis of later psychopathology.

All of these key features have received substantial support from empirical research (Belsky & Cassidy, 1994; Rajecki et al., 1978; Rutter, 1981, 1991) and have had very important implications for both theory (Sroufe & Rutter, 1984) and practice (Holmes, 1993a, 1993b; Schaffer,

1990). Of course, the early specification of attachment theory did not prove correct in all its details. Four main changes have taken place over the years. First, in his early writings, Bowlby drew parallels between the development of attachments and imprinting (Bowlby, 1969/1982). It became apparent that there were more differences than similarities and this parallel was dropped later on (Bowlby, 1988) and is no longer seen as helpful by most writers on attachment. Second, and similarly, early accounts emphasized the need for selective attachments to develop during a relatively brief "sensitive period" in the first 2 years of life, with the implication that even very good parenting that is provided after this watershed is too late. In keeping with the changes that have taken place in thinking about sensitive periods more generally, it has become clear that this all or nothing view required modification. There is a sensitive period during which it is highly desirable that selective attachments develop, but the time frame is probably somewhat broader than initially envisaged and the effects are not as fixed and irreversible as once thought. The third change concerns abandonment of the notion of "monotropy." Bowlby's early writings were widely understood to mean that there was a biological need to develop a selective attachment with just one person and that the quality of this relationship differed from that of all others. The hypothesis of a high degree of selectivity (so that there is not an interchangeability among relationships) has been amply confirmed. What is now clear, however, is that although there are very definite hierarchies in selective attachments, it is usual for most children to develop selective attachments with a small number of people who are closely involved in child care. Finally, it came to be appreciated that social development was affected by later, as well as earlier, relationships (Bowlby, 1988). Nevertheless, these modifications aside, the major tenets of attachment theory have been broadly confirmed. Of course, that is not to say that there is not a host of crucial questions remaining to be answered. There is. Let me deal with these by considering a round baker's dozen of issues.

UNRESOLVED QUESTIONS

Behavioral Control System

From the outset, a central feature of attachment theory concerned the proposition that attachment was under the control of a biologically based behavior system. For a long time, there was a major problem in terminology, as the same word "attachment" was used to refer to discrete patterns of behavior (such as proximity seeking), to a dyadic relationship, to a postulated inbuilt predisposition to develop specific attachments to individuals, and to the hypothesized internal controlling mechanisms for this predisposition (see Hinde, 1982). Few would doubt the need to invoke some such control system, and helpful guidelines are available in the evidence on the conditions that promote proximity-seeking behavior in young children. Thus, one of the important early observations was that fear intensifies proximity seeking and that, if there is no one else to turn to, infants will cling even to an abusing parent. The monkey studies undertaken by Harlow and his colleagues (see, e.g., Harlow & Harlow, 1969) also indicated that this tendency to cling was not a function of feeding. The psychoanalytic and behavioral secondary drive views could be rejected firmly. Bowlby (1969/1982) argued that three types of features tended to activate attachment: tiredness or distress of the child; threatening features in the environment; and absence or moving away of the attachment figure. Experimental work over the last two decades has shown also that there are neuroendocrine and neurobiological accompaniments of attachment responses (Hofer, 1994; Kraemer, 1992; Levine, 1982). Nevertheless, substantial uncertainty remains on the sort of control system to be envisaged (should this be in neurobiological terms or in cognitive functioning?) and there is continuing uncertainty as to quite how the hypothesized system might actually work. It seems likely that the mechanisms involved in determining that *proximity seeking* takes place in a particular way and at a particular time may not be the same as the mechanisms involved in determining the *qualities* of a selective attachment relationship.

Measurement of Attachment Security

A major step forward in the study of attachment relationships came with Ainsworth's recognition that the security or insecurity of an attachment relationship constituted a crucial aspect of individual differences in such relationships, together with her development of the Strange Situation procedure for assessing attachment security (Ainsworth, Blehar, Waters, & Wall, 1978). It has worked remarkably well and has become the standard form of measurement in attachment research. Nevertheless, it is by no means free of limitations (see Lamb, Thompson, Gardner, Charnov, & Estes, 1984). To begin with, it is very dependent on brief separations and reunions having the same meaning for all children. This may be a substantial constraint when applying the procedure in cultures, such as that in Japan (see Miyake, Chen, & Campos, 1985), in which infants are rarely separated from their mothers in ordinary circumstances. Equally, separations from the main caregiver may not constitute the same stressor for children reared in institutions in which child care is shared among multiple, changing adults (see below). Also, because older children have the cognitive capacity to maintain relationships when the other person is not present, separations may not provide the same stress for them. Modified procedures based on the Strange Situation have been developed for older preschool children (see Belsky & Cassidy, 1994; Greenberg et al., 1990; Stevenson-Hinde & Shouldice, 1995) but it is much more dubious whether the same approach can be used in middle childhood. Moreover, despite its manifest strengths, the procedure is based on just 20 minutes of behavior, with the categories mainly reliant on the brief period following reunion. It can scarcely be expected to tap all the relevant qualities of a child's attachment relationships. Q-sort procedures based on much longer naturalistic observations in the home and interviews with mothers now exist, extending the data base (see Vaughn & Waters, 1990). This approach has advantages but also it has the important limitation that the observations extend well beyond the stress situations postulated to elicit attachment behaviors. A further constraint is that the Strange Situation coding procedure results in discrete categories rather than in continuously distributed dimensions. Not only is this likely to provide boundary problems, but also it is not at all obvious that discrete categories best represent the concepts that are inherent in attachment security. It seems much more likely that infants vary in their degrees of security and there is a need for measurement systems that can quantify this individual variation.

Qualities of Attachment

Following Ainsworth's extremely important and influential lead (Ainsworth, 1967; Ainsworth et al., 1978), attachment relationships have been classified as showing security, avoidant insecurity, and resistant insecurity. During the last decade, however, it became apparent that some children's behavior did not fit readily into any of these three patterns and, moreover, that some children with a known history of abuse and neglect were classified as secure, although their behavior outside the Strange Situation suggested abnormalities. This led to the development of an avoidant/ambivalent or disorganized category (Crittenden, 1988; Main & Solomon, 1990; Radke-Yarrow, Cummings, Kuczynski, & Chapman, 1985). Even with this additional category it remains quite uncertain whether the concept of insecurity, and its classification, is adequate to cover individual variations in attachment relationships (Rutter, 1980). Thus, for example, in two studies (Rogers, Ozonoff, & Maslin-Cole, 1991; Sigman & Ungerer, 1984) children with autism, who show severe relationship deficits, did not stand out in terms of their responses to the Strange Situation, at least as traditionally measured. In a third study (Capps,

Sigman, & Mundy, 1994) all the autistic children showed disorganized attachment but 40% of those were subclassified as securely attached, and the overall pattern was not well captured by any of the categories. Also, children reared in institutions with an ever-changing roster of numerous caregivers tend to show patterns of indiscriminant proximity seeking that is obviously abnormal, but with qualities not well captured by measures of insecurity (see Goldberg, Chapter 6, this volume).

The Role of Temperament

For a long time, attachment theorists were very reluctant to accept the possibility that the infant's own temperamental characteristics might influence the qualities of attachment security (Sroufe et al., 1983). They emphasized that the concept applied to a dyadic relationship and not to an individual feature and that, empirically, the security shown in a child's relationship with one parent bore only a weak association with the quality shown in the relationship with the other parent (Fox, Kimmerly, & Schafer, 1991). The evidence on the connections between temperament and attachment security are limited, but it now seems apparent that a temperamental dimension reflecting negative emotionality is associated with insecure attachment, although it is only one of many factors that influence children's responses to separation and reunion (Goldsmith & Alansky, 1987; Thompson, Connell, & Bridges, 1988; Vaughn et al., 1992).

Transformation of a Dyadic Quality into an Individual Characteristic

The process by which a relationship quality becomes transformed into an individual characteristic remains a crucial unanswered question. There is no doubt that attachment security starts as a dyadic relationship feature, as shown by the repeated finding that the quality of a child's relationship with one person is only weakly related to the quality of relationships with other people. On the other hand, attachment theory has always argued that later relationships are strongly affected by early attachment relationships. Also, empirical findings indicate that there are continuities with later peer relationships, so that some reflection of attachment quality must be carried forward within the individual unless the continuity is merely a consequence of continuity in environmental influences (Belsky & Cassidy, 1994; Rutter, 1991). The latter cannot be a sufficient explanation in all circumstances, if only because Hodges and Tizard's (1989a, 1989b) follow-up of residential nursery children showed that the links between relationships persisted in spite of a change of environment. But if, as has been shown, children's relationships with key figures in their environment vary in their security qualities, how are discrepant relationships dealt with in the transformation into an individual characteristic? Does the most important relationship predominate, is there a balance between differing relationships, or does one secure relationship compensate for insecurities in others? No very satisfactory explanation has been found and tested.[1]

Internal Working Models

The prevailing view at the moment, however, is that the process resides in some form of internalized representation or working model of relationships (Bretherton, 1987, 1990; Sroufe & Fleeson, 1986; Stern, 1985). At some level, this must be the case because children are thinking, feeling beings who actively process their experiences. Necessarily, they will bring to any relationship both memories of past interactions and expectations of future ones. The difficulty comes in translating this general notion into something more specific that can lead to testable hypotheses. At the moment, the notion of internal working models is too all encompassing to have much testable explanatory power (Hinde, 1988). Furthermore, at least insofar as the processes in infancy are concerned, it would seem that the cognitive competence required to represent both sides of discrepant relationships are beyond the abilities of, for example, 12-month-old infants (Dunn, 1988, 1993). The attraction of internal working models lies in its explicit recognition of the role of active thought processes in the mediation of the effects of experiences and in its providing a mechanism for both continuity and change. Nevertheless, although it is clear that internal working models represent a reality in what is happening, so far they have failed to give any increased precision to our understanding of the processes involved.

Manifestations of Attachment Postinfancy

One of the hallmarks of attachment theory is its claim that attachment security remains a key feature of relationships throughout the whole of life. The claim is bold, but it is supported by the extensive body of evidence showing that bereavement or loss of a love relationship constitutes a potent stressor throughout life (after early infancy) and that the presence of a close, confiding relationship is protective against stress in adults of all ages, as well as in children (Hazan & Shaver, 1994; Parkes et al., 1991; Rutter & Rutter, 1993). The issue that is only partially resolved concerns how to measure attachment qualities, after the first few years of life. The findings certainly suggest that confiding and emotional exchange index attachment relationships during adolescence and adult life in a way that they do not in early childhood. Those features indicate which relationships include important attachment qualities, but they provide a less satisfactory index of the quality of the attachment. Hazan and Shaver (1994) have provided a useful review of the features of adult relationships that are thought to reflect insecure attachment. These include both a lack of self-disclosure and indiscriminant, overly intimate, self-disclosure; undue jealousy in close relationships; feelings of loneliness even when involved in relationships; reluctance to commitment in relationships; difficulty in making relationships in a new setting, and a tendency to view partners as insufficiently attentive. These characteristics make sense conceptually and they provide a good basis for further research but it remains to be determined whether these have the same meaning as the qualities of insecurity as observed in infancy.

How One Relationship Affects Another Relationship

It is not just a matter of how attachment security is shown in varied ways over the lifespan, but also a question of how one relationship affects another relationship (Hinde & Stevenson-Hinde, 1988). Thus, strong claims have been made about the ways in which insecurity in a person's attachment relationship with parents in early childhood influences their relationships in adult life (Main, 1991; Main & Hesse, 1990; Main, Kaplan & Cassidy, 1985). This has led to Mary Main's development of the Adult Attachment Interview (Main et al., 1985; van IJzendoorn, 1995; van IJzendoorn & Bakermans-Kranenburg, Chapter 5, this volume). The Adult Attachment Interview comprises a series of apparently straightforward questions to elicit an account of childhood from which inferences are drawn about attachment and about the person's evaluation of those experiences. Attachment insecurity is identified on the basis of a tendency to deny negative experiences, to be unable to reevoke the feelings associated with negative experiences; presentation of an overidealized picture of parents; or a continuing preoccupation with parents associated with confused, incoherent concepts, and unresolved anger. The postulate is that it is important for healthy personality development to have access to memories of painful experiences, to come to terms with them, and to integrate them into a positive view of the self. One intriguing aspect of the connections between relationships concerns the evidence that measures of maternal attachment insecurity obtained during pregnancy predict the insecurity of the infant's attachment relationships with the mother as measured later (Fonagy, Steele, & Steele, 1991; Fonagy, Steele, Steele, Higgitt, & Target 1994).

Nevertheless, it would be a mistake to seek to view all connections between relationships in terms of a persistence of attachment qualities. As both Hinde and Stevenson-Hinde (1988) and Sameroff and Emde (1989) emphasized, there are many other features that require explanation. Why, for example, do some women in a discordant marital relationship show more involvement (albeit with less sensitivity) with their babies than do mothers in a harmonious relationship (Engfer, 1988); why do marital relationships tend to alter after the birth of a first child (Belsky & Isabella, 1988); why do dyadic interactions tend to be different when a third party is present (Clarke-Stewart, 1978; Corter, Abramovitch, & Pepler, 1983); and why do children who have a very close relationship with their mothers tend to develop a hostile relationship with their next-born sibling (Dunn & Kendrick, 1982)? Whereas these compensatory and rivalry effects are in no way incompatible with the attachment theory, the theory certainly does not provide an adequate explanation on its own (Rutter, 1991). There is a need both to consider dyadic relationships in terms that go beyond attachment concepts, and to consider social systems that extend beyond dyads (Dunn, 1993; Hinde, 1976, 1979; Nash, 1988; Sameroff & Emde, 1989).

Moreover, there is a problem in the wish of many adult attachment theorists to extend attachment concepts to sexual relationships and to parents' relationships with their young children. Thus, an absolutely key feature of secure attachment relationships in early childhood is that they provide security. This is not obviously present with respect to parent–child relationships. Thus, mothers and fathers do not usually feel more secure when their young children are with them. They *provide* security but do not *receive* it (Rutter & Rutter, 1993). Nevertheless, their early *experience* of selective attachment seems to be associated with a greater capacity to be well-functioning parents. The link seems important, but it is by no means inevitable, and it is not obvious that it makes sense to equate this with an infant's attachment to its parents. Of course, the relationship is a strong, committed one and it does have many features in common with attachments, but it is not identical. Similarly, sexual relationships may show strong attachment qualities, but they do not necessarily do so. Thus, a person may have a strong sexual longing for someone else in the absence of a committed relationship and without that relationship bringing any sense of security. Rather than view a sexual relationship as a variety of attachment relationships, it may be more useful to ask which sexual relationships show attachment qualities and which ones do not, and why there are differences between the two.

Boundaries of Attachment

That question leads on to the somewhat related issue of the boundaries of attachment. One of the major achievements of the initial attachment concept was the careful distinction between attachment qualities and other features of relationships. Unfortunately, the attractiveness of attachment theory has meant that there has been rather a neglect of these other features, together with an implicit tendency to discuss relationships as if attachment security was all that mattered. Both Sameroff and Emde (1989) and Dunn (1993) have drawn attention to the evidence that children's relationships with other people are complex and involve a range of different dimensions and functions. These include connectedness, shared humor, balance of control, intimacy, and shared positive emotions. If we are to understand the interconnections between relationships, it will be necessary for us to take into account the range of dimensions that seem to be involved. It seems unlikely that these will be reducible to a single process involving attachment security or any other postulated quality.

There are at least two other difficulties with the way in which attachment concepts tend to be used. First, there is a tendency to refer to relationships as if they did, or did not, reflect attachment, and as if each relationship had to be one thing or another. It is clear from the evidence that this is nonsense. To begin with, as already noted, most people have several relationships involving a strong attachment. They differ in the importance and strength of the attachment, but it is a quantitative variation and not a categorical distinction. Also, however, it is obvious that any one relationship may include several different qualities. Thus, parents usually have an attachment relationship with their children but that relationship also includes caregiver qualities, disciplinary features, playmate characteristics, and other aspects. Each of these may predominate in different contexts but the overall relationship involves a complex mix of all these different features.

The second major problem with the use of attachment concepts concerns the tendency to use them to refer to an individual, rather than to a particular relationship (Kobak, 1994). Thus, the Adult Attachment Interview classifies *individuals* as secure or insecure, rather than classifying that person's relationships with different people. This seems to have some validity in that Fonagy et al. (1991, 1994) found a significant association between parental attachment security and their children's attachment security. Nevertheless, as Dunn (1993) pointed out, it is evident that parents have different relationships with different children; that children have different relationships with each of their parents; that the associations between relationships among different dyads within and outside the family are of only modest strength; and that patterns of relationships show reciprocity, rivalry, and compensation as well as generalization.

Associations with Later Functioning

One specific issue with regard to boundaries on attachment theory concerns the predictive claims in relation to later functioning. Sroufe (1988) emphasized the need to resist the tendency to overextend predictive claims to widespread aspects of personal functioning in later life. He argued that the specific claims of attachment theory concern the child's developing sense of inner confidence, efficacy, and self-worth, together with aspects of intimate personal relationships, such as the capacity to be emotionally close, to seek and receive care, and to give care to others. Thus, he suggested that attachment had no direct connections with cognitive development and that, although anxious attachment was a risk factor for psychopathology, it did not directly cause later psychiatric disorders. The empirical research findings support this caution. Significant associations have been found between insecure attachment in infancy and various forms of later psychopathology in both childhood and adult life (Belsky & Cassidy, 1994) but the associations are of only moderate strength and the findings are by no means entirely consistent across studies (see Goldberg, Chapter 6, this volume). The findings are such as to make it necessary to consider carefully the nature of the processes involved.

Belsky and Cassidy (1994) contrasted three alternative models. First, there is a narrow, domain-specific model in which maternal sensitivity to attachment signals forecasts attachment security in the child, which itself predicts only outcomes directly involving the attachment system (such as later intimate relationships). According to this model, parental qualities may be related to a much broader range of outcomes, but the mechanisms involved in, for example, competence in play or cognitive development are quite different and are not part of attachment processes. At the other extreme, a broad general model would postulate that attachment security is directly responsible for fostering development across a wide range of domains. A third model expects to find some generality, but only because of third variables that are involved in a variety of different developmental processes. It is important to recognize that the adverse environments that predispose to attachment insecurity usually include a wide range of risk features that may have nothing much to do with attachment as such. Thus, the Harlow monkeys reared on wire surrogates showed gross problems in later sexual and parenting behavior. But these monkeys were reared in conditions of social isolation and it cannot be assumed that the later sequelae were a result of attachment insecurity or attachment failure. Similarly, the adverse outcomes associated with an institutional rearing or child abuse are a function of environments that appear deleterious in a variety of different connections. There are good reasons for supposing that abnormalities in the development of attachment relationships play a role in these adverse outcomes but it has to be admitted that their importance in relation to alternative mediating processes has not been put to the test in rigorous fashion as yet.

The Role of Parenting Qualities and Patterns of Caregiving

A central tenet of attachment theory has always been that the quality of parenting is strongly influential in shaping the security of an infant's attachment relationships with parents. There is now an abundance of evidence showing the existence of significant associations. Rates of inse-cure attachment are raised substantially in maltreated children and in those reared by depressed mothers. Within normal samples, too, measures of parental sensitivity are associated with security of attachment in the infant. Also, a therapeutic intervention in a high-risk group of Dutch mothers showed that gains in maternal sensitivity were associated with a reduction in patterns of insecurity (van den Boom, 1990). Clearly, there are associa-tions between patterns of parenting and qualities of attachment security. Yet, it has to be said that most of the associations that have been found have been of only moderate strength. We have still to gain a full under-standing of how parenting qualities interact with other variables in the development of attachment relationships.

Perhaps the greatest uncertainty concerns child care outside the home. Following Bowlby's WHO report (1951), claims were made that group daycare caused infants grave psychological damage (WHO Expert Com-mittee on Mental Health, 1951). It is now clear that that view was seriously mistaken. Most infants who experience good quality group daycare with continuity in caregiving show no detectable ill effects (Zigler & Gordon, 1982). On the other hand, there is some suggestion (albeit disputed; Clarke-Stewart, 1989; McCartney & Galanopoulos, 1988) that there *may* be elevated rates of insecurity in the case of children with early and extensive daycare experience (Belsky & Rovine, 1988). To a substantial extent, such risks as there are clearly derive from the poor quality of care rather than from the fact that it has been provided on a group basis. Nevertheless, it may be that group daycare may pose difficulties for some babies under a year old when it is on a full-time basis and when the babies also have other experiences that put them at risk (Belsky & Rovine, 1988). Resolution of the issue awaits further evidence.

Adaptive Value of Secure Attachment

Because, in ordinary circumstances, a majority of infants show secure attachments, and because insecure attachments are associated with a somewhat increased risk of later psychopathology, there has been a tendency to assume that only secure attachment is normal and that it is fundamentally more adaptive in a biological sense. This represents a misunderstanding of biology, as Hinde (1982) has noted. As he commented, mothers and babies will be programmed by evolution to form a range of possible relationships that vary according to circumstances. Natural selection will tend to favor individuals with a range of potential styles, rather than those with just one style (see Crittenden, Chapter 3, this volume). Statistical considerations point to the same conclusion. Although secure attachments predominate in most general population samples, they are far from universal. In American samples, they average about 60% (Campos et al., 1983). It would not seem sensible to regard 40% of infants as showing biologically abnormal development. Moreover, further research is needed to determine the extent to which attachment insecurity constitutes a diagnosis-specific or a general risk factor, and to delineate the mechanisms involved. The category of insecure attachment cannot be equated with psychopathology or disorder (Belsky & Nezworski, 1988).

Disorders of Attachment

Nevertheless, there are disorders in which abnormalities in attachment features seem to constitute the predominant characteristics (Sameroff & Emde, 1989; Zeanah & Emde, 1994). Both DSM-IV (American Psychiatric Association, 1994) and ICD-10 (World Health Organization, 1992) include attachment disorders of childhood in their classification systems. Systematic evidence on these attachment disorders is distinctly limited but it appears that they may take two main forms. First, there is a variety that tends to be associated with parental abuse or neglect. There is a combination of strongly contradictory or ambivalent social responses that may be most evident at times of partings and reunions; there is emotional disturbance as evident in misery or lack of emotional responsiveness, withdrawal, or aggression; and there may be fearfulness and hypervigilance. Secondly, there is a pattern that is more commonly associated with an institutional upbringing (see Chisholm, Carter, Ames, & Morison, 1995) in which the children show an unusual degree of diffuseness in selective attachments during the preschool years accompanied by generally clinging behavior in infancy and indiscriminantly friendly, attention-seeking behavior in early or middle childhood. Usually there is difficulty in forming close confiding relationships with peers. There is no doubt that these patterns occur, but Richters and Volkmar (1994) have pointed to the fact that the disorders extend beyond attachment qualities and they raise queries as to whether it is helpful to put the diagnosis in terms of a disorder of attachment per se.

In addition to these two postulated attachment disorders, researchers have sought to apply attachment concepts to conduct problems (Goldberg, Chapter 6, this volume; Greenberg, DeKlyen, Speltz, & Endriga, Chapter 7, this volume; Greenberg & Speltz, 1988; Greenberg, Speltz, & DeKlyen, 1993; Waters, Posada, Crowell, & Keng-Ling, 1993), to patterns of social withdrawal (Rubin & Lollis, 1988), and to borderline personality disorders (Fonagy et al., Chapter 8, this volume; Patrick, Hobson, Castle, Howard, & Maughan, 1994), as well as to a range of other conditions (Parkes et al., 1991). The ideas are provocative and heuristically useful in focusing attention on the possible role of underlying relationship disturbances in conditions apparently characterized by quite different phenomenology (such as delinquent acts or depression). Further research will be needed to show how far attachment concepts are useful in gaining a better understanding of the mechanisms involved in the genesis of these disorders.

CLINICAL IMPLICATIONS OF ATTACHMENT THEORY AND FINDINGS

Let me conclude by seeking to draw together the ideas and findings that I have reviewed to draw inferences about the clinical implications of attachment concepts and findings.

Psychoanalytic Theories of Development

Perhaps the first implication to note is that the findings decisively reject the traditional psychoanalytic theory of development as put forward by either Freud or Klein. At first sight, that may seem a curious inference to make because in the first volume of the attachment trilogy, Bowlby (1969/1982) stated that his frame of reference had been that of psychoanalysis and that his own early thinking on attachment had been inspired by psychoanalytic work. Also, Sroufe (1986) argued that attachment concepts had done much to advance psychoanalytic theory. Bowlby's own view, as expressed in his later papers (Bowlby, 1988), was quite different. He stated firmly that "although psychoanalysis is avowedly a developmental discipline it is nowhere weaker, I believe, than in its concepts of development" (p. 66). He went on to maintain that attachment theory differed fundamentally from psychoanalytic theory in its rejection of the model of development in which an individual is held to pass through a series of stages in any one of which he may become fixated or to which he may regress. He also rejected the psychoanalytic idea that emotional bonds were derivative from drives based on food or sex. He concluded that systematic and sensitive studies of human infants have rendered the psychoanalytic model of development "untenable". If the evidence requires a rejection of the psychoanalytic postulates of drive, of psychosexual stages, and of fixation and regression, there would seem to be little point in persisting with the fiction that psychoanalysis offers any useful understanding of developmental processes. It is time that the theory be given a respectful burial, but be dismissed with respect to its contemporaneous value.[2]

The respect should be given, however, because historically psychoanalysis was very important. Bowlby was right in giving it credit for its role in the origins of attachment theory. Thus, it was important in suggesting a focus on relationships, despite the fact that it was hopelessly wrong in the mechanisms proposed for their development. It was also important in pointing to the role of early childhood features (although wrong in giving precedence to fantasies over real life experiences; see also Stern, 1989). The focus on early life was also explicit in ethology (which played an even greater role in the development of attachment theory). But, in keeping with research findings, Bowlby in his later writings placed a much greater emphasis on the role of later, as well as earlier experiences, and on the complex ways in which early adversities have indirect effects because of the tendency for one adversity to increase the likelihood of occurrence of another. Psychoanalytic theory also was important in its emphasis on the central role of mental mechanisms. Bowlby very firmly rejected the psychoanalytic view that childhood experiences were of only secondary importance (and the evidence supports that rejection) but he did accept that the cognitive processing of experiences played a key role in their effects (see van IJzendoorn & Bakermans-Kranenburg, Chapter 5, this volume). Of course, that notion is by no means confined to psychoanalysis. For example, Kagan (1984) emphasized the same process (i.e., cognitive processing) on entirely different grounds, and internal working models are a central feature of cognitive–behavioral therapies (Beck, Rush, Shaw, & Emery, 1979; Robins & Hayes, 1993; Teasdale, 1993). Although it is important not to throw out the baby with the bathwater, there is an awful lot of psychoanalytic water that needs to go down the plughole and we also need to appreciate that psychoanalysis is only one of the parents of the baby and that the growing infant differs in very important ways from its progenitors.

Patterns of Residential Care for Children

The most immediate and obvious impact of attachment concepts was on patterns of residential care for children. Children's wards in hospitals began to allow parents to visit on a more regular basis, and to stay overnight when children were young, and there was a turning away from large, institutional orphanages providing caregiving on a group basis with multiple, rotating caregivers. All is not well in patterns of residential care but undoubtedly there is now a much better appreciation of children's needs. At first, there was an unfortunate emphasis on the trauma of separations so that some residential staff sought to avoid forming relationships with the children so that they would not be so upset when the staff had to change. It is now appreciated that that is not the main concern. Separations may indeed be stressful (Rutter, 1979) but the lack of an opportunity to form selective attachments is likely to be more damaging (Rutter, 1981). There also is a recognition of the need to provide continuity in caregiving for young children. Nevertheless, the problem of how to provide that is very far from solved. It is still usual in many residential nurseries for children to experience an extraordinarily large number of caregivers. In Tizard's studies (Tizard, 1977), for example, the children experienced over 50 caregivers during the preschool years.

Provision of Child Care

It might be thought that attachment concepts should have their most direct application in the field of child care, but their application here has not been free of difficulties. At first, a misleadingly concrete application of the notion of monotropy (which in itself turned out to be partially mistaken) led to recommendations that mothers should not go out to work and that all forms of group day care are necessarily harmful. It is now clear that these recommendations were misplaced (Rutter, 1991; Schaffer, 1990). Human societies have always involved several adults caring for children, as reflected in the title of Emmy Werner's (1984) excellent book *Child Care: Kith, Kin and Hired Hands*. Nevertheless, attachment ideas have been important in indicating some of the features that make for quality in child care and also in pointing to the importance of consistency in daycare arrangements. Children cope well with having several adults look after them, provided that it is the same small number of adults over time and provided that the individuals with whom they have a secure attachment relationship are available at times when they are tired, distressed, or facing challenging circumstances. That much is generally accepted. What is less clear is the extent to which the considerations that apply to the main caregivers also apply to subsidiary caregivers. Consistency in caregiving is clearly important, but does it have the same importance with respect to help with caregiving when one or other of the parents constitutes the main caregiver? A satisfactory answer to that question is not yet available.

Assessment of Parenting

Attachment concepts, and the features involved in the use of the Strange Situation, have been very helpful in alerting clinicians regarding how to assess children's relationships with their caregivers at a time when decisions are needed about possible child abuse, about foster placements, and about adoption. We are now aware that just because children cling to someone when they are stressed does not necessarily mean that they have a secure relationship with them. It also has become apparent that separations, and especially reunions, provide a good opportunity to assess relationships and that we need to focus rather more on the children's use of parental presence to have the confidence to explore than on the level of distress at the time of separation. It has also been helpful to appreciate the difficulties experienced by young children when having to change parents in the first few years of life, although it has been important to appreciate that they can form new selective attachments at that age. Nevertheless, three caveats are needed.

1. As noted already, the Strange Situation itself does not constitute a diagnostic tool and the assessment of selective attachments in older children is less straightforward than it is with infants.

2. The original notion that children could not form initial selective attachments after the supposed sensitive period of the first 2 years has proved mistaken. Hence, late adoption may be more beneficial than was once thought (although clearly there should be a general policy of "the earlier, the better").

3. The degree of commitment of the adoptive parents seems an important factor in success and also it is helpful for parents to have an awareness of the types of problems that may constitute sequelae of early adverse attachment experiences. A recognition that these need to be understood in relationship terms (see Sameroff & Emde, 1989) and not just as signs of "naughtiness," is important.

One specific issue concerns decisions regarding how and when children need to be removed from their biological parents when they are being abused or neglected. All would accept that it is extraordinarily difficult to decide when the qualities of parental care are so bad that it is necessary to remove the child. Considerations of parent–child relationships are important, but it is clear that considerations concerning safety, security, and the adequacy of care are also crucial. Appreciation of the difficulties of providing all that is needed in good parenting in conditions of foster care and residential care need to be taken into account. Nevertheless, what is important is attention to the child's relationships with those who constitute his social family and not concern with some hypothetical "blood bond."

Parental Divorce and Family Breakup

Early writings on the risks associated with parental divorce and family breakup focused on the role of "loss" because it had received such an emphasis in early writings on attachment. Empirical findings have made clear, however, that the main risks do not stem from loss as such, but rather from the discordant and disrupted relationships that tend to precede or follow the loss (see Bretherton, Walsh, Lependorf, & Georgeson, Chapter 4, this volume). That is so with respect to risks in childhood (Block, Block, & Gjerde, 1986; Cherlin et al., 1991; Rutter, 1994a) and it is so with longer-term risks in relation to vulnerability to depressive disorders in adult life (Harris, Brown, & Bifulco, 1986; Kendler, Neale, Kessler, Heath, & Eaves, 1992). These findings are, of course, entirely in line with attachment concepts. The problem lay in taking the notion of loss out of context and giving it a greater emphasis than it warranted. Loss is a risk indicator but it is not the major player in most risk mechanisms. The distinction is an important one and applies widely in the difficulties of moving from statistical associations to recommendations on policy and practice (Rutter, 1994b).

"Maternal Bonding" to Infants

One of the more unfortunate misapplications of attachment theory came with Klaus and Kennell's (1976) claim that mothers "bonded" with their babies during a critical period in the first few days of life and that skin to skin contact was necessary for this to take place. The empirical evidence in support of this suggestion was always weak and it did not reflect a proper understanding of attachment processes. A mother's relationship with her child is not the same thing as a child's initial selective attachments and in neither case are they dependent on a single sensory modality operating over a very short time period. Kennell and Klaus (1984), in line with numerous others (Goldberg, 1983; Sluckin, Herbert, & Sluckin, 1983), have now accepted that parental relationships develop over time and that there is more than one route involved. The simplistic "superglue" notion of maternal bonding has fortunately passed into oblivion. Nevertheless, it is necessary that we do not lose sight of the various important factors that may foster and facilitate the development of parents' relationships with their babies (Rutter, 1989; Rutter & Rutter, 1993).

Psychotherapy

Thoughtful psychotherapists have sought to consider how psychotherapy may be improved by attention to attachment concepts (Holmes, 1993a, 1993b). There is, as yet, no general agreement on the psychotherapeutic implications of attachment concepts but certain possible implications may be suggested. On the positive side, an attention to real life experiences, and not just fantasies about them, is obviously important. Equally, however, the cognitive models about such experiences and the mental models of relationships need to be a focus. The chief shift from a traditional psychoanalytic position lies, perhaps, in attention to interpersonal, as distinct from intrapersonal, defenses. Obviously, too, a recognition of the importance of the factors involved in good relationships is crucial and Holmes (1993a) suggested that this applies to the therapeutic relationship as well as to other relationships. On the negative side, as already discussed, it is important to put aside a misguided reliance on psychosexual stages and on notions of fixation and regression. These suggestions are closely related to those put forward by the psychoanalyst Peter Lomas (1987) in his book *The Limits of Interpretation: What's Wrong with Psychoanalysis?* He pointed to what he called the "dreadful, pessimistic and bizarre" (p. 34) Freudian notion of primary narcissism and argued that it was encouraging that psychotherapists were moving, however painfully and gradually, toward a less mechanistic idea of infantile experiences and to a greater appreciation of the importance of loving relationships. Although he was careful to note the differences between good parenting and good psychotherapy, he suggested that both need to be based on mutual warmth, respect, and trust and that an undue reliance on the uninvolved, dispassionate interpretation of defenses may not constitute the best way forward.

Disorders of Attachment

Finally, it is necessary to consider the implications for psychopathological disorders. I have noted already the importance of attachment theory in drawing attention to disorders primarily characterized by abnormalities in selective attachment—so-called "reactive attachment disorders." However, three cautions are necessary. First, it is most unfortunate that DSM-IV (American Psychiatric Association, 1994) has chosen to specify pathogenic child care as one of the diagnostic criteria. It is true that the condition came to notice in circumstances of abnormal care, but the evidence is not yet available for decisions on whether the same behavioral pattern can be found in the absence of gross neglect or abuse. Second, as Richters and Volkmar (1994) pointed out, the syndrome includes a variety of psychopathological features that seem to extend well outside the bounds of an abnormality in selective attachment. Third, great care needs to be taken in the assessment of attachment qualities in children from backgrounds that are unusual with respect to the children's experiences of continuous relationships with, but also brief separations from, a limited number of caregivers and/or in which they have psychopathological or physical disorders (Main & Solomon, 1990; Vaughn et al., 1994). This is especially so with respect to use of the Strange Situation. Clinicians need to be aware of the necessity of not basing assessments of relationships on this one procedure, despite its many strengths (see Goldberg, Chapter 6, this volume). A wider range of interview and observational data are needed.

Attachment concepts have also been important in alerting clinicians to the possible role of relationship difficulties in a wider range of psychopathological disorders, but perhaps especially conduct disorders (Greenberg & Speltz, 1988; Greenberg et al., 1993; Greenberg et al., Chapter 7, this volume), antisocial and borderline personality disorders (Fonagy et al., Chapter 8, this volume; Patrick et al., 1994; Quinton, Pickles, Maughan, & Rutter, 1993; Zoccolillo, Pickles, Quinton, & Rutter, 1992), and social withdrawal (Rubin & Lollis, 1988). This fits in with the empirical evidence of the importance of poor peer relations in psychopathological disorders (Asher, Erdley, & Gabriel, 1994; Parker & Asher, 1987). Clearly, in some cases, abnormalities in early selective attachments with parents have played a role in etiology. Once again, however, a caution is necessary. As both Sameroff and Emde (1989) and Dunn (1993) have emphasized, attachment is not the whole of relationships and still we have much to learn about the interconnections between parent–child relationships, peer relationships, sibling relationships, and sexual relationships in adult life. Attachment concepts are clearly useful in thinking about relationship disturbances but it is important that we should not be unduly constrained by thinking only in attachment terms.

It would be reasonable to suppose that an understanding of the role of attachment difficulties in psychopathology should have implications for therapeutic interventions. We may accept that there are such implications but what is much less clear is just how attachment concepts should shape treatment (see Belsky & Nezworski, 1988; Sameroff & Emde, 1989; Zeanah & Emde, 1994). It is necessary that we take seriously the need to develop therapeutic approaches that build on what is known about the role of attachment disturbances but, equally, it is important that we do not obtain premature closure on treatment strategies.

CONCLUSIONS

In looking back on the years since the first volume of Bowlby's trilogy on attachment, it is obvious that the field has changed out of all recognition. From the early days when he was criticized by academic psychologists and ostracized by the psychoanalytic establishment, attachment concepts have become generally accepted. That they have become so is a tribute to the creativity and perceptiveness of Bowlby's original formulations and to the major conceptual and methodological contributions of Ainsworth. It is also a function, however, of the role of research in modifying attachment concepts. Inevitably, there have been instances in which attachment concepts have been overgeneralized or misinterpreted in a naive and simplistic fashion. That is unavoidable with ideas that are intellectually provocative and so obviously relevant to public policy and clinical practice. As I have sought to indicate, we are very far from having reached an understanding of the development of relationships or of the ways in which distortions in relationships play a role in psychopathology. Attachment theory has been hugely helpful in bringing about progress in both areas and doubtless it will continue to do so in the future. But, if knowledge is to advance in the way that we all hope that it will, it will be necessary that we pay attention to one of the first features of attachment theory, namely that attachment is not the whole of relationships. What is needed now is a bringing together of attachment concepts and other formulations of relationships so that each may profit from the contributions of the other.

ACKNOWLEDGMENT

This chapter constitutes a slightly modified version of a paper with the same title published in the *Journal of Child Psychology and Psychiatry* (1995), *36*, 549–571. Adapted by permission.

NOTES

1. In seeking an explanation, we need to appreciate that the security of attachments to professional caregivers may be as important as those to parents (see e.g., Aviezer, van IJzendoorn, Sagi, & Schuengel, 1994; Howes, Rodning, Galluzzo, & Myers, 1988; Oppenheim, Sagi, & Lamb, 1988)

2. Bowlby (1988) was far from alone in considering that psychoanalytic concepts of development require radical revision (see, e.g., Emde, 1992; Zeanah, Anders, Seifer, & Stern, 1989). Psychoanalysts are prone to claim that psychoanalysis paved the way in pointing to the importance of early experiences, but as various reviewers have noted (see, e.g., Emde, 1992; Holmes, 1993a, 1993b; Stern, 1989), the reverse is the case. Many Kleinian analysts still argue that object relations derive from the ontogeny of fantasy life and not from actual interactions in the family. Of course, that would not be true of most post-Freudian psychoanalytic conceptualizations. Various psychoanalytic writers (e.g., Dare, 1985; Shapiro & Esman, 1992; Wallerstein, 1988) have rightly pointed to the plurality of psychoanalytic theories, some of which are not reliant on the traditional concepts as expressed by either Freud or Klein. Nevertheless, as Wallerstein (1988) noted, the current theories do not agree on the processes involved in development (there is greater consistency on some of the key clinical concepts). Moreover, accounts of psychoanalytic views on development, in major psychiatric textbooks (e.g., Kaplan, Sadock, & Grebb, 1994), in developmental textbooks (Miller, 1993), and in books for a wider public (Wolff, 1981, 1989), continue to refer to the outmoded concepts listed here.

REFERENCES

Ainsworth, M. D. S. (1967). *Infancy in Uganda: Infant care and the growth of love.* Baltimore: Johns Hopkins Press.
Ainsworth, M. D. S., Blehar, M. C., Waters, E., & Wall, S. (1978). *Patterns of attachment: A psychological study of the Strange Situation.* Hillsdale, NJ: Erlbaum.
American Psychiatric Association. (1994). *Diagnostic and statistical manual of mental disorders* (4th ed.). Washington, DC: Author.
Asher, S., Erdley, C. A., & Gabriel, S. W. (1994). Peer relations. In M. Rutter & D. Hay (Eds.), *Development through life: A handbook for clinicians* (pp. 456–487). Oxford: Blackwell Scientific.
Aviezer, O., van IJzendoorn, M. H., Sagi, A., & Schuengel, C. (1994). "Children of the dream" revisited: 70 years of collective early child care in Israeli kibbutzim. *Psychological Bulletin, 116,* 99–116.
Beck, A. T., Rush, A. J., Shaw, B. F., & Emery, G. (1979). *Cognitive therapy of depression.* New York: Guilford Press.
Belsky, J., & Cassidy, J. (1994). Attachment: Theory and evidence. In M. Rutter & D. Hay (Eds.), *Development through life: A handbook for clinicians* (pp. 373–402). Oxford: Blackwell Scientific.

Belsky, J., & Isabella, R. (1988). Maternal, infant, and social–contextual determinants of attachment security. In J. Belsky & T. Nezworski (Eds.), *Clinical implications of attachment* (pp. 41–94). Hillsdale, NJ: Erlbaum.

Belsky, J., & Nezworski, T. (Eds.). (1988). *Clinical implications of attachment.* Hillsdale, NJ: Erlbaum.

Belsky, J., & Rovine, M. J. (1988). Nonmaternal care in the first year of life and the security of infant-parent attachment. *Child Development, 59,* 157–167.

Block, J. H., Block, J., & Gjerde, P. F. (1986). The personality of children prior to divorce: A prospective study. *Child Development, 57,* 827–840.

Bowlby, J. (1951). *Maternal care and mental health* (WHO Monograph Series, No. 2). Geneva: World Health Organization.

Bowlby, J. (1982). *Attachment and loss: Vol. 1. Attachment* (2nd ed.). New York: Basic Books. (First edition published 1969)

Bowlby, J. (1973). *Attachment and loss: Vol. 2. Separation, anxiety and anger.* London: Hogarth Press.

Bowlby, J. (1980). *Attachment and loss: Vol. 3. Loss, sadness and depression.* London: Hogarth Press.

Bowlby, J. (1988). *A secure base: Clinical implications of attachment theory.* London: Routledge & Kegan Paul.

Bretherton, I. (1987). New perspective on attachment relations: Security, communication, and internal working models. In J. D. Osofsky (Ed.), *Handbook of infant development* (2nd ed., pp. 1061–1100). Chichester: Wiley.

Bretherton, I. (1990). Open communication and internal working models: Their role in the development of attachment relationships. In R. A. Thompson (Ed.), *Nebraska Symposium on Motivation: Vol. 36. Socioemotional development* (pp. 57–113). Lincoln: University of Nebraska Press.

Bretherton, I., & Waters, E. (Eds.). (1985). Growing points in attachment theory and research. *Monographs of the Society for Research in Child Development, 50*(1–2, Serial No. 209).

Campos, J. J., Barrett, K., Lamb, M. E., Goldsmith, H. H., & Stenberg, C. (1983). Socioemotional development. In M. M. Haith & J. J. Campos (Eds.), *Mussen handbook of child psychology: Vol. 2. Infancy and developmental psychobiology* (4th ed., pp. 783–915). New York: Wiley.

Capps, L., Sigman, M., & Mundy, P. (1994). Attachment security in children with autism. *Development and Psychopathology, 6,* 249–261.

Casler, L. (1968). Perceptual deprivation in institutional settings. In G. Newton & S. Levine (Eds.), *Early experience and behavior: The psychobiology of development* (pp. 573–626). Springfield, IL: Charles C Thomas.

Cherlin, A. J., Furstenberg, F. F. Jr., Chase-Lansdale, P. L., Kiernan, K. E., Robins, P. K., Morrison, D. R., & Teitler, J. O. (1991). Longitudinal studies of effects of divorce on children in Great Britain and the United States. *Science, 252,* 1386–1389.

Chisholm, K., Carter, M. C., Ames, E. W., & Morison, S. J. (1995). Attachment security and indiscriminately friendly behavior in children adopted from Romanian orphanages. *Development and Psychopathology, 7,* 283–294.

Clarke-Stewart, K. A. (1978). And Daddy makes three: The father's impact on mother and young child. *Child Development, 49,* 466–478.

Clarke-Stewart, K. A. (1989). Infant daycare: Malignant or maligned? *American Psychologist, 44,* 266–274.

Corter, C., Abramovitch, R., & Pepler, D. (1983). The role of the mother in sibling interactions. *Child Development, 54,* 1599–1605.

Crittenden, P. M. (1988). Relationships at risk. In J. Belsky & T. Nezworski (Eds.), *Clinical implications of attachment* (pp. 136–174). Hillsdale, NJ: Erlbaum.

Dare, C. (1985). Psychoanalytic theories of development. In M. Rutter & L. Hersov (Eds.), *Child and adolescent psychiatry: Modern approaches* (2nd ed., pp. 204–215). Oxford: Blackwell Scientific.

Dunn, J. (1988). *The beginnings of social understanding.* Cambridge, MA: Harvard University Press.

Dunn, J. (1993). *Young children's close relationships: Beyond attachment.* (Individual Differences and Development Series, Vol. 4). Newbury Park, CA: Sage.

Dunn, J., & Kendrick, C. (1982). *Siblings: Love, envy, and understanding.* Cambridge, MA: Harvard University Press.

Emde, R. N. (1992). Individual meaning and increasing complexity: Contributions of Sigmund Freud and René Spitz to developmental psychology. *Developmental Psychology, 28,* 347–359.

Engfer, A. (1988). The interrelatedness of marriage and the mother–child relationship. In R. A. Hinde & J. Stevenson-Hinde (Eds.), *Relationships within families: Mutual influences* (pp. 104–118). Oxford: Clarendon Press.

Fonagy, P., Steele, H., & Steele, M. (1991). Maternal representations of attachment during pregnancy predict the organization of infant–mother attachment at one year of age. *Child Development, 62,* 891–905.

Fonagy, P., Steele, M., Steele, H., Higgitt, A., & Target, M. (1994). The Emanuel Miller Memorial Lecture 1992: The theory and practice of resilience. *Journal of Child Psychology and Psychiatry, 35,* 231–257.

Fox, N. A., Kimmerly, N. L., & Schafer, W. D. (1991). Attachment to mother/attachment to father. A meta-analysis. *Child Development, 62,* 210–225.

Goldberg, S. (1983). Parent–infant bonding: Another look. *Child Development, 54,* 1355–1382.

Goldsmith, H. H., & Alansky, J. A. (1987). Maternal and infant temperamental predictors of attachment: A meta-analytic review. *Journal of Consulting and Clinical Psychology, 55,* 805–816.

Greenberg, M. T., Cicchetti, D., & Cummings, M. (Eds.). (1990). *Attachment in the preschool years: Theory, research and intervention.* Chicago: University of Chicago Press.

Greenberg, M. T., & Speltz, M. L. (1988). Attachment and the ontogeny of conduct problems. In J. Belsky & T. Nezworski (Eds.), *Clinical implications of attachment* (pp. 177–218). Hillsdale, NJ: Erlbaum.

Greenberg, M. T., Speltz, M. L., & DeKlyen, M. (1993). The role of attachment in the early development of disruptive behavior problems. *Development and Psychopathology, 5,* 191–213.

Grosskurth, P. (1986). *Melanie Klein: Her world and her work.* London: Hodder & Stoughton.

Harlow, H. F., & Harlow, M. K. (1969). Effects of various mother–infant relationships on rhesus monkey behaviours. In B. M. Foss (Ed.), *Determinants of infant behaviour* (Vol. 4, pp. 15–36). London: Methuen.

Harris, T., Brown, G. W., & Bifulco, A. (1986). Loss of parent in childhood and adult psychiatric disorder: The role of lack of adequate parental care. *Psychological Medicine, 16,* 641–659.

Hazan, C., & Shaver, P. R. (1994). Attachment as an organizational framework for research on close relationships. *Psychological Inquiry, 5,* 1–22.

Hinde, R. A. (1976). Interactions, relationships and social structure. *Man, 11,* 1–17.

Hinde, R. A. (1979). *Towards understanding relationships.* London: Academic Press.

Hinde, R. A. (1982). *Ethology.* Oxford: Oxford University Press.

Hinde, R. A. (1988). Continuities and discontinuities: Conceptual issues and methodological considerations. In M. Rutter (Ed.), *Studies of psychosocial risk: The power of longitudinal data* (pp. 367–383). Cambridge: Cambridge University Press.

Hinde, R., & Stevenson-Hinde, J. (Eds.). (1988). *Relationships within families: Mutual influences.* Oxford: Clarendon Press.

Hodges, J., & Tizard, B. (1989a). IQ and behavioural adjustment of ex-institutional adolescents. *Journal of Child Psychology and Psychiatry, 30,* 53–75.

Hodges, J., & Tizard, B. (1989b). Social and family relationships of ex-institutional adolescents. *Journal of Child Psychology and Psychiatry, 30,* 77–97.

Hofer, M. A. (1994). Hidden regulators in attachment, separation, and loss. In N. A. Fox (Ed.), The development of emotion regulation: Biological and behavioral considerations. *Monographs of the Society for Research in Child Development, 59*(1–2, Serial No. 240), 192–207.

Holmes, J. (1993a). Attachment theory: A biological basis for psychotherapy? *British Journal of Psychiatry, 163,* 430–438.

Holmes, J. (1993b). *John Bowlby and attachment theory.* London/New York: Routledge.

Howes, C., Rodning, C., Galluzzo, D. C., & Myers, L. (1988). Attachment and child care: Relationships with mother and caregiver. *Early Childhood Research Quarterly, 3,* 403–416.

Kagan, J. (1984) *The nature of the child.* New York: Basic Books.

Kaplan, H. I., Sadock, B. J., & Grebb, J. A. (1994). *Kaplan and Sadock's synopsis of psychiatry* (7th ed.). Baltimore: Williams & Wilkins.

Kendler, K. S., Neale, M. C., Kessler, R. C., Heath, A. C., & Eaves, L. J. (1992). Childhood parental loss and adult psychopathology in women: A twin study perspective. *Archives of General Psychiatry, 49,* 109–116.

Kennell, J. H., & Klaus, M. H. (1984). Mother–infant bonding: Weighing the evidence. *Developmental Review, 4,* 275–282.

Klaus, M. H., & Kennell, J. H. (1976). *Maternal–infant bonding: The impact of early separation or loss on family development.* Saint Louis, MO: Mosby.

Kobak, R. (1994). Adult attachment: A personality or relationship construct? *Psychological Inquiry, 5,* 42–44.

Kraemer, G. W. (1992). A psychobiological theory of attachment. *Behavioral and Brain Sciences, 15,* 493–541.

Lamb, M. E., Thompson, R. A., Gardner, W., Charnov, E. L., & Estes, D. (1984). Security of infantile attachment as assessed in the "Strange Situation": Its study and biological interpretations. *Behavioral and Brain Sciences, 7,* 127–147.

Levine, S. (1982). Comparative and psychobiological perspectives on development. In W. A. Collins (Ed.), *Minnesota Symposia on Child Psychology: Vol. 15. The concept of development* (pp. 29–63). Hillsdale, NJ: Erlbaum.

Lomas, P. (1987). *The limits of interpretation: What's wrong with psychoanalysis?* Harmondsworth, Middlesex: Penguin.

Maccoby, E., & Masters, J. C. (1970). Attachment and dependency. In P. H. Mussen (Ed.), *Carmichael's manual of child psychology* (Vol. 2, 3rd ed., pp. 73–157). New York: Wiley.

Main, M. (1991). Metacognitive knowledge, metacognitive monitoring, and singular (coherent) vs multiple (incoherent) models of attachment: Findings and directions for future research. In C. Parkes, J. Stevenson-Hinde, & P. Morris (Eds.), *Attachment across the life cycle.* London: Tavistock/Routledge.

Main, M., & Hesse, E. (1990). Parents' unresolved traumatic experiences are related to infant disorganized attachment status: Is frightened and/or frightening parental behavior the linking mechanism? In M. T. Greenberg, D. Cicchetti, & E. M. Cummings (Eds.), *Attachment in the preschool years: Theory, research and intervention* (pp. 161–184). Chicago: University of Chicago Press.

Main, M., Kaplan, N., & Cassidy, J. (1985). Security in infancy, childhood, and adulthood: A move to the level of representation. In I. Bretherton & E. Waters (Eds.), Growing points in attachment theory. *Monographs of the Society for Research in Child Development, 50*(1–2, Serial No. 209), 66–106.

Main, M., & Solomon, J. (1990). Procedures for identifying disorganized/disoriented infants in the Ainsworth Strange Situation. In M. T. Greenberg, D. Cicchetti, & E. M. Cummings (Eds.), *Attachment in the preschool years: Theory, research and intervention* (pp. 121–160). Chicago: University of Chicago Press.

McCartney, K., & Galanopoulos, A. (1988). Child care and attachment: A new frontier the second time around. *American Journal of Orthopsychiatry, 58,* 16–24.

Miller, P. (1993). *Theories of developmental psychology* (3rd ed.). New York: Freeman.

Miyake, K., Chen, S., & Campos, J. J. (1985). Infant temperament, mother's mode of interaction, and attachment in Japan: An interim report. In I. Bretherton & E. Waters (Eds.), Growing points of attachment theory and research.

Monographs of the Society for Research in Child Development, 50(1–2, Serial No. 209), 276–297.

Nash, A. (1988). Ontogeny, phylogeny and relationships. In S. W. Duck (Ed.), *Handbook of personal relationships* (pp. 121–141). Chichester: Wiley.

O'Connor, N., & Franks, C. M. (1960). Childhood upbringing and other environmental factors. In H. J. Eysenck (Ed.), *Handbook of abnormal psychology* (pp. 393–416). London: Pitman.

Oppenheim, D., Sagi, A., & Lamb, M. (1988). Infant–adult attachments on the kibbutz and their relation to socio-emotional development four years later. *Developmental Psychology, 24,* 427–433.

Parker, J. G., & Asher, S. R. (1987). Peer relations and later personal adjustment: Are low-accepted children at risk? *Psychological Bulletin, 102,* 357–389.

Parkes, C. M., Stevenson-Hinde, J., & Morris, P. (Eds.). (1991). *Attachment across the life cycle.* London: Tavistock/Routledge.

Patrick, M., Hobson, P., Castle, D., Howard, R., & Maughan, B. (1994). Personality disorder and the mental representatives of early social experience. *Development and Psychopathology, 6,* 375–388.

Quinton, D., Pickles, A., Maughan, B., & Rutter, M. (1993). Partners, peers, and pathways: Assortative pairing and continuities in conduct disorder. *Development and Psychopathology, 5,* 763–783.

Radke-Yarrow, M., Cummings, E. M., Kuczynski, L., & Chapman, M. (1985). Patterns of attachment in two- and three-year-old normal families and families with parental depression. *Child Development, 56,* 884–893.

Rajecki, D. W., Lamb, M. E., & Obmascher, P. (1978). Toward a general theory of infantile attachment: A comparative review of aspects of the social bond. *Brain and Behavioral Sciences, 1,* 417–464.

Richters, M. M., & Volkmar, F. R. (1994). Case study: Reactive attachment disorder of infancy or early childhood. *Journal of the American Academy of Child and Adolescent Psychiatry, 33,* 328–332.

Robins, C. J., & Hayes, A. M. (1993). An appraisal of cognitive therapy. *Journal of Consulting and Clinical Psychology, 61,* 205–214.

Rogers, S. J., Ozonoff S., & Maslin-Cole, C. (1991). A comparative study of attachment behavior in young children with autism or other psychiatric disorders. *Journal of the American Academy of Child and Adolescent Psychiatry, 30,* 483–488.

Rubin, K. H., & Lollis, S. P. (1988). Origins and consequences of social withdrawal. In J. Belsky & T. Nezworski (Eds.), *Clinical implications of attachment* (pp. 219–252). Hillsdale, NJ: Erlbaum.

Rutter, M. (1979). Separation experiences: A new look at an old topic. *Journal of Pediatrics, 95,* 147–154.

Rutter, M. (1980). Attachment and the development of social relationships. In M. Rutter (Ed.), *Developmental psychiatry* (pp. 267–279). Washington, DC: American Psychiatric Press.

Rutter, M. (1981). *Maternal deprivation reassessed* (2nd ed.). Harmondsworth, Middlesex: Penguin.

Rutter, M. (1989). Intergenerational continuities and discontinuities in serious parenting difficulties. In D. Cicchetti & V. Carlson (Eds.), *Child maltreatment* (pp. 317–348). New York: Cambridge University Press.

Rutter, M. (1991). A fresh look at 'maternal deprivation.' In P. Bateson (Ed.), *The development and integration of behaviour* (pp. 331–374). Cambridge: Cambridge University Press.

Rutter, M. (1994a). Family discord and conduct disorder: Cause, consequence or correlate? *Journal of Family Psychology, 8,* 170–186.

Rutter, M. (1994b). Beyond longitudinal data: Causes, consequences, changes and continuity. *Journal of Consulting and Clinical Psychology, 62,* 928–940.

Rutter, M., & Rutter, M. (1993). *Developing minds: Challenges and continuities across the lifespan.* Harmondsworth, Middlesex: Penguin; New York: Basic Books.

Sameroff, A. J., & Emde, R. N. (Eds.). (1989). *Relationship disturbances in early childhood: A developmental approach.* New York: Basic Books.

Schaffer, H. R. (1990). *Making decisions about children: Psychological questions and answers.* Oxford: Basil Blackwell.

Shapiro, T., & Esman, A. (1992). Psychoanalysis and child and adolescent psychiatry. *Journal of the American Academy of Child and Adolescent Psychiatry, 31,* 6–13.

Sigman, M., & Ungerer, J. (1984). Attachment behaviors in autistic children. *Journal of Autism and Development Disorders, 14,* 231–244.

Sluckin, W., Herbert, M., & Sluckin, A. (1983). *Maternal bonding.* Oxford: Blackwell Scientific.

Sroufe, L. A. (1983). Infant–caregiver attachment and patterns of adaptation in the preschool: The roots of maladaptation and competence. In M. Perlmutter (Ed.), *Minnesota Symposia on Child Psychology: Vol. 16. Development and policy concerning children with special needs* (pp. 41–83). Hillsdale, NJ: Erlbaum.

Sroufe, L. A. (1986). Bowlby's contribution to psychoanalytic theory and developmental psychology. *Journal of Child Psychology and Psychiatry, 27,* 841–849.

Sroufe, L. A. (1988). The role of infant–caregiver attachments in development. In J. Belsky & T. Nezworski (Eds.), *Clinical implications of attachment* (pp. 18–38). Hillsdale, NJ: Erlbaum.

Sroufe, L. A., & Fleeson, J. (1986). Attachment and the construction of relationships. In W. Hartup & Z. Rubin (Eds.), *Relationships and development* (pp. 51–71). Hillsdale, NJ: Erlbaum.

Sroufe, L. A., Fox, N., & Pancake, V. (1983). Attachment and dependency in developmental perspective. *Child Development, 54,* 1615–1627.

Sroufe, L. A., & Rutter, M. (1984). The domain of developmental psychopathology. *Child Development, 55,* 17–29.

Stern, D. N. (1985). *The interpersonal world of the infant: A view from psychoanalysis and developmental psychology.* New York: Basic Books.

Stern, D. N. (1989). The representation of relational patterns: Developmental considerations. In A. J. Sameroff & R. N. Emde (Eds.), *Relationship distur-bances in early childhood: A developmental approach* (pp. 52–68). New York: Basic Books.

Stevenson-Hinde, J., & Shouldice, A. (1995). Maternal interactions and self-re-ports related to attachment classifications at 4.5 years. *Child Development, 66,* 583–596.

Teasdale, J. (1993). Emotion and two kinds of meaning: Therapy and applied cognitive science. *Behaviour Research and Therapy, 31,* 339–354.

Tizard, B. (1977). Varieties of residential nursery experience. In J. Tizard, I. Sinclair, & R. V. G. Clark (Eds.), *Varieties of residential experience* (pp. 102–121). London: Routledge & Kegan Paul.

Thompson, R. A., Connell, J. P., & Bridges, L. J. (1988). Temperament, emotion, and social interactive behavior in the Strange Situation: An analysis of attachment system functioning. *Child Development, 59,* 1102–1110.

van den Boom, D. (1990). Preventive intervention and the quality of mother–infant interaction and infant exploration in irritable infants. In W. Koops, H. J. G. Soppe, J. L. van der Linden, P. C. M. Molenaar, & J. J. F. Schroots (Eds.), *Developmental psychology behind the dikes* (pp. 249–270). Delft: Uitgeverij Eburon.

van IJzendoorn, M. H. (1995). Adult attachment representations, parental respon-siveness, and infant attachment: A meta-analysis on the predictive validity of the Adult Attachment Interview. *Psychological Bulletin, 117,* 387–403.

Vaughn, B. E., Goldberg, S., Atkinson, L., Marcovitch, S., MacGregor, D., & Seifer, R. (1994). Quality of toddler–mother attachment in children with Down Syndrome: Limits to interpretation of strange situation behavior. *Child Development, 65,* 95–108.

Vaughn, B. E., Stevenson-Hinde, J., Waters, E., Kotsaftis, A., Lefever, G. B., Shouldice, A., Trudel, M., & Belsky, J. (1992). Attachment security and temperament in infancy and early childhood: Some conceptual clarifications. *Developmental Psychology, 28,* 463–473.

Vaughn, B. E., & Waters, E. (1990). Attachment behavior at home and in the laboratory. *Child Development, 61,* 1965–1973.

Wallerstein, R. S. (1988). One psychoanalysis or many? *International Journal of Psycho-Analysis, 69,* 5–21.

Waters, E., Posada, G., Crowell, J., & Keng-Ling, L. (1993). Is attachment theory ready to contribute to our understanding of disruptive behavior problems? *Development and Psychopathology, 5,* 215–225.

Werner, E. E. (1984). *Child care: Kith, kin and hired hands.* Baltimore: University Park.

Wolff, S. (1981). *Children under stress* (2nd ed.). Harmondsworth, Middlesex: Penguin.

Wolff, S. (1989). *Childhood and human nature: The development of personality.* London/New York: Routledge.

World Health Organization. (1992). *The ICD-10 classification of mental and behavior disorders: Clinical descriptions and diagnostic guidelines.* Geneva: Author.

World Health Organization Expert Committee on Mental Health (1951). *Report of the second session 1951.* Geneva: WHO.

Zeanah, C. H., Anders, T. F., Seifer, R., & Stern, D. M. (1989). Implications of research on infant development for psychodynamic theory and practice. *Journal of the American Academy of Child and Adolescent Psychiatry, 28,* 657–668.

Zeanah, C. H., & Emde, R. N. (1994). Attachment disorders in infancy and childhood. In M. Rutter, E. Taylor, & L. Hersov (Eds.), *Child and adolescent psychiatry: Modern approaches* (3rd ed., pp. 490–504). Oxford: Blackwell Scientific.

Zigler, E. F., & Gordon, E. W. (Eds.). (1982). *Day care: Scientific and social policy issues.* Boston: Auburn House.

Zoccolillo, M., Pickles, A., Quinton, D., & Rutter, M. (1992). The outcome of childhood conduct disorder: Implications for defining adult personality disorder and conduct disorder. *Psychological Medicine, 22,* 971–986.

3

Patterns of Attachment and Sexual Behavior: Risk of Dysfunction versus Opportunity for Creative Integration

PATRICIA McKINSEY CRITTENDEN

Successful species must solve two problems: staying safe and reproducing. Bowlby's attachment theory is focused on the effect of the first on human functioning, whereas Freud's theory of psychosexual development is focused on the second. Although much of Freud's thinking is outdated empirically, such that even most psychanalytic theorists have modified it in favor of approaches that are more similar to attachment theory (i.e., object relations, ego psychology, self psychology), Freud nevertheless correctly identified one of the essential components of species survival and thus, one of two central organizers of adaptive functioning (Crittenden, 1994a, 1995). In this chapter, I offer some thoughts on individual differences in the way the issues of protection and reproduction are solved.

I find the model for individual differences in Ainsworth's three patterns of attachment in infancy—that is, Types A, B, and C (Ainsworth, 1979)—with the addition of a fourth pattern, A/C (Crittenden, 1985a, 1985b, 1988; Radke-Yarrow, Cummings, Kuczynski, & Chapman, 1985). Because my thinking about the patterns has changed over the last few years, I first describe what I mean by the A and C patterns, in terms both of the organization of the attachment and exploratory behavior systems and also of mental functioning.[1] Regarding mental functioning, I consider the sorts of information available to the brain as well as the sophisticated organization of this information in memory systems (Crittenden, 1995).

Before beginning, let me describe where this discussion is headed. Some time ago, when discussing the risks for psychopathology associated with anxious attachment, I was asked: *If being a Type B is so good, why didn't evolution hard-wire it into our brains?* Accepting for a moment the metaphorical premise that "evolution" is capable of reasoning, I think the reason may be that using a "B" strategy (of open and direct communication of intentions and feelings together with negotiation and compromise) can be a disadvantage, *especially under dangerous circumstances*. Indeed, the A (defended/disengaged) and C (coercive/enmeshed) strategies have unique advantages that assist individuals to cope with dangerous circumstances. Of course, it is true that either the A or C strategy alone can skew perception and behavior, leaving individuals vulnerable to dysfunction under some conditions. But together, in the A/C strategy, they can yield individuals who are vulnerable under all conditions, vulnerable under almost no conditions, or responsive to changes in threats to safety and the opportunity to reproduce.

A/Cs, in other words, may be both especially prone to dysfunction under conditions that carry little threat to safety or reproduction and, at the same time, uniquely able to adapt in ways that promote both safety and reproduction under conditions of serious threat. As a side effect of their strategy and of the conditions that foster its development, I argue that A/Cs sometimes are able to construct models of reality that are outstandingly creative and meaningful.

AN EVOLUTIONARY PERSPECTIVE ON BRAIN DEVELOPMENT AND THE MENTAL PROCESSING OF INFORMATION

Let me begin with an evolutionary perspective on staying safe and reproducing. The human brain has evolved to organize incoming sensory information in ways that promote our safety and ability to reproduce. There are four ways in which this occurs.[2]

Privileged Information and Perception

First, information relevant to safety and to reproduction is privileged; that is, we attend to such information in preference to other information (Gallistel, Brown, Carey, Gelman, & Keil, 1991). Such information includes information from and about other humans, especially attachment figures and potential sexual partners, as well as information directly tied to safety and danger.

The Reptilian Brain, Temporal/Cognitive
Information, and Sexual Behavior

Second, species that are as evolved as reptiles are able to infer meaning from the temporal order of events (Luria, 1973; Ornstein & Thompson, 1984). That is, when preceding events are predictably linked to subsequent events, organisms respond as though they presumed, in a sensorimotor way, that the preceding event caused the subsequent event. If the subsequent event is reinforcing, the preceding event will be repeated frequently. If the subsequent event is punitive, the preceding event will be avoided or inhibited. Moreover, the "events" and responses can be complex sets of conditions or sequences of events. The midbrain, in other words, enables organisms to use information regarding the temporal order of events to infer causal relations that can be used to modify behavior predictively. The principles of such learning are represented in Skinnerian and Pavlovian learning theory. I refer to this sort of information as "cognition."

Note, however, that the causal inference can be erroneous; events that precede other events do not necessarily cause them. Especially when only one instance of temporal relation is observed, the conclusion of causality may be false. Nevertheless, when the single instance has perceived implications for safety and survival, it may be too dangerous to risk a second attempt at trial learning. In such cases, one instance may effectively change behavior in ways that would appear irrational if the original learning conditions were not known. A familiar example of this is aversion to foods that, on a single occasion, are followed by feeling nauseous (Gustavson, Garcia, Hankins, & Rusiniak, 1974). Such foods are treated as though they were poisonous, although in fact they may not actually have caused the nausea. Regardless of the accuracy of the inference, information about causality is generated by the midbrain and is used to regulate future behavior.

The midbrain also regulates courting behavior (MacLean, 1973). Although little, if any, of this potential is used in immature organisms, after puberty species-specific patterns of sexual behavior (mental and physical) become powerful influences on behavior.

The Limbic System, Contextual Information, and Affect

Third, the brains of mammals have evolved to include various forms of a limbic system. Put overly simplistically, the limbic system processes information relevant to dangers that have not yet been experienced (MacLean, 1990). Stimuli indicative of dangerous contexts, for example, darkness, entrapping conditions, and being alone, elicit feelings of anxiety (Bowlby,

1973; LeDoux, 1986; Seligman, 1971). This anxiety is not tied to something specific that is known to be dangerous; rather, it is experienced as
unfocused, "free-floating" anxiety. When we feel this anxiety, we feel we
must "get out of here." If we cannot flee, we prepare to defend ourselves
(Selye, 1976). Although we cannot attribute the feeling to a specific danger,
in fact, as both Bowlby and Seligman noted, contexts that elicit feelings of
anxiety carry a higher risk of danger than do others. Conversely, we feel
comfort when we are in light, open spaces, and with other people. Indeed,
of all the people we could have, we prefer someone who is stronger, wiser,
and committed to our welfare; we prefer an attachment figure.

I call information derived from feelings "affect." Its function is to
provide contextual cues that alert us to the possibility of danger. Like
cognitive information, with experience we expand our perception of
dangerous and safe contexts. Conditions that are frequently associated
with unconditioned elicitors of anxiety come themselves to evoke a conditioned affective response, thus reflecting Pavlovian learning principles.
In mammalian species conditioned stimuli are most quickly associated
with affective responses when several natural elicitors co-occur with the
conditioned stimulus (Mowrer & Gordon, 1983; Mowrer, 1988). Again,
the more dangerous the context is perceived to be, the more likely it is that
the association will be made in a single trial. In addition, dangerous
outcomes become associated with perceptual aspects of context. Thus,
contextual learning (that is experienced as affect) can facilitate or hinder
display of cognitive learning, based on the perceived cues of danger in
contexts (Gordon, Mowrer, McGinnis, & McDermott, 1985).

Like information about causality, affective information may be in
error. That is, there can be cues of danger and one can feel anxious when,
in fact, there is no danger. Similarly, one can feel comfortable when there
is danger. Because feeling adds meaning to simple sensory information in
ways that are not conscious, it can be quite difficult to calm anxiety when
there is no danger. Like erroneous cognitive information, erroneous affective information can modify behavior in ways that are incomprehensible
to onlookers who perceive the dangerousness of the situation differently
and who are unaware of the original learning experience.

The limbic system also regulates unlearned feelings of sexual arousal
and satisfaction that promote successful reproduction. With the advent of
puberty, sexual stimuli elicit sexual arousal and a focusing of attention in
ways that are quite similar to the effects of anxiety (Cantor, Zillmann, &
Einsiedel, 1978). Particularly when the source of arousal is neither immediate nor intense, lingering nonsexual arousal may be readily associated
with later-occurring sexual stimuli, leading to a misattribution of sexual
arousal (Cantor, Zillmann, & Bryant, 1975). Similarly, sexual climax
elicits feelings of satisfaction that are quite similar to the comfort associ-

ated with reduced anxiety. Thus, chronically anxious individuals may be prone to misattribution of sexual desire, whereas those experiencing episodes of focused and intense anxiety would have reduced elicitation of sexual desire (Zillmann, 1984). Furthermore, when the desire for comfort is expressed as sexual behavior that leads to sexual satisfaction, a conditioned misattribution may be operantly reinforced. One consequence may be the clinically observed relation between anxiety and sexual behavior (Barlow, Sakheim, & Beck, 1983; Hale & Strassberg, 1990).

Cortical Integration

Finally, mammals, especially primates, and most especially *Homo sapiens*, have an evolved cortex. The cortex integrates information coming from the lower brain. One function of the cortex is to evaluate the accuracy of information by comparing and contrasting different inputs. When there is no discrepancy, responding progresses unimpeded; indeed, it rarely becomes conscious (Lashley, 1958/1960). Although this leads to efficient responding, it also has serious implications if the information or the habitual response is inappropriate.

When there is a discrepancy among the sources of information, the mind is capable of alerting in ways that foster the construction of more accurate representations of what is "out there" and greater refinement of behavioral responses. In infants, this can be observed as surprise and curiosity (Kagan, 1970); in toddlers and older humans, it may be experienced consciously. At any age, however, the more threatening the potential danger is perceived to be, the more likely the mind is to generate protective action without full cortical evaluation of the information or the response.

A related function of the cortex is to resolve ambiguous information. Often this requires that several bits of information be considered in concert. For example, sexually arousing stimuli may elicit both courtship behavior and sexual feelings. Information about previous experience or the context, however, may be used to inhibit action on these potentials. For a male, such inhibitory contextual information could be the presence of another, more dominant male, the recognition that the sexually attractive object is not a sexually mature member of one's own species, or that the female is likely, once again, to reject one's overtures.

In conclusion, I want to propose that the human brain has evolved to organize sensory information in ways that promote protection and reproduction. The brain does so (1) by attending preferentially to information relevant to protection and reproduction, (2) by attributing causation to temporally organized information so as to modify behavior in ways that increase desired outcomes and reduce undesirable ones, (3) by eliciting feelings of anxiety and sexual excitement and of comfort and satisfaction when we experience probable dangerous or safe contexts or conditions conducive to reproduction, and (4) by integrating information cortically. These processes are genetically transmitted and universal to our species (Tooby & Cosmides, 1990).

INDIVIDUAL DIFFERENCES IN MENTAL AND BEHAVIORAL FUNCTIONING IN INFANCY

Patterns of Attachment

Type B: Securely Attached Infants

Both experience and mental maturation change the way cognitive and affective information are cortically integrated to yield mental representations of reality[3] and organized patterns of behavior (Crittenden, 1994b). When caregivers respond to infants' signals, they provide infants with information about the effects of their behavior. Because of differences in caregivers' behavior, some infants learn that the effects are prompt, predictable, and soothing. For these infants, expression of anxiety or discomfort leads to caregiving that, in turn, leads to comfort. In learning theory terms, these infants are on a schedule of predictable, positive reinforcement of affective signals. Further, parents' ability to differentiate infants' needs and signals enables infants to better differentiate their signals, thus, leading to clearer, less ambiguous communication (Stern, 1985). By 1 year of age, we call such infants secure, Type B (B1–4) (Ainsworth, 1979). (See Figure 3.1.)

Type A: Avoidantly Attached Infants

Other infants learn that the effects of their affective behavior are prompt, predictable, and unpleasant. For example, some mothers are exasperated by infant crying or infants' demands to be picked up; these mothers reject, withdraw from, or punish their infants. In such cases, expression of anxiety leads to maternal behavior that elicits discomfort, thus exacerbating the infant's distress. Such infants are on a schedule of predictable punishment of affective signals. Consequently, they learn in a sensorimotor way to inhibit display of affect. Infants who inhibit expression of feelings of fear, desire for the caregiver, and anger at their mothers' unavailability are called avoidant, Type A (A1–2) (Ainsworth, 1979; Main, 1981). Note, however, that it is expression of negative affect that most Type A caregivers do not reward. Such caregivers are protective and give appropriate care to their infants. Indeed, most of their infants learn to trust that their caregivers will protect them, without the prod of negative affect. (See Figure 3.1.)

Type C: Ambivalently Attached Infants

Infants in a third group learn that the effects of their behavior are unpredictable; for these infants, caregivers respond sometimes and not at other times, or they respond in ways that are soothing only sometimes (Ainsworth et al., 1978; Cassidy & Berlin, 1994). These infants are on a schedule of intermittent, unpredictable reinforcement. Such a schedule is very powerful in terms of eliciting and maintaining behavior at intense levels for long periods of time in spite of punishment, reinforcement of incompatible behavior, or lack of response. Infants who experience con-current and unsoothed feelings of anger, fear, and desire for comfort come to associate both the feelings and concurrent conditions with possible danger. When these feelings are directed toward the same attachment figure, the infants are called ambivalent, Type C (C1–2). Unlike Type A infants, Type C infants have little basis for predicting the protective availability of their caregivers. (See Figure 3.1.)

Type A/C: Avoidant/Ambivalent Infants

Some infants whose home environments are complex and varied switch between the inhibition of Type A functioning and the distress of Type C

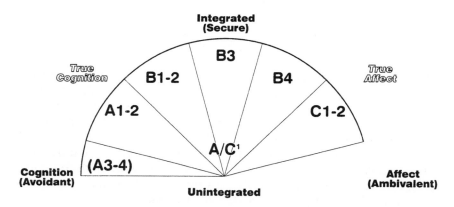

FIGURE 3.1. Patterns of attachment in infancy as a function of type of information and degree of integration of information. I = avoidant/ambivalent. From Crittenden (1995). Reprinted by permission.

functioning. Most A/C infants experience poor caregiving, such as that from mothers who both abuse and neglect their children (Crittenden, 1985a, 1985b, 1988) or who themselves have bipolar depression (Radke-Yarrow et al., 1985). Put another way, infants with an A/C pattern experience both unpredictable and dangerous environments. The A/C pattern itself represents an attempt to adapt to a varied and varying reality; as such it represents an achievement that fosters infants' protection at the same time that infants' subjective experience is one of considerable anxiety and discomfort.

In each of these four cases, caregivers teach infants, through their pattern of responses to infants' affective signals, how to use the affective and cognitive information available to their minds (Vygotsky, 1987). In the case of predictably sensitive responding, infants learn to use both cognitive and affective information. Infants whose affective signals are punished learn that cognitive predictions can be trusted, but that affect misleads; consequently, they tend to discard (i.e., defend against) information about their own feelings in organizing their behavior. Infants of inconsistent caregivers learn that affect is neither consistently reinforced, nor consistently punished; such infants are unable to organize their behavior effectively around either affect or cognition. They tend to be very distressed.

By 1 year of age, these four groups of infants are easily differentiated.[4] Two of them, avoidant and ambivalent infants, face particular problems that cannot be resolved with sensorimotor mental functioning. Specifically, inhibited infants know how to prevent unwanted rejection and punishment, but not how to elicit desired caregiving, whereas infants of inconsistent mothers do not know how to influence caregiver behavior predictably.

Sexuality in Infancy

Although infants have gender and respond to sensual contact, current empirical work does not support the notion of infant sexuality. There is, however, no question that mothers are sexual. This presents an asymmetry that appears to have left both theorists and the societies that they reflect uncomfortable. Freud solved the problem by sexualizing infants and focusing on sexuality as the primary organizer of human adaptive and dysfunctional behavior throughout the lifespan. Bowlby both identified the importance of protection and also saw the fallacy of sexualizing infants and children. His theory, however, desexualized mothers.

In the thinking that I offer here, I am presuming that, although prepubertal humans have gender and immature sexual organs, they normally do not respond preferentially to sexual stimuli, have sexual feelings, or have functional sexual organs. Their parents, on the other hand, are fully sexual and may have sexual responses to their infants. Patterns of adult integration of information may be relevant to whether and how adults act on sexual feelings that are elicited by children. Because the patterns are the result of individual differences in adults' ontological experiences, together with their mental activity around those experiences, adults' patterns of attachment may be relevant not only to infants' patterns of attachment, but also to sexual behavior with children and to children's sexual development (for clinical case example, see Lieberman, Chapter 9, this volume).

THE PRESCHOOL YEARS

After the period of rapid neurological change at the end of the second year of life, children gain new mental competencies. These increase the ways in which cognitive and affective information can be integrated (Crittenden, in press). The range of preschoolers' attachment relationships expands to include multiple hierarchical (i.e., asymmetrical), nonreciprocal[5] relationships with caregiving adults such as daycare providers and grandparents. Having a range of models promotes flexibility of behavior wherein the distortions of one relationship are reduced by experience with other attachment figures. Finally, cultural differences noticeably influence children's behavior. In this chapter, culture is viewed as information that other members of our species, who have lived in similar contexts, have learned about how to stay safe and reproduce *in that context*. This information is passed from adult to child, thus reducing the need for experiential learning and increasing the probability that well-proven patterns of behavior will protect the child. In the preschool years, cultural influences reflect biases emphasizing affective or cognitive organization of information and behavior and gender-based differences in patterns.

Patterns of Attachment

Type B and Balanced Representation

With the advantage of linguistic representation and intuitive logic, preschool-aged children are able to communicate with caregivers regarding future events (Marvin, 1977). Of particular interest is adults' availability to children should children need help and protection. When adults and children are able to exchange accurate information about feelings and intentions, they can be apart without either parents or children feeling anxious. This facilitates children's safe exploration of their environment. This, in turn, fosters children's ability to learn about the world, to develop affiliative relationships with other people, and to learn the skills necessary to care for themselves. As a consequence, the internal representational models of such children reflect both their own observations and the more sophisticated knowledge of their caregivers. Children who mentally integrate both cognitive and affective information are called "balanced/secure," with subgroups that range from *reserved* to *comfortable* to *reactive* (Crittenden, 1992a).[6]

Because balanced/secure children are able both to communicate the range of their feelings and also to reason intuitively with caregivers about the danger of situations, they often feel comfortable, even when they do not get their way. Preliminary studies, however, suggest that boys and girls may not experience this outcome equally. To the contrary, boys may be more often classified as secure than girls (Crittenden & Claussen, 1994; Fagot & Pears, 1996; Teti, Gelfand, Messinger, & Isabella, 1995; Moore, Crawford, & Lester, 1994). This may reflect both cultural and physiological influences that promote the inhibition of display of anger among girls.

Dominance and Submission

Preoperational[7] children use coy behavior to negotiate dominance disputes. Coy behavior is composed of behaviors used by other mammals to terminate others' aggression, for example, baring the belly and the neck, and to elicit nurturance, for example, glancing eye contact and an openmouth smile with teeth covered (Eibl-Eibesfeldt, 1979). These signals (which, when used together, are called coy behavior) enable children to disarm parental anger and transform it into parental nurturance. Coy behavior, together with the sophisticated intellectual competencies of the preoperational mind, enables preschool children to organize and implement a coercive behavioral strategy (Crittenden, 1992a).

This strategy involves displaying angry threats and/or aggression at high intensity until parents respond. Although this reduces the problem of parental unavailability, the nature of the response remains uncertain. If the parent's response is appeasing, the display of anger usually escalates. If, on the other hand, the parent's response is angry, the child switches to coy behavior. Coy, feigned helplessness is used to "bribe" the parent until he or she becomes exasperated with that also; then the child switches back to threatening aggressiveness. For example, in a grocery store check-out line, a child demands a candy bar. The parent ignores this. The child begins to whine and rapidly escalates to crying, then screaming, and possibly to a full tantrum. At some point, the parent takes notice. If the parent tries to figure out what the child wants and to give it to him or her, the child is likely to maintain the angry display. The child may even reject the offered candy bar and demand a different one. This will continue until the parent is fed up and becomes angry. The child then switches to coy behavior. The child looks meek and innocent, with head cocked to the side, sweet little glances to the angry parent, tummy pushed forward, and a tender little smile (without evidence of aggressive teeth). The parent is likely to melt and the expected punishment for the child's previous outrageously angry behavior is reduced or foregone altogether. The child then continues to act dependent and incompetent until the parent becomes exasperated with the feigned helplessness of the coy display and again shows anger. Then the child switches back to displays of anger. Most parents, fearing another tantrum, try to placate the child, who then demands more. And so on, in an entangling pattern from which many parents are unable to extricate themselves.

All preschool-aged children discover this strategy. Among young children, the threatening and disarming halves of the pattern are displayed approximately equally and in quite rapid alternation. With development, the displays become more discrete and, often, one becomes dominant. Cultural gender values appear to influence this selection such that boys and girls show different predominant patterns, with boys displaying more threatening/dominant behavior and girls more disarming/submissive behavior (Block, Block, & Gjerde, 1986; Emery, 1982; LaFreniere & Sroufe, 1985; Lewis, Feiring, McGuffog, & Jaskir, 1984; Renken, Egeland, Marvinney, Mangelsdorf, & Sroufe, 1989). All of the referenced studies, however, use the infant patterns of attachment as opposed to the preschool patterns (and distributions) being referred to here. With the latter, gender differentiation might well be clearer.

Type C and the Coercive Strategy with Its Obsessive Subpatterns

Although the coercive strategy is discovered by all children, it becomes characteristic of children of inconsistent caregivers because it increases the predictability of caregiver behavior. Mentally, it involves splitting feelings of anger, fear, and desire into separate display packages that are alternately displayed in exaggerated form. Affect, in other words, is emphasized (through intense display of feelings) in order to get cognitive predictability. Preschool-aged children who use this strategy on a regular basis as their primary means of regulating relationships are called "coercive" (Type C). (See Figure 3.2.)

Coercive children effectively transform their situation of not being able to predict what the parent will do into a situation in which parents cannot predict what children will do. Because parents find this both entrapping and frustrating, many try to extricate themselves by using false cognition. That is, they behave in ways that mislead their children with regard to their intentions. If they want to do something that will displease their child, they mislead the child into believing that they will do as the child wants. When the child trustingly relaxes his or her guard, the parent does what the child did not want. Parents who do this teach their children not to trust cognitive information and instead to stick to intensely affective demands. In the mild (normative) form of the coercive strategy, the two halves of the patterns are called "threatening" (C1) and "disarming" (C2), whereas in the more severe forms that carry greater risk of dysfunction, they are called "aggressive"[8] (C3) and "feigned helpless" (C4). Because the coercive strategy functions only in the presence of the attachment figure, coercive children are excessively clingy; in the more extreme subpatterns, this becomes an obsession with maintaining access to the attachment figure. Although boys and girls differ in the dominant display pattern, there is no difference in the number of boys and girls who are classified as

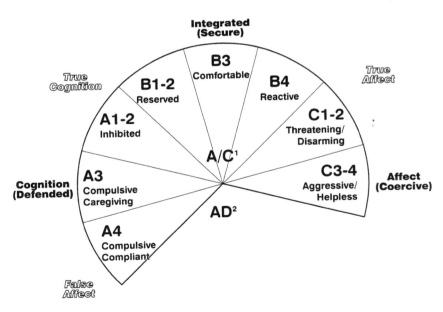

FIGURE 3.2. Patterns of attachment in the preschool years as a function of type of information and degree of integration of information. 1 = defended/coercive; 2 = anxious depressed. From Crittenden (1995). Reprinted by permission.

"coercive" (Crittenden & Claussen, 1994; Fagot & Pears, 1996; Moore et al., 1994; Teti et al., 1995).

Type A and the Defended Strategy with Its Compulsive Subpatterns

Children whose caregivers punish affective displays dare not, and need not, use a coercive strategy. Nevertheless, they need a way to elicit caregiver support. Use of coy behavior quickly demonstrates that caregivers like smiles and sweetness from children. Consequently, many children with rejecting and intrusive caregivers learn to act happy when they are actually frightened and angry. They learn, in other words, to falsify the display of affect to obtain the nurturant response that they desire from attachment figures (Crittenden, 1992a; Winnicott, 1958). Preschool-aged children who use false affective display to elicit desired caregiving are called "defended" (Type A). (See Figure 3.2.)

For "inhibited" (A1–2) children, this behavior is used in a mild form that distorts their reality only a little; indeed, a bit of false positive affect can smooth interpersonal relationships, thus making them more satisfying to both parties. Other children, however, have more difficult circumstances. When caregivers are, themselves, withdrawn, that is, psychologically unavailable (Erickson & Egeland, 1987), children learn to use false positive affect to elicit attention without making any demands that might cause the parent to retreat (psychologically) further. Caregiving behavior ranges from simply entertaining the parent to actual role reversal (see Lieberman, Chapter 9, this volume, for a clinical case example). Such children are in a subgroup of defended children labeled "compulsive caregiving" (A3; Bowlby, 1980; Crittenden, 1992a). At the other extreme, there are caregivers who are hostilely aggressive when their demands are not met. Their children learn to hide their real desires and preferences and to do immediately that which their parents desire. Such children are called "compulsively compliant" (A4; Crittenden & DiLalla, 1988). In the preschool years, there appears to be a higher proportion of girls than boys who are classified as defended, especially defended/compulsive caregiving.

Type A/C

The A/C pattern of the preschool years is far more developed than in infancy. This is in part because the coercive strategy is organized to effectively modify caregivers' behavior and in part because, with greater mental flexibility, children are able to combine not only the A and C

patterns, but also specific subpatterns. In addition, they can selectively
display varied subpatterns within a strategy, for example, switching from
simple inhibition of affect (A1–2) to compulsive caregiving (A3). Although,
technically, this is not an A/C strategy, it functions similarly. Finally,
children may use a defended strategy with one parent and a coercive one
with the other, thus, constructing an A/C pattern that is tied to specific
interactants. In any of these cases, the A/C pattern implies a mental change
in the attention given to information, a change in which some information
is ignored or distrusted under one set of circumstances, followed by
changed circumstances in which the opposite sort of information is ignored
or distrusted. Such mental agility is both adaptive in changing and dangerous circumstances and also predictive of risk for later disorder, including,
in some cases, dissociative mental processes (Putnam, 1995).

Anxious Depressed Children

For a small number of children, especially children of nonthreatening,
unipolar depressed and neglecting parents, nothing that the children do
changes the probabilities of their parents' behavior. These children appear
to use scraps of the strategies in a self-soothing strategy (Crittenden, 1992a,
1995) that resembles aspects of both learned helplessness (Seligman, 1975)
and distorted self-development (Kohut, 1992). Children of unipolar depressed mothers often show this pattern of "anxious depression" (see
Figure 3.2) or the compulsive caregiving pattern (Teti et al., 1995).

Summary

Defended children learn to use cognitive information to organize their
behavior, to inhibit display of true feelings, and to falsely display positive
feelings. Doing so enables them to experience more satisfying relationships
with caregivers and to reduce the isolation of the infant avoidant pattern.
Coercive children learn to split their mixed feelings and display them with
exaggeration in an alternating coercive pattern of angry threats and
disarming bribes. In addition, some children whose parents behave in
rejecting and punitive ways on some occasions and in inconsistently
responsive ways on other occasions learn both the defended and coercive
strategies and use them selectively, depending upon caregivers' behavior.
Children of parents with bipolar depression and children whose parents
both abuse and neglect them often show this strategy (Crittenden, 1985a,
1985b; Radke-Yarrow et al., 1985). Although all three groups of children
show behavioral and mental distortion, all have learned effective behav-

ioral strategies that increase their safety, given the way their parents behave. Children classified as anxious depressed have not found a strategy that changes the probabilities on caregiver behavior; instead, they organize around soothing themselves.

Memory Systems

Among the new cortical abilities available to preoperational children is the ability to encode information that is more sophisticated than preconscious sensorimotor schema, that is, procedural memory (Tulving, 1972, 1985). One type of information (that probably appears in infancy) is tied closely to contexts that elicit feelings of anxiety (including desire for comfort, anger, and fear) and comfort. This information exists in the form of perceptual sensory images[9] (Lazarus, 1982; Leventhal, 1984; Plutchik, 1980), for example, the sight of huge threatening hands looming over oneself, the special sound of a bomber, and the smell accompanying death—or a dentist's office. Comfort might be imaged as the fragrance of a father's smooth cheek, the yielding warmth of a woman's breasts, or the soft smelliness of a favored teddy bear. Such aspects of dangerous or safe situations become associated with affective responses and function to elicit the associated feelings in future situations, i.e., they are conditioned elicitors of unconditioned affects. Images of danger tend to reflect distal sensory information (sight, sound, smell) whereas images of comfort tend to be proximal (touch, quiet sounds, intimate odors). Imaged information enables one to estimate, preconsciously and rapidly, the threat of a situation, based on past experience with similar situations.

Another, more sophisticated, sort of information, labeled semantic memory, contains verbal generalizations (i.e., propositions) that facilitate prediction of how people or situations will be in the future (Bowlby, 1980). Semantic memory is cognitive in nature and regulates problem-solving behavior (Crittenden, 1992b). Episodic memory, on the other hand, refers to information about specific events. Both affective and cognitive information are integrated such that events unfold in memory in temporal order and with sensory information from multiple modalities. The information needed to construct episodes is stored at numerous sites within the brain; as a consequence, a high level of integration is needed to retrieve episodes (Tulving, 1985, 1995). Elsewhere I have argued that the relatively small number of experiences that are retained as episodes tend to be those that contain unresolved, mixed, and arousing affects tied to danger (Bowlby, 1980; Crittenden, 1994b). I have also proposed that episodic memory regulates behavior when affective arousal is too high for cool, cognitive problem solving; often the outcome is the unwitting replication of past failed responses. If, however, one is able to keep all sorts of information conscious, the mind has the maximum opportunity to resolve new problems without repeating past failed solutions. Because each of the memory systems is biased to detect certain information at the expense of other information, each distorts the representation of reality in predictable ways (Bowlby, 1980; Crittenden, 1994b). Together, however, they can provide a complex, textured model of what is "out there" and the options that one has for responding. This sort of integration, however, exceeds the ability of preoperational children.

Preschoolers and Sexuality

Recent attention to sexual abuse of children has highlighted the issue of children's sexuality. Moreover, much has been made in psychoanalytic theory of preschoolers' sexuality, particularly of masturbation and the "oedipal phase." The perspective being developed here is somewhat different.

Preschoolers' "masturbation" seems better conceptualized as self-soothing behavior that uses stroking of highly innervated parts of the body, that is, the fingers, mouth, and genitals, to facilitate a change from an aroused and distressed state to a calmer, more comfortable state. This is quite different from sexual masturbation that uses stroking to facilitate a change from a calm state to a sexually aroused and focused one. The comparison of these processes serves as a reminder that identifying the function of behavior is essential to understanding its meaning and that most organs can serve more than one function. With regard to the oedipal phase, I have offered an interpretation of this in terms of the challenge to children of realizing that people of great importance to themselves can, nevertheless, have intimate and satisfying relationships with other people. For further discussion of this, see Crittenden (1994a).

Finally, recent public awareness of sexual abuse of children makes it clear that children, especially children over 2 years of age, can be perceived by adults as potential sexual partners. Although explaining this response in adults exceeds the scope of this chapter, it is relevant to note that coy behavior is morphologically very similar to flirtatious behavior. Indeed, its roots in dominance and submission may be the same. The fact that infants do not display coy behavior may help to account for the substantially lower rates of sexual abuse of infants as compared with preschool-aged children (U.S. Department of Health and Human Services, 1994).

Again, it is important to note that adults who integrate information poorly or who deal with erroneous information are least likely to be able to regulate their behavior appropriately, including their sexual behavior. In the preschool years, Type A children learn to inhibit and falsify their feelings and to organize their consciously regulated behavior around adults' generalizations about how one should behave. Nevertheless, episodic memory may regulate their behavior when they are highly aroused. If this is carried forward to later developmental stages, it creates risk that feelings may sometimes motivate behavior that cannot be explained or acknowledged consciously. Type C children learn to exaggerate their affective display and to demand its satisfaction immediately and with little cortical interference from semantic regulation. After puberty, when feelings become sexual, this pattern may reduce adults' inhibition to sexual activity with children, particularly when children exhibit coy behavior and the desire for nurturance. A/C adults (and the children in their care) experience both risks.

MENTAL INTEGRATION AND THE SCHOOL YEARS

In the school years, children gain additional mental skills. Among the many implications of concrete logical functioning, I consider two: false cognition and mental integration of information from different memory systems. In terms of attachment, school-aged children develop best friend relationships. These can be considered the first step in the process of developing attachments to peers. Thus, the attachment figures of school-aged children include not only adults (with whom they have hierarchical, nonreciprocal relationships; see Youniss, 1992), but also best friends with whom they have symmetrical but nonreciprocal relationships; that is, the children are of equivalent status and each treats the other, in low stress situations, as an attachment figure, but neither thinks of themselves as an attachment figure.

False Information

One implication of concrete mental operations is that school-aged children learn to use false cognition to deceive others with regard to their intentions. This is not simply lying; it is organizing one's behavior so as to lead other people to false predictions about what one is intending to do. Doing so prevents others from protecting themselves from the individual's action. It also distorts others' predictive, cognitive information. For example, when children feel threatened by caregivers' behavior, they use false cognition, for example, feigned helplessness, to elicit caregiving. Of course, this mental and behavioral strategy may be diverted to other, more antisocial ends as, for example, when a child enters a store and looks like a shopper but, in fact, is stealing.

Coercive children are both the most likely to add false cognition to their strategy for regulating access to attachment figures and the most likely to engage in antisocial, "punitive" (C5) behavior. That is, some extremely aggressive children may become preoccupied with retribution, obsessed with revenge against those who have offended them and may use deception in the service of punitive behavior. Other coercive children may integrate deception with disarming behavior to create a "seductive" (C6) pattern of misleading others with regard to one's need for rescue and willingness to submit to the other. The false cognition of the coercive pattern, together with the false affect associated with the defended pattern, expands symmetrically my model of types of information associated with the Ainsworth's ABC strategies. The A/C strategy, of course, uses both false affect and false cognition. (See Figure 3.3.)

Mental Integration of Information

A second implication of concrete mental functioning is that, in the school years, children begin to integrate information from the various memory

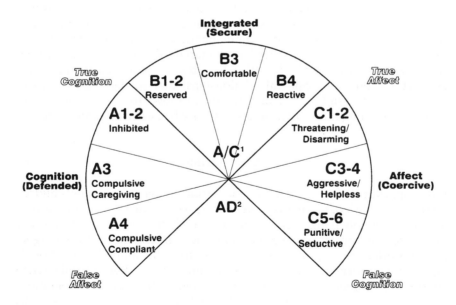

FIGURE 3.3. Patterns of attachment in the school years as a function of type of information and degree of integration of information. I = defended/coercive; 2 = anxious depressed. From Crittenden (1995). Reprinted by permission.

systems (Crittenden, 1992b, 1994a). Put another way, school-aged children are able to hold information from more than one memory system conscious at one time and to compare this information. This is reflected in school-aged children's fascination with riddles and jokes in which a situation has one meaning when viewed form one perspective and another meaning from a different perspective. Moreover, school-aged children recognize the simultaneous relatedness and incongruence of the perspectives.

By analogy, integration of information from different memory systems functions as though children had several distorted lenses through which to view reality. By peering through first one and then another, children are able to construct more complete and accurate representational models of reality. Of course, both reality and the integrated model are often less purely secure, defended, or coercive than the ABC patterns of infancy or even of the preschool years. As a consequence, many children construct both complex representational models that mix A and C characteristics and also complex patterns of behavior that reflect more subtle differences in caregivers' behavior. Often the models are organized in a conditional hierarchy, for example, "My mother is usually supportive, but, if she is tired, then she can be rejecting."

Differentiation within a Pattern

In some cases, a major pattern merely becomes differentiated. For example, some C2 boys become "sissies" whereas others behave as clowns. Although both subpatterns are "disarming" in the sense that they avoid conflict, nevertheless, the use of humor in the clowning pattern creates the potential for the child to recognize, with neither complete integration nor complete denial, two discrepant aspects of reality. Thus, this pattern may provide a new gradient between coercive and balanced children. Similarly, the defended subpatterns become further differentiated with some inhibited children putting on the false smile of popularity, whereas others retreat into isolation or compensatory and private interests, that is, early compulsive self-reliance (Bowlby, 1979).

Differentiation within the A/C Pattern

In other cases, patterns are blended but without equal weight, for example, A3/c2. More balanced children learn to use the defended and coercive strategies when conditions are such that these strategies will be the most effective. They do so, however, without distorting how their minds process information. Particularly in peer relations, including best friend attachments, children learn that other people sometimes use false affect or false cognition to gain advantage. Having this knowledge is highly adaptive, presuming that it does not create doubt that communication can be honest and relationships trustworthy. The goal, of course, is to learn how to distinguish between true and false communication.

Multiple Representational Models

Finally, in the school years, children become able to articulate integrations of representational models of relationships with more than one person. Thus, children can characterize their mother as compared with their father and can describe how to act with regard to each (something they have known preconsciously since infancy; Main & Weston, 1981). For example, a child can be consciously aware that if he wants affection or sympathy, then he should go to Mom, whereas Dad is an easy mark for money. The more balanced a child's mental processing, the more likely it is that a child will be able to construct differentiated models of both self and others. Such models will represent both usual functioning and variations. For example, a child might be able to describe his or her father as caring and patient, except when he has had a hard day at work; then it is wise to stay out of his way. Similar models of one's self enable children to perceive themselves as unified wholes, even though they are aware of acting differently with different people or on different occasions. Children who are less balanced with regard to affect and cognition and who are less able to access different memory systems are less likely to develop hierarchical, conditional models of self and others. For them, some aspects of themselves and others may be denied or split off (Case, 1992; Fischer, 1980).

Reorganization

The outcome of the integrative processes of the school years is the development of patterns of behavior and internal representational models of self and others that are less purely balanced, defended, or coercive. Such models more nearly reflect the range of real experiences that each of us has with others. In addition, such models expand the range of A/Cs from the not fully organized models of infants and the split, dichotomous models of preschoolers to (1) "softer," A/C-like integrative models among relatively balanced children, (2) split and complex unintegrated models among more troubled children, and (3) the more ominous emergence of highly distorted integrations of false affect with false cognition. Although the last of these does not fully form in the school years, with the advent of false cognition some children in highly threatening environments can be expected to use both false affect and false cognition and to embark on pathways with higher than usual probabilities of social dysfunction.

Gender Distributions

Although there are few empirical data on school-aged children that are derived from the theoretical perspective used here, it seems likely that, during the school years, boys would be subjected to cultural biases stressing the strength and invulnerability of males. This should be expressed as an increase in defended classifications for boys when the defense is specifically against the display of vulnerability, that is, fear of abandonment and desire for comfort. Anger would not be defended against by such boys because it is a gender-acceptable feeling. There are corroborating data from adolescence (Kobak, Cole, Ferenz-Gillies, & Flemming, 1993).

Sexuality

Sexuality and Mental Integration

It is significant, I think, that the process of mental integration of multiple internal representational models begins at a time when (1) children do not yet have sexual feelings and (2) they are becoming quite competent at caring for themselves under ordinary circumstances. These conditions would tend to lower affective arousal to manageable levels that would facilitate the integrative process.

Under these conditions, the process of mentally integrating information may itself enable some children with Type A or C internal representational models and behavioral strategies to self-correct their mental and behavioral functioning, thus enabling them to become more balanced. Such a process of reorganization implies that the child has recognized a discrepancy between expected and experienced conditions, has generated an alternate model of reality, and has tested the alternate model and found that it fits experience better than does the original model. If, however, the environment remains threatening or is perceived as too threatening to risk testing of alternate hypotheses, children may be unable to engage in the integrative process. Moreover, it should be noted that, for some children, a formerly supportive environment may become threatening, thus increasing the probability of a shift in functioning from balanced to defended, coercive, or A/C. In any of these cases, the process of integration may be delayed until after puberty, when it must then occur in the more complex intra- and interpersonal environment of sexuality.

Sexuality and Intimacy

Although I argue that most prepubertal children are not yet sexual, school-aged children are aware of others' sexuality. This includes both the relative importance of sexuality to adults and the social attitudes associated with it. Because school-aged children do not themselves have experience of sexual intimacy, they are unlikely to be able to differentiate intimacy from secrecy or to understand the importance of sexuality to parental relationships, including the importance of parental sexual bonds to protection of children. Nevertheless, school-aged children learn a great deal about their culture's and their family's attitudes toward sex, including what is thought to be "sexy" and what is thought of people who display interest in sexuality. In many cultures, this means learning that males display sexual interest more openly than do females, that females are often the object of males' dominance disputes, and that females often are subjected to sexual advances that are not desired or reciprocated. Similarly, children may observe that females can gain status through selection of a sexual partner and that they use sexual signals to accomplish this. Possibly because children cannot fully understand sexuality, many experience discomfort with sexual behavior.

ADOLESCENCE, SEXUALITY, AND MENTAL INTEGRATION

There are two major maturational advances in adolescence that are relevant to this discussion. The first is the ability of the adolescent mind to engage in abstract mental operations, that is, sophisticated cortical integration of information, including conscious integration of information about the self and others. Even more than in the school years, humor becomes one means by which the not fully integrated mind can make use of discrepant sources of information without either achieving full integration or discarding one set of information. For Type A adolescents and adults, dry humor permits feelings to be implied without being stated; for the Type C adolescent, humor permits acknowledgment that surfaces of power or submission may cover opposite conditions, that is, that the overtly powerful are covertly manipulated by the apparently powerless. Humor permits these contradictions to coexist without either integrative resolution or the resolution of denial or submission. The second involves the maturational achievement of sexual maturity and the integration of sexuality into strategies for managing relationships with others.

Cortical Integration of Personal Values

Adolescents actively examine their own values and behavior (Erikson, 1950). These are compared and contrasted with those of other important people, including parents, peers, and public figures. The outcome is the resolution of two issues: "Who am I?" and "Are others what they appear to be?"

In Western cultures, the issue of self-identity often is perceived in terms of the contrast of self to others (Erikson, 1968; Mahler, Pine, & Bergman, 1975; Neisser, 1991). Eastern cultures may experience uniqueness as the greater challenge (Geertz, 1984; Markus & Kitayama, 1990; Roland, 1988; Rosaldo, 1984). In either case, the process is a recursion of the process of "clarification by dichotomization" that began in infancy and proceeded in more sophisticated ways at each successive maturational stage (Fischer, 1980). In adolescence, the challenge is to reconcile aspects of self that are shared with important others with aspects that are not shared. Because important others are never in full agreement (among themselves) regarding values and appropriate behavior, adolescents face the risk of alienating some important people, for example, parents and peers, with each selection that they make. Those who fear loss of essential parental support may yield self-development for the advantage of parental protection (Marcia, 1988) or, conversely, despair of ever finding acceptability (Marold, 1987). This highlights once again the issue of security. Adolescents who feel confident of their ultimate acceptability to others and of their own competence often feel more comfortable making personal choices than do less secure adolescents (Kroger, 1985). Ironically, secure adolescents are also likely to experience the least discordant and most supportive networks, thus making their choices actually less threatening.

Of particular interest to adolescents is the nature of "true" information. Having intuitively discovered false affect and false cognition in the preschool and school years, adolescents consciously discern discrepancies between what others communicate and what they do. Put another way, adolescents are concerned with the possibility that others do not always mean what they communicate (Erikson, 1968). Consequently, adolescents place great value on explicit and consistent communication. Hypocrisy and lack of sincerity become the cardinal crimes of adolescence. Adults, of course often are perceived as stating (piously) one value while, nevertheless, behaving in another (often self-serving) manner. This elicits derision and distrust from adolescents. Again, however, there is a tendency to overdraw and polarize models of reality such that others are identified as always sincere or always suspect. As a result, adolescents' own perspectives may become naively trusting and gullible or bitterly cynical (Chandler, Boyes, & Ball, 1990). The true condition of conflict among values yielding varied behavior across occasions is difficult for adolescents (and many adults) to grasp. In particular, it is difficult for adolescents to conceptualize "character" as an interaction of self and context that must necessarily yield some uncertainty regarding behavior on any specific occasion.

Nevertheless, adolescents, like humans at all other ages, seek guides to behavior that accurately predict future events, that is, representational models that reduce uncertainty and risk. The reality is that, with development, such models become better, but never perfect. It is at the point of unfulfilled expectations that the alert mind discovers the missing information that is essential for a reorganized and more accurate model. If very threatened, however, the mind may give up search for truth in favor of a distortion that increases the probability of safety.

Puberty and Individual Differences in Reproductive Strategies

The second major maturational advance associated with adolescence has to do with sexuality. The advent of puberty presents the issue of reproduction. For the first time, important intimate relationships (with girl- and boyfriends) combine the function of protection with the function of reproduction. This combined focus suggests a functional reason for the power of adolescent love relationships to support or threaten adolescents' personal identity and for the enduring quality of later-forming spousal bonds. After the limited physical relationships of the school years, heterosexual peer attachments recall the sensual, physical closeness of the mother–infant dyad.

Sexuality ultimately transforms the ABC patterns to which it is added. There are substantial individual differences in how this is accomplished. For example, with sexuality, the C2 boy who earlier was a vulnerable "wimp" may now become a charmingly seductive adolescent, "a ladies' man" in an outdated parlance or a boy "with a killer style" in today's slang. Such a boy, who is relatively unable to protect himself and has low status in the male dominance hierarchy, may nevertheless find ways to attract desirable females and, as a consequence, to reproduce effectively. The boy's overt behavior, however, belies hidden feelings of anger, fear of abandonment, and desire for comfort. Ironically, part of his attractiveness may be tied to girls' feeling of comfort in the seductive boy's presence; such feelings would be most motivating among girls who themselves felt vulnerable. Sexual feelings, in other words, may easily become confused with the protective function of attachment feelings (Zillmann, 1984). The overlap of attachment and sexual functions, feelings, and behavioral systems probably promotes survival, with each system as serving as a backup to the other such that pair and family bonds are maintained, thus promoting the survival of children. (For an expansion if these ideas, see Crittenden, 1997a.)

The defended patterns of attachment may be transformed differently by sexuality. For example, isolated (A5), defended adolescents who are uncomfortable with intimacy may find that promiscuity (A6) both eases their loneliness, enabling them to "dance" the dance of intimacy (even if only through physical reflexes), and, at the same time, increases their probability of reproduction. Other defended adolescents may sublimate sexual feelings into sports activities, academic excellence, or peer leadership. Again, irony underlies some of the transformations. Popularity achieved through false social facades may both keep the popular individual in contact with many admiring peers and, at the same time, actually limit access to intimate relationships. Although it appears that the popular adolescent could "have" anyone, in fact, he or she may have no one.

The full patterning of these transformations exceeds the scope of this chapter. There is, however, empirical evidence in the work of the Blocks (1980) and Caspi, Elder, and Herbener (1990) on Americans, of Kroger (1985) on New Zealanders, and of Pulkkinen and Ronka (1994) on Finns that these transformations reflect both continuity and change from school age to adulthood and also that there are gender-differentiated patterns.

Mate Selection in Attachment Terms

Boy- and girlfriend relationships provide the pattern for selection of a spouse. Based in part on the emerging integration of individual differences in attachment and sexuality, adolescents choose partners. Unlike the best friend relationships of childhood, these love relationships are both symmetrical and reciprocal. That is, each of the partners is aware of incurring some responsibility for nurturing the other. The selection process can be informative for adolescents who attend to information about discrepancies. For example, most adolescents at some time respond to the initiatives of a seductive peer. Once in such relationships, however, many are hurt and puzzled by the partner's self-interest, lack of reciprocity, and inability to share intimacy. The promise of the seductive behavior is unfulfilled. In more extreme cases, the partner's vulnerability and expectation of deceit can lead to obsessive desire for contact and unfounded jealousy; similarly, underlying anger can lead to violence, particularly when there is a perceived threat to the relationship. Experience with such partners can be valuable for mentally alert adolescents who are willing to explore the boundary between appearance and reality; in the future, they may be less dazzled by appearance and more valuing of other character traits.

Mate selection probably also depends upon the "fit" between the partners' existing mental and behavioral patterns (Crittenden, 1997a; Crittenden, Partridge, & Claussen, 1991). Often partners will have similar or compatible patterns in which each frequently meets the other's expectations; that is, we select partners who are similar to ourselves. It is also true, however, that opposites attract. When partners' patterns do not fit, the outcomes are varied and, sometimes, dramatic. Some potential partners will be rejected because of the incongruence, whereas others will be accepted because they fill in "gaps" in personality or mental functioning. Such partnerships can be thought of as A/C dyads in which each partner takes half of the pattern. As with the A/C individual, this increases the range of adaptability of the partnership. It also increases the probability of conflict as each experiences repeated failed expectations by the other and lack of understanding from the other. The adaptiveness of the attraction of opposites may depend upon circumstances surrounding the couple, their ability and willingness to respond with mental and behavioral flexibility, and their conscious awareness and acceptance of the differences between themselves. Where these are absent, the partners each may behave in ways that are unexpected and painful to the other. When this occurs frequently, suspicion and doubt may characterize the relationship and lead to emotional and physical contention that, in the extreme, can create both physical and psychological danger.

Gender Differences

In adolescence, physical gender differences become more distinct and take on psychological meanings. Males become larger and stronger than do females and females become capable of bearing children. Both of these changes can function to promote or to destroy intimacy. Specifically, the strength of men can be used to protect spouses and children or to dominate and terrorize them. Similarly, the power of conceiving children can be used to promote men's reproductive opportunity or to cuckold them. Finally, in sexual intercourse itself, the man can overwhelm with physical power and the woman can deny psychological participation. In each of these cases, mutual trust is needed. Without the trust, each partner becomes at risk for losing something important in the now dangerous environment of intimate relationships.

ADULTHOOD, INTERPERSONAL INTEGRATION, AND PARENTHOOD

Adulthood is characterized by relative competence in the ability to protect oneself physically and by a focus on opportunities to reproduce, protect one's progeny, and expand one's range of competence. Individuals' relationships range across the full spectrum of intimacy, including the remnants of the hierarchical, nonreciprocal attachment to one's parents, the symmetrical and reciprocal attachment to one's spouse (and best friends), and the hierarchical, nonreciprocal attachment of one's children to oneself. Mentally, adulthood is marked by sophisticated and ongoing mental integration. The first two of these are considered briefly, followed by a more comprehensive perspective on adult mental functioning.

Reproduction and Protection of Self and Progeny

Although it may seem that the issue of self-protection is largely resolved by adulthood, this is limited to narrow, physical definitions of "self." In adulthood, humans face challenges to their psychological self-identity as partners, as parents, and as members of adult communities (Erikson, 1950). In each of these roles, they must function in new and unfamiliar ways which create opportunities for personal growth as well as risk of failure. In facing these risks, they turn to attachment figures for support (Bowlby, 1979). When they reach too far or have too little psychological safety in their relationships, they risk becoming fearful or angry. Management of feedback about their behavior and feelings tied to these experiences reflects past mental and behavioral strategies as well as current reorganizations of models for managing challenging circumstances. Of course, it is the reorganizations in adults' zones of proximal development (Vygotsky, 1987) that provide opportunities for growth.

Another major task in adults' "zone of proximal development" is protection of one's progeny. Management of this task often reflects the pattern used in other relationships. In some cases, however, parents' conscious desire not to repeat their childhood history leads to inversions when the opposite pattern is shown with children (Crittenden et al., 1991). For example, a formerly rejected parent who is defended may become the hovering, overinvolved parent of a coercive child. By attempting to protect the child from unpleasant experiences, especially feelings of anxiety and rejection, the parent may fail to permit the child to rely on his or her emerging competencies. This, in turn, is likely to create self-doubt in the child and fear of the unseen threat from which the caregiver is offering protection. Moreover, because the threat is unseen, there is no safety signal for the child. Thus, the child is likely to employ a coercive strategy of immature, dependent behavior (that pleases the defended parent) while displaying unfocused, diffuse anxiety and fearfulness. Ironically, defended adults, who have little experience with displaying and regulating feeling, would be relatively unprepared to recognize and protect against a strategy based on exaggeration and lack of regulation of affect.

There are several reasons why parents might have partners or children whose strategy is the opposite of their own. First, both defended and coercive adults have limited experience with regulation of affect and integration of affect and cognition; this reduces their ability to be balanced with regard to their children's affective signals. Further, each trusts the very sort of information that the opposite pattern falsifies. For example, coercive adults trust the predictive value of affect; they are, therefore, most easily mislead by defended individuals who falsify affect. Together, these lead to the probability that some anxiously attached adults will choose partners with an opposite pattern and/or that their children will use the opposite pattern. Finally, as noted above, adults who are conscious of their limitations may seek correction in their partner and children and, in the process, overcorrect.

Managing Multiple and Varied Intimate Relationships

Because adulthood is characterized by a range of attachments in which one's role varies, it is important that adults have available hierarchically organized meta-models of attachment. Such models reflect both the differences in type of relationship (e.g., attachment to one's parents, attachment to one's spouse, and attachment of one's children to oneself) as well as unique differences in the quality of each relationship (e.g., a secure relationship with one's mother, but a coercive relationship with one's father). Relationships that differ in type make different and often competing demands on oneself. Both balancing loyalties to different family members and also meeting the needs of (1) children for protection, (2) spouses for protection and sexual intimacy, and (3) aging parents for protection requires well integrated mental functioning. In addition, it is helpful if others trust that one eventually will be available, even if with some delay, unless protection is essential, in which case one will be available immediately.

For some adults, this integration is seriously incomplete. The effects on behavior can be very disturbing and include a range of disorders; for a fuller discussion, see Crittenden (1995). For A/Cs, there is a particular risk of bipolar depression and of compression of relationships in which limitations in one relationship are satisfied in another or are resolved by using behavior appropriate to another. Sexual behavior with children reflects such compression and may result from either of these processes, that is, seeking from a child satisfaction that is missing with one's spouse or offering sexual behavior to a child when one feels incompetent with other forms of intimacy. In the first case, the reproductive function has become distorted, whereas in the second case protective behavior is distorted. In both cases, integration of information has been insufficient to inhibit the inappropriate behavior. I think, however, that it is worth noting that there may be a relative advantage to species survival (as opposed to personal happiness) when there are overdetermined protective and reproductive responses and when these overlap both functionally and behaviorally. The alternative is missed opportunities for protection and reproduction. To conclude, a major task of adulthood is to find ways to meet the range of needs and desires of important others while still being true one's self. Hierarchical meta-models help one to organize and choose among competing demands in a flexible and varied manner that promotes the well-being of all family members.

Similarly, meta-models assist one in responding to relationships of differing quality. Although one might presume that all of an individual's relationships would be of the same quality, opposite relationships may be sought or created among As and Cs. Balanced adults also may have varied relationships. For example, one's parent may not have been balanced or sensitively responsive. Nevertheless, through one's own mental integration, one may have become a balanced individual who, thus, has an insecure relationship with one or both parents. In addition, for all people, no two relationships are identical. Thus, failure to differentiate among relationships is both maladaptive (in that it leads to ineffective strategies) and indicative of a distortion in the processing of information.

Finally, even within a single relationship, there is variation across time and contexts. Hierarchically organized meta-models provide conditional information that enables one to adjust one's behavior to fit variations in conditions while nevertheless maintaining balance in mental processing of information. When the pattern of changes is predictable, it can be modeled in ways that yield coherency of self and others as well as variation in the behavior of both self and others. When prediction is poor, either the model requires revision to better fit a predictable reality, or if the behavior of important others is unpredictable, the model is likely to be less fully organized. Disorganization has, of course, been a topic of considerable attention within attachment (Carlson, Cicchetti, Barnett, & Braunwald, 1989; Crittenden, 1992a; Lyons-Ruth, Repacholi, McLeod, & Silva, 1991; Main & Hesse, 1990; Main & Solomon, 1986). By adulthood, disorganization is probably a dimension (rather than a state or trait) and may vary with regard to the portion of the meta-model that is disorganized or the conditions under which it is disorganized. This would be reflected in behavioral variation.

Mental Functioning in Adulthood

Intimacy becomes a central issue in adulthood as individuals seek various sorts of union with others, including parents, spouses, and children.

Ironically, achievement of perfect unity creates the discomfort of giving up essential aspects of self, whereas failure to achieve perfect intimacy, unity, or understanding creates the discomfort of unfulfilled relationships and isolation. Similarly, adults become aware that few things can be determined to be entirely true at all times and for all people (Chandler et al., 1990). With their new integrative capacity, some adults begin to be aware of these limits to truth and intimacy and of the paradoxical limits of any one source of information or representational model of reality (Crittenden, 1997b, in press).

For example, imaged memory provides enduring indicators of contexts associated with affectively rousing occurrences; it reflects temporally invariant truth. Such images facilitate rapid, self-protective action. The images, however, are "disembodied" from the temporal and interpersonal contexts in which they occurred. Temporally, they exclude information about eliciting events and consequences. Interpersonally, they limit the imaged person to one fragmented aspect of behavior. Moreover, both people and images can have more than one function and these are not apparent from the image itself. For example, the image of hands can refer to the fear and dread associated with being hit as well as the comfort of hands that caress, make biscuits, or smooth Vaporub on a sore chest. Finally, images are applied to other people for whom they may or may not be relevant. Such images can keep fear and anger alive long after the threatening events have lost their power to harm oneself. This not only ties one to the past; it also precludes recognition of the full humanity of the other person, including their ability to feel, and elicit in others, a range of feelings. Under these conditions, neither intimacy nor truth are fulfilled. To be fully accurate and to form the basis for an intimate understanding of the other person (and of the self), the image must be set in an interpersonal context and experienced in the changing dimension of time. Thus, accuracy of meaning requires the integration of the image with other information. The outcome of such integration is a useful, but less fully protective, construction that is a temporally ordered, contextually bounded, and schematized whole that represents the interaction of self and other. As such, it is no longer an image.

Images express intimacy when a shared image captures the nature of a relationship similarly for two people. For example, couples often associate a melody ("our song") with the romantic early phase of their relationship that is recalled fondly by both. Ironically, as years go by, the melody often serves as a reminder not only of the past shared love, but also of the less enchanting experience of the relationship in the present. Recognition that the partner has somehow changed, thereby failing to fulfill the promise of the image, leaves some people resentful. The problem, of course, is that temporally invariant truth captures the affective essence of one aspect of a relationship by constraining reality to a single dimension that is temporally frozen. People and relationships do change. Put another way, truth in relationships must necessarily change; without change, it is false for all but one moment, and even that moment is restricted to one aspect of the relationship. Its promise deceives with regard to the future.

Procedural behavior yields intimate unity with another person when each behaves in the same manner. Its "truth" is effective coordination of behavior. It may be experienced in moments as simple as mutual gaze or in the complex process of evading maternal anger by smiling an unfelt joy and comforting the feared, but grinning mother. Interpersonally, unity of relationship is experienced procedurally when the infant's body sinks in against the receptive mother's body or when lovers arrive at the same point at the same moment for a kiss of matching intensity. But when one's behavior is *exactly* mirrored by another person's, such that it cannot be transformed into a dyadic dance, the effect is of mockery, a parody of one's self (as any child who parrots a parent's words knows). Perfect unity destroys the whole. This, of course, is frustrating and angering (as parents discover). What is needed is a subtle mismatch, a meshing of the behavior of one person with that of another. Maternal soothing of infant crying and sexual intercourse between a man and a woman provide examples of procedural meshing that does not match, but can yield sublime harmony.

Semantic models provide a similar paradox. The truest semantic prediction is that something will be itself. Such a prediction is a perfect match; nevertheless, it is an uninformative, tautological, circular argument. It could hardly be called "information" or knowledge that could lead to wisdom. Put philosophically, the generalization that is *always* true does not fit any situation perfectly and, consequently, is never true except in sterile, constructed worlds, such as mathematics. In other words, true things are vacuous and meaningful things are false. Ironically, there must be some error for the semantic conclusions to fit the specifics of other people and relationships; semantic models must be (more or less) false in general to be true in specific.

Individuals who depend excessively on semantic memory and representational models tend to structure information logically and to experience relationships as shared beliefs and values. Such people seek "truth" in the logical coherence, propositional quality of generalized principles in semantic memory/models. They also distance themselves from "living" affect by treating feelings as nouns to be analyzed independently from the person experiencing affect. Thus, they tend to exclude affect as a primary or "true" motivation for behavior. In order to avoid dealing with discrepancies between experience and semantic beliefs, they tend to (1) exclude discrepant information from perception, (2) distort it to yield semantic coherency, or (3) hold it in unconscious memory. (Together, these yield idealization.)

For most Type As, right thinking and right behaving (i.e., dogmatism as described by Chandler et al., 1990) are sought as ways to avoid punitive outcomes, especially anger from and abandonment by caregivers.[10] The earlier this is begun, however, the more likely it is that infants and children will superstitiously learn to associate some randomly occurring events with desired outcomes. Thus, there will be hypervigilance, constant self-monitoring, and, sometimes, compulsive behavior of both rational and irrational sorts. In terms of relationships, interpersonal unity is achieved when there is agreement on logical principles; it is a sublime and cool unity, a unity that feels neither close, nor personal and that has no intimacy. The absence of self-relevant intimacy (see Crittenden, in press) ultimately leads to dissatisfaction, feelings of isolation, and the search for alternatives.

Episodic memory, on the other hand, encodes autobiographical incidents. It represents the attempt to recreate in memory an exact replica of a particular moment in time, that is, it represents correspondent truth. The paradox for episodic memory is that, because no perfectly remembered experience will fit any other occasion, perfect episodic models can model only the past and have no value for the future. Some error in the model is needed for generalization. Relationships are established episodically when individuals share memory of the same experience. The more the memories correspond to one another, the closer the feeling of shared experience. This explains, I think, the endless squabbles between family members over the details of shared past experiences; for example, was it on Tuesday or Wednesday that your mother arrived for Christmas? These details, however, are not the central unifying feature of episodic memories. If they were, we could not experience unity with persons who were not participants of the remembered experience. Rather, it is the affect experienced that unifies speaker and listener. Thus, the squabbles over details can be curtailed if the speakers can agree on the affective meaning to them both of the experience. If they cannot, the symbolic dispute over who remembers accurately will continue. Further, a nonparticipant listener can experience close relationship with the speaker if he or she captures the affective essence of the experience to the speaker. This, of course, is empathy, the point at which the listener can truly say "I understand." But, when the listener understands entirely ("truly"), the listener feels the feeling; indeed, he or she feels it exactly as the speaker does. This, however, is not empathy; it is affect contagion. It "steals" the speaker's affect, making it the listener's affect. Now the speaker feels robbed of his unique self and abandoned by the listener. Moreover, the listener now needs the soothing response that the speaker had hoped to receive. Intimacy that is too close fails.

Like semantic memory, episodic memory is ultimately paradoxical. To the extent that a memory accurately corresponds to the remembered event, it is "true." But if it is entirely true, it fits only that one instance and no others. For all others, the true episodic memory is (more or less) untrue. Thus, episodic models must necessarily be false in the specific to be true in general. Of course, true and false used in this way are now relative terms rather than absolutes. For those who are conscious of these things, this paradox, following on the heels of the semantic paradox, must be quite unsettling. Moreover, to the extent that it is experienced, but not consciously understood, it may remain a disturbing, disruptive, and maddening aspect of failed relationships.

Each memory system is biased and represents "truth" differently. Imaged memory captures affect, but its cause and effects are lost, as is its variability over time. Procedural memory and models are biased toward temporally ordered behavior; unenacted affect is lost to this system (so the procedural self may have no way to represent feelings that are experienced, but whose display is inhibited.) Semantic memory is biased by the "truths" that caregivers tell children. Episodic memory is biased to reflect experiences that recall strong, unresolved feelings. Together, however, these memory systems give the mind multiple perspectives on reality.[11] When they are integrated, humans have the best opportunity to identify and correct discrepancies with new, more sophisticated behavior and more complex, integrative internal representational models. Indeed, I propose that people with conscious access to all memory systems can most fully identify and correct discrepancies between imaged feelings, actions, beliefs, and recalled experiences. Only these people can behave with personal and interpersonal integrity.

Thus, across sources of information, memory systems, internal representational models, and relationships, adults must to learn to find the balance between unity and isolation. To use a musical analogy, if harmony is achieved by forcing every voice to be identical, the result is both boring and wasteful of the unique characteristics of each. On the other hand, a cacophony of unrelated sounds is only noise. Instead, fulfilling music involves different sounds joined in concordant ways. The point is that at the very moment when our minds seem capable of full integration and our bodies seek sexual union with another person, we discover that unity is not possible, that paradoxically, unity destroys intimacy. To contribute a meaningful aspect of ourselves to relationships, we must necessarily and to some extent be uniquely alone.

Integration

What would cause one to engage in the difficult process of integration? Failed expectations. At any given moment, interpersonal behavior is based on one's model of self and others. From procedural models, a variant of sensorimotor procedural schemata is drawn. If enacting this schema leads to the expected outcome, one moves (mentally) to the next situation. All of this is preconscious; it is like the way we drive down familiar roads without hitting cars, ultimately arriving at our expected destination (often with no memory of driving there.) If the procedural schema leads to unexpected outcomes (e.g., there is a detour sign), the process may become conscious and trigger mental problem solving. Procedural models, thus, regulate daily behavior under familiar conditions. If the unexpected occurs, one may access semantic memory/models to see if there is useful information about oneself, the other person, or the context that will allow adjustment of one's behavior. A new or revised procedural schema is tried. In other words, semantic memory/models regulate problem-solving behavior and function to promote more sophisticated responses than the individual has previously used.

On the other hand, if the situation is highly emotionally arousing, people are unlikely to be able to engage in the cool, "cognitive," problem-solving process. Instead, a matching of present affect with previous occasions during which the same or a similar affect has been experienced (i.e., affect resonance) initiates recall of an image or an episodic memory. This memory then supplies the model for current behavior. Such memories, however, represent previous behavior that is less mature than present behavior. This, of course, accounts for the perception that the individual has "regressed."

Unmet expectations, thus, instigate the process of conscious integration. The successful resolution of this process, however, requires recognition of both affect and cognition. When the individual has learned to distrust one or the other, there may be no way to manage the integration. If affect is not intense, one can assert the semantic "truth" and deny (mentally exclude from perception) contradictory information. If affect is intense, one responds on the basis of it and constructs false logic (inverted reasoning driven by affect) to rationalize it. Because both of these strategies simplify the complexity of reality, there is an innate tendency to adopt them, as long as they lead to satisfactory outcomes.

A/Cs, Bs, and "Earned" Bs

Where does that leave our A, B, C, and A/C patterns? Individuals using the defended (A) and coercive (C) strategies have each adapted to particular environments and function effectively within them. Each also is more or less limited if the environment changes considerably. Theoretically, the most challenging change would be that of the opposite pattern. Thus, As and Cs each would be least well fitted to the environment of the other.

Type Bs present an interesting dilemma. It seems easy to presume that they could shift their behavior to accommodate normative A and C environments (without distorting the functioning of their minds), but what about adaptation to the environments that generate the compulsive and obsessive patterns or the A/Cs? Such adaptation requires awareness of, even some expectation of, false affect and false cognition. Furthermore, it would be helpful to have experience with differentiating these from true information as well as being able to integrate this knowledge into smooth patterns of adaptive behavior. Possibly, Bs growing up in an integrated environment would have little experience with false information or with integration of discrepant information. (See Melzak & Scott, 1957, for a similar notion with regard to pain.) If we consider a secure child with a sensitive attachment figure, we could say that, because the child experienced an integrated, supportive reality, he or she now has trusting relationships characterized by open and clear communication of true feelings and intentions. Note, however, that it is reality that is integrated and not necessarily the child's mind. To be fully integrated, the adult mind must be aware of false information (both cognitive and affective), manipulative relationships, and the possibility of treachery. For trustingly naive individuals, treacherously threatening environments may pose very great danger.

On the other hand, in adulthood, integrative A/Cs become a possibility in a way that they were not at younger ages. Conceptualized as one type of "earned" B (Main & Goldwyn, in press), they have achieved their balanced status as a result of previous integration of harsh realities. This may provide the advantage of adaptation under a great range of conditions. In addition, because adults must manage to accept the uncertainty of not always knowing how others will behave (without feeling vulnerable at all times), integrative A/Cs may be able to accept the risk of acting even when the outcome cannot be certain. Having experienced both trusting relationships and their minds' competence, they, more than others, may be able to take this leap of hope.

Thus, I would argue that it would be this achieved mental balance in the context of a sometimes dangerous reality that creates adaptive behavior under the widest range of conditions. Viewed from this perspective, the "earned" B category is a special sort of A/C that is not merely protective and reproductive. Rather, it can open a window to self-determination and self-made reality within the constraints (even very severe constraints) of external reality.

At the other extreme, however, there is a different sort of integrative A/C, an "AC" (without the "/"). The psychopath presumes all information to be potentially false and threatening and blends false affect with false cognition to yield a distorted reality in which nothing is certain to be safe and everything is potentially dangerous. (See Haapasalo, 1994, for an overview of these characteristics.) The behavior shown by a psychopath is a composite of all the A and C subpatterns—the seductive charm of the C2, the caregiving of the A3, the compliance of the A4, etcetera—all presented to match the desires and expectations of the naive and gullible victim. Once there is no threat, however, all of the dangerous underside of the A and C patterns become apparent in the fear and lethal rage of the psychopath. (See Figure 3.4.)

Between these two poles is an assortment of A/Cs. Such individuals recognize, more or less, that both false and true information exists. Furthermore, they are more or less able to discern correctly the dangerousness of situations. Some are blended A/Cs whereas others are oscillating A/Cs. They range from those whose behavior is carefully organized and regulated to meet changing realities to those whose mental functioning becomes internally driven such that external reality has little to do with their changing perspectives and behavior. Some are As or Cs in the process

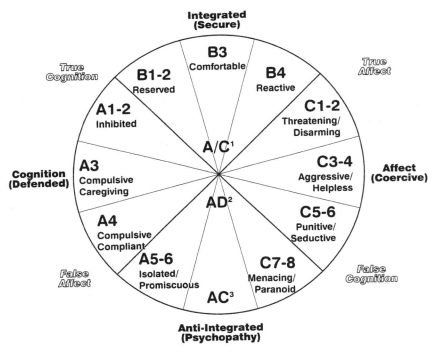

FIGURE 3.4. Patterns of attachment adolescence and adulthood as a function of type of information and degree of integration of information. I = defended/coercive; 2 = anxious depressed; 3 = anti-integrated AC. From Crittenden (1995). Reprinted by permission.

of a not-yet-complete course of therapy. For most, however, there is the frequent and unsettling experience of a working model that clashes against a different reality. Such clashes hold the potential, I think, to destroy the personality or to facilitate integrative solutions that may be the seed of brilliant creativity—creativity that makes apparent truths that the rest of us have known all along, but could not articulate. For all, however, there is a tenuous balance between imagined harmony and actual functioning.

The Risk of Creativity

One reason that I am intrigued by A/Cs is that, unlike As or Cs who have only half the needed information, A/Cs have all of it. But unlike Bs who are balanced in their use of information, A/Cs cannot integrate it; at any given moment, they are in the A or the C state and only dimly aware (if they are aware at all) of any other state. For them, life is a constant process of swinging between sets of unmet expectations that require access to the missing, defended-against information for resolution. Thus, the A/C exists in a near-constant state of tension caused by the collision of two separate world views that are not integrated. Each clash, however, provides a new opportunity for the mind to access and hold concurrently both views and, possibly, to use each source of information to correct and modify the other, thus, achieving an integration.

Compared with the integration of the balanced, but naive, Type B individual, the integration of an A/C has the possibility of being more profound. A/Cs are aware of false cognition and false affect in a way that few Bs are; in addition, they experience the paradoxes of truth and unity in ways that are unexpected and painful. Thus, their experience with the range of human experience is both greater and more disturbingly intense. (Although it could be argued that they have little experience with supportive, honest environments, I think they can envision such reality with greater insight than the unthreatened B can envision falseness, treachery, and desertion. Their failure to achieve the imagined harmony is the source of tragedy.) Thus, A/Cs have the range of experience for creativity as well as repeated discordant moments that challenge one to remodel or reenvision reality. When A/Cs are intelligent (and intelligence, i.e., the mind's ability to make associations, seems to me to be an important and independent dimension), there is the potential for creative genius. Historically, it seems that expression of this genius often follows periods of intense disappointment.

Such periods also carry a risk of depression. Type As are at risk for affective depression, the failure to genuinely feel, to participate affectively with others. Moreover, without information about affect, As may find themselves in unresolvable situations. When this is pervasive such that progress toward goals deemed essential to the self is impossible and when affect cannot be accessed to correct distorted models and behavior, depression is one possible outcome. Flight into an artificial, private world of constructed truth may be another; because such a world would collapse if shared, it cannot be permitted to be penetrated by others.

The reverse is true for Cs. Without access to cognition, they can act only on feeling. When that is insufficient, they escalate their activity, but the escalation only makes the situation worse. They become agitated and frantic. Without access to cognition (or trust of it), they too fail to resolve problems. If they refuse to recognize the limits of their feelings to guide behavior, they may become uncontrollably destructive. If they do sense their limitations, they may experience the opposite face of the affective–cognitive disorder of depression.

A/Cs who lack access to both affect and cognition (at different times), who distrust both sources of information, and who perceive the discrepancy between expectation and outcome, may find many situations unresolvable. Their risk of depression is very great. When, in addition, they experience the paradoxical nature of truth, life itself may seem futile and reality the ultimate, cruel joke. Thus, those A/Cs who become aware of the impossibility of "Truth" in either the temporally invariant, coordinated, coherent, or correspondent senses experience the basis for despair. On the other hand, creative solutions may provide the life-saving integration. If so, the line between depression and creative achievement, between genius and sterile (Type A) and enraged (Type C) madness, thus becomes thin.

Paradox and irony underlie the perspective being offered here. If what I have written is more or less accurate, then the achievement of the secure Type B individual is not perfect harmony in relationships (because that is impossible), but rather both a tolerance for ambiguity and imperfection and also a means by which perfect harmony can be approximated with increasing accuracy—without ever being achieved. Mathematically, security can then be expressed as an asymptotic curve. Emotionally, life and relationships are experienced as being "good enough" (Winnicott, 1958). Relationships enable one to experience enough empathic harmony to *feel* relatively safe and understood and enough intellectual harmony to *be* understood relatively well. Both forms of harmony are, however, less than perfect, leading to a constant tension. In this way, secure, balanced Type Bs are like A/Cs. Their tension, however, is not tinged with fear of destruction or abandonment; rather, it is mild enough to be invigorating without being terrorizing. Consequently, change is a gradual and smooth process in which dissonance is barely perceptible, readily tolerated, and used to transform inaccurate internal representational models into less inaccurate internal representational models. In visual terms, where As, Cs, and A/Cs flail against failed black and white, balanced Bs enjoy the perception of soft shades of gray. For them, satisfaction in relationships comes from the process of getting there together, whereas for individuals with less balanced patterns of mental integration, relationships are evaluated in terms of achievement of the goal. Because the goals of truth and unity always elude, relationships evaluated in these ways must always fail. The secure, balanced individual, in other words, finds beauty in a flawed world expressed inexactly. For them, empathy and intimacy become almost possible most of the time. By not demanding perfect unity, they can relax in nearly realized, soft gray, and fuzzy perfection (see Kosko, 1993).

Their comfort, however, may not as often lend itself to the brilliant insights and creative constructions of some of the A/Cs. Between the madness and terror of ACs, the sterility of As, the fantasy of Cs, and the comfort of Bs lie the A/Cs. It is those who have earned at least a toehold on security, without giving up the awareness of dysynchrony, paradox, and pain, who may have the greatest opportunity for creative integrations that promote harmonious activity, productive analysis, and compassionate awareness of others. Those unable to achieve a balanced integration face greater-than-usual risks of psychopathology (Chandler et al., 1990).

CONCLUSIONS

To conclude, I am offering a dimensional approach to Ainsworth's patterns of attachment and attempting to concatenate basic mental and behavioral processes across a series of maturational changes. In addition, I am seeking a way to integrate Freud's emphasis on sexuality (i.e., reproduction) with Bowlby's emphasis on protection and noting that these are the two essential functions for any species. Developmentally, I am construing the mind as actively interacting with reality, with attachment figures providing a scaffold (Bruner, 1984; Stern, 1985; Vygotsky, 1987). Attachment figures can assist and buffer children by giving them an integrated, supportive reality or they can fail to protect children, leaving them to their own insufficient resources. Other attachment figures distort reality and themselves threaten their children, thus assisting in the creation of a skewed reality. By adulthood most of us have experienced some combination of these conditions and, depending upon the combination and upon our innate characteristics (especially intelligence), we organize in ways that are adaptive in a greater or narrower range of circumstances. For those in the most challenging circumstances, the outcome can be profoundly comforting or intensely distressing.

This is a reminder that attachment is not a theory about happiness; it is about protection and, as I am construing it here, successful reproduction. Happiness is desirable, but it is not essential to these ends; moreover, it can limit adaptive functioning under some conditions. Thus, I find that the naive B pattern of attachment is adaptive under some, but not all, conditions and that it can carry substantial risk under conditions of danger. The integrated patterns of adulthood provide both the means for adults to achieve balance, even under difficult circumstances, and the opportunity for them to create the sorts of environments in which their children can develop safely. Culture reflects patterns of childrearing practices that represent the outcome of generations of such person–environment interactions. From this perspective, each of the patterns (and each cultural variation in distribution of patterns) has an adaptive value under some circumstances, as well as carrying risk under others. It is the function of the maturing mind to increase each individual's breadth of adaptability. The excitement and the impetus to growth, however, remain at the points of incongruence and discrepancy between new information and existing internal representational models.

It is at these points of incongruence that the elements of individual personality reorganize to reflect new and deeper understandings. Because A/Cs both have access to all the information and also frequently experience the discomfort of discrepancy, their personalities sometimes contain the essential ingredients of creative genius. For there is no profound art that does not have shadows and a vanishing point, nor great music without counterpoint and minor keys, nor exquisite dance without the distance that makes closeness poignant. Indeed, John Bowlby devoted two of his three volumes on attachment to separation and loss, not because they were to be avoided, but because they cannot be avoided. Humans, unlike any other species, both remember past separations and losses and also anticipate those of the future. Attachment is not about happiness. Rather, it is about individual differences in coping with a reality that contains both safety and threat, joy and sorrow. Nevertheless, occasionally, when the elements of personality are offered to the fire of experience, the light that is released can be almost blinding and can almost pierce the darkness beyond.

ACKNOWLEDGMENTS

I wish to thank Andrew Brink for his support, helpful comments, and catalytic dialogue during the development of the ideas in this chapter. In addition, several colleagues, including Lorenzo Cionini, Hellgard Rauh, Maria von Salisch, and Jari Sinkkonin, have provided helpful comments on earlier versions of this chapter.

NOTES

1. Because the ABC patterns are used in many different ways, it is necessary to be specific. I refer to the patterns of processing information that are described below. I choose this definition because patterns of behavior, e.g., avoidant, aggressive, change with development.

2. After completion of this chapter, a review of recent neurological findings both provided support for the constructs of privileged information, affect, and cognition and also contributed biological detail to the maturational and neurological processes that yield these constructs (see Crittenden, in press).

3. Mental representations of reality (i.e., internal representational models) are defined here as mental structures that allow one to predict the probable outcomes of behavior prior to acting. Although they represent reality, they must necessarily do so inaccurately by reflecting perceptions and interpretations of reality. Both cognitive and affective information inform such models. See Crittenden (in press) for a neurological discussion of representation.

4. Although the effects of individual differences in genetic potential (i.e., temperament) are not a focus of this chapter, brief mention is relevant. Certainly there are such differences and certainly they are reflected in behavioral differences among infants. I suggest that the interaction of universal mental processes with experience yields individual differences in mental and behavioral strategy (i.e., quality of attachment), whereas personality results from a second interaction, that of strategy with unique genetic variation in nonessential characteristics (Tooby & Cosmides, 1990). Also see Crittenden (in press).

5. I use reciprocal to refer to reciprocity of what each partner gives and receives from the relationship. Thus, spouses often have reciprocal relationships, whereas parents and children do not. Symmetrical relationships are those in which the participants have the same hierarchical rank (e.g., two adults or two children, both of equal power).

6. Although Marvin's work on preschool children is central to the theory discussed here, the classificatory system is not that which he developed with Cassidy (Cassidy & Marvin with the MacArthur Working Group, 1992). Moreover, the predictions from these two classificatory systems reflect substantial theoretical differences and yield empirical differences.

7. The terms preoperational, concrete, and formal operations are borrowed from Piaget's theory of cognitive development. Piaget's use of the word "cognitive" is similar to my use of "cortical integration," whereas my use of "cognitive" refers to a particular sort of predictive information. Cortical functioning, in my terms, integrates cognitive information with affective information in increasingly complex ways. See Crittenden (in press) for further elaboration of these ideas in terms of neurological structures and maturation.

8. In earlier papers and *Preschool Assessment of Attachment* manuals, I have labeled the C3 preschool subpattern "punitive" because the pattern seemed similar to the "controlling punitive" subpattern of Main and Cassidy (1988) and Cassidy

and Marvin (1992). In this chapter, the term "aggressive" is substituted because it describes the angry, aggressive quality of preschool children's behavior. The term "punitive" is reserved for a proposed C5 pattern that develops in the school years and that describes children who are obsessed with revenge.

9. I have said previously that there are at least three memory systems. I offer a possible fourth here. In all cases, I am referring to types of information that first become salient at different ages, are encoded and retrieved differently, and serve different functions. The physiological evidence supporting memory systems is discussed in Crittenden (in press).

10. The alternative to dogmatism is skepticism, that is, doubt of any certainty. Thus, skepticism is closely related to the notion of false cognition.

11. For a more detailed discussion of truth and distortions of truth, see Crittenden (1997b).

REFERENCES

Ainsworth, M. D. S. (1979). Infant–mother attachment. *American Psychologist, 34,* 932–937.
Ainsworth, M. D. S., Blehar, M., Waters, E., & Wall, S. (1978). *Patterns of attachment: A psychological study of the Strange Situation.* Hillsdale, NJ: Erlbaum.
Barlow, D. H., Sakheim, D. K., & Beck, J. G. (1983). Anxiety increases sexual arousal. *Journal of Abnormal Psychology, 92,* 49–54.
Block, J. H., & Block, J. (1980). The role of ego-control and ego-resiliency in the organization of behavior. In W. A. Collins (Ed.), *Minnesota Symposium on Child Psychology* (Vol. 13, pp. 39–70). Hillsdale, NJ: Erlbaum.
Block, J. H., Block, J., & Gjerde, P. F. (1986). The personality of children prior to divorce: A prospective study. *Child Development, 57,* 827–840.
Bowlby, J. (1973). *Attachment and loss: Vol. 2. Separation.* New York: Basic Books.
Bowlby, J. (1979). *The making and breaking of affectional bonds.* London: Tavistock.
Bowlby, J. (1980). *Attachment and loss: Vol. 3: Loss.* New York: Basic Books.
Bowlby, J. (1982). *Attachment and loss: Vol. 1. Attachment.* New York: Basic Books. (Original work published 1969)
Bruner, J. S. (1984). Vygotsky's zone of proximal development: The hidden agenda. *New Directions for Child Development, 23,* 93–97.
Cantor, J. R., Zillmann, D., & Bryant, J. (1975). Enhancement of experienced sexual arousal in response to erotic stimuli through misattribution of unrelated residual arousal. *Journal of Personality and Social Psychology, 32,* 69–75.
Cantor, J. R., Zillmann, D., & Einsiedel, E. F. (1978). Female responses to provocation after exposure to aggressive and erotic films. *Communication Research, 5,* 395–412.
Carlson, V., Cicchetti, D., Barnett, D., & Braunwald, K. (1989). Disorganized/dis-

oriented attachment relationships in maltreated infants. *Developmental Psychology, 25,* 525–531.

Case, R. (1992). The role of the frontal lobes in the regulation of cognitive development. *Brain and Cognition, 20,* 51–73.

Caspi, A., Elder, G. G., & Herbener, E. S. (1990). Childhood personality and thee prediction of life-course patterns. In L. Robins & M. Rutter (Eds.), *Straight and devious pathways from childhood to adulthood* (pp. 13–35). Cambridge, England: Cambridge University Press.

Cassidy, J., & Berlin, L. J. (1994). The insecure/ambivalent pattern of attachment: Theory and research. *Child Development, 65,* 971–991.

Cassidy, J., & Marvin, R. S., with the Working Group of the John D. and Catherine T. MacArthur Foundation on the Transition from Infancy to Early Childhood (1992). *Attachment organization in three- and four-year olds: Coding guidelines.* Unpublished manuscript, University of Virginia.

Chandler, M., Boyes, M., & Ball, C. (1990). Relativism and stations of epistemic doubt. *Journal of Experimental Child Psychology, 50,* 370–395.

Crittenden, P. M. (1985a). Maltreated infants: Vulnerability and resilience. *Journal of Child Psychology and Psychiatry, 26,* 85–96.

Crittenden, P. M. (1985b). Social networks, quality of parenting, and child development. *Child Development, 56,* 1299–1313.

Crittenden, P. M. (1988). Relationships at risk. In J. Belsky & T. Nezworski (Eds.), *Clinical implications of attachment* (pp. 136–174). Hillsdale, NJ: Erlbaum.

Crittenden, P. M. (1992a). Quality of attachment in the preschool years. *Development and Psychopathology, 4,* 209–241.

Crittenden, P. M. (1992b). Treatment of anxious attachment in infancy and early childhood. *Development and Psychopathology, 4,* 575–602.

Crittenden, P. M. (1994a). Peering into the black box: An exploratory treatise on the development of self in young children. In D. Cicchetti & S. Toth (Eds.), *Rochester Symposium on Developmental Psychopathology: Vol. 5. The self and its disorders* (pp. 79–148). Rochester, NY: University of Rochester Press.

Crittenden, P. M. (1994b). Brain, mind, and intimate relationships: An evolutionary perspective on mental health. *Bulletin of the New Zealand Psychological Society, 83,* 44–50.

Crittenden, P. M. (1995). Attachment and psychopathology. In S. Goldberg, R. Muir, & J. Kerr (Eds.), *Attachment theory: Social, developmental, and clinical perspectives* (pp. 367–406). Hillsdale, NJ: Analytic Press.

Crittenden, P. M. (1996). Language, attachment, and behavior disorders. In N. J. Cohen, J. H. Beitchman, R. Tannock, & M. Konstantareaus (Eds.), *Language, learning, and behavior disorders: Emerging perspectives* (pp. 119–160). New York: Cambridge University Press.

Crittenden, P. M. (1997a). The effect of early relationship experiences on relationships in adulthood. In S. Duck (Ed.), *Handbook of personal relationships* (2nd ed., pp. 99–119). Chichester, England: Wiley.

Crittenden, P. M. (1997b). Truth, error, omission, distortion, and deception: The application of atachment theory to the assessment and treatment of psychological disorder. In S. M.C. Dollinger & L. F. DiLalla (Eds.), *Assessment and intervention across the lifespan* (pp. 35–76). Hillsdale, NJ: Erlbaum.

Crittenden, P. M. (in press). Toward an integrative theory of trauma: A dynamic–

maturational approach. In D. Cicchetti & S. Toth (Eds.), *Rochester Symposium on Developmental Psychopathology: Vol. 10. Risk, trauma, and memory processes.* Rochester, NY: University of Rochester Press.

Crittenden, P. M., & Claussen, A. L. (1994, June). *Quality of attachment in the preschool years: Alternative perspectives.* Paper presented at the symposium "Quality of Attachment in the Preschool Years," P. M. Crittenden, chair, International Conference on Infant Studies, Paris, France.

Crittenden, P. M., & DiLalla, D. (1988). Compulsive compliance: The development of an inhibitory coping strategy in infancy. *Journal of Abnormal Child Psychology, 16,* 585–599.

Crittenden, P. M., Partridge, M. F., & Claussen, A. H. (1991). Family patterns of relationship in normative and dysfunctional families. *Development and Psychopathology, 3,* 491–512.

Eibl-Eibesfeldt, I. (1979). Human ethology: Concepts and implications for the sciences of man. *Behavior and Brain Sciences, 2,* 1–57.

Emery, R. (1982). Interparent conflict and the children of discord and divorce. *Psychological Bulletin, 92,* 310–330.

Erickson, M., & Egeland, B. (1987). A developmental view of the psychological consequences of maltreatment. *School Psychology Review, 16,* 156–168.

Erikson, E. H. (1950). *Childhood and society.* New York: Norton.

Erikson, E. H. (1968). *Identity, youth, and crisis.* New York: Norton.

Fagot, B., & Pears, K. (1996). From infancy to seven years: Continuities and change. *Development and Psychopathology, 8,* 325–344.

Fischer, K. W. (1980). A theory of cognitive development: The control and construction of hierarchies of skills. *Psychological Review, 87,* 477–531.

Gallistel, C. R., Brown, A. L., Carey, S., Gelman, R., & Keil, F. C. (1991). Lessons from animal learning for the study of cognitive development. In S. Carey & R. Gelman (Eds.), *The epigenesis of mind: Essays on biology and cognition* (pp. 3–36). Hillsdale, NJ: Erlbaum.

Geertz, C. (1984). On the nature of anthropological understanding. In R. A. Schweder & R. A. Levine (Eds.), *Cultural theory: Essays on mind, self, and emotion.* New York, MA: Cambridge University Press.

Gordon, W. C., Mowrer, R. R., McGinnis, C. P., & McDermott, M. J. (1985). Cue-induced memory in the rat. *Bulletin of the Psychonomic Society, 23,* 233–236.

Gustavson, C., Garcia, J., Hankins, W., & Rusiniak, K. (1974). Coyote predation control by aversive stimulus. *Science, 184,* 581–583.

Haapasalo, J. (1994). Types of offenses among the Checkley psychopaths. *International Journal of Offender Therapy and Comparative Criminology, 38,* 59–68.

Hale, V. E., & Strassberg, D. S. (1990). The role of anxiety in sexual arousal. *Archives of Sexual Behavior, 19,* 569–581.

Kagan, J. (1970). Attention and psychological change in the young child. *Science, 170,* 826–832.

Kobak, R., Cole, H., Ferenz-Gillies, R., & Flemming, W. (1993). Attachment and emotion regulation during mother–teen problem solving: A control theory analysis. *Child Development, 64,* 231–245.

Kohut, H. (1992). The disorders of the self and their treatment. In D. Capps &

R. K. Finn (Eds.), *Individualism reconsidered: Readings bearing on the endangered self in modern society* (pp. 315–327). Princeton, NJ: Princeton Theological Seminary Press.

Kosko, B. (1993). *Fuzzy thinking: The new science of fuzzy logic.* New York: Hyperion.

Kroger, J. (1985). Separation–individuation and ego-identity in New Zealand university students. *Journal of Youth and Adolescence, 14,* 133–147.

LaFreniere, P. J., & Sroufe, A. (1985). Profiles of peer competence in the preschool: Interrelations between measures, influence of social ecology, and relation to attachment history. *Developmental Psychology, 21,* 56–66.

Lashley, K. S. (1960). Cerebral organization and behavior. In F. A. Beach, D. O. Hebb, C. T. Morgan, & H. W. Nissen (Eds.), *The neuropsychology of Lashley* (pp. 529–543). New York: McGraw-Hill. (Original work published 1958)

Lazarus, Z. (1982). Thoughts on the relation between emotion and cognition. *American Psychologist, 37,* 1019–1024.

LeDoux, J. E. (1986). The neurobiology of emotion. In J. E. LeDoux & W. Hirst (Eds.), *Mind and brain: Dialogues in cognitive neuroscience* (pp. 301–354). Cambridge, England: Cambridge University Press.

Leventhal, H. (1984). A perceptual–motor theory of emotion. In L. Berkowitz (Ed.), *Advances in experimental social psychology: Vol. 17. Theorizing in social psychology: Special topics* (pp. 117–182). New York: Academic Press.

Lewis, M., Feiring, C., McGuffog, C., & Jaskir, J. (1984). Predicting pathology in six-year-olds from early social relations. *Child Development, 55,* 123–136.

Luria, A. R. (1973). *The working brain: An introduction to neuropsychology.* London: Penguin.

Lyons-Ruth, K., Repacholi, B., McLeod, S., & Silva, E. (1991). Disorganized attachment behavior in infancy: Short-term stability, maternal and infant correlates, and risk-related subtypes. *Development and Psychopathology, 3,* 377–396.

MacLean, P. D. (1973). *A triune concept of brain and behavior.* Toronto: University of Toronto Press.

MacLean, P. D. (1990). *The triune brain in evolution: Role in paleocerebral functions.* New York: Plenum Press.

Mahler, M., Pine, F., & Bergman, A. (1975). *The psychological birth of the human infant.* New York: Basic Books.

Main, M. (1981). Avoidance in the service of attachment: A working paper. In K. Immelmann, G. Barlow, L. Petrinovich, & M. Main (Eds.), *Behavioral development: The Bielfeld interdisciplinary project* (pp. 651–693). New York: Cambridge University Press.

Main, M, & Cassidy, J. (1988). Categories of response to reunion with the parent at age six: Predictability from infant attachment classifications and stable across a one-month period. *Developmental Psychology, 24,* 415–426.

Main, M., & Goldwyn, R. (in press). Adult attachment classification system. In M. Main (Ed.), *A typology of human attachment organization: Assessed in discourse, drawing, and interviews.* Cambridge, England: Cambridge University Press.

Main., M., & Hesse, P. (1990). Lack of resolution of mourning in adulthood and its relationship to infant disorganization: Some speculations regarding causal mechanisms. In M. Greenberg, D. Cicchetti, & E. M. Cummings (Eds.), *Attachment in the preschool years* (pp. 161–182). Chicago: University of Chicago Press.

Main, M., & Solomon, J. (1986). Discovery of an insecure disorganized/disoriented attachment pattern: Procedures, findings, and implications for the classification of behavior. In M. Yogman & T. B. Brazelton (Eds.), *Affective development in infancy* (pp. 121–160). Norwood, NJ: Ablex.

Main, M., & Weston, D. (1981). The quality of toddlers' relationship to mother and father: Related to conflict behavior and readiness to establish new relationships. *Child Development, 52,* 932–940.

Marcia, J. E. (1988). Common processes underlying ego identity, cognitive/moral development, and individuation. In D. Lapsky & F. C. Power (Eds.), *Self, ego, and identity: Integrative approaches* (pp. 211–225. New York: Springer-Verlag.

Markus, H., & Kitayama, S. (1990). *Culture and the self: Implications for cognition, emotion, and motivation.* Unpublished manuscript.

Marold, D. (1987). *Correlates of suicidal ideation among young adolescents.* Unpublished doctoral dissertation, University of Denver.

Marvin, R. S. (1977). An ethological–cognitive model for attenuation of mother–child attachment behavior. In T. M. Alloway, L. Kramer, & P. Pliner (Eds.), *Advances in the study of communication and affect: Vol. 3. The development of social attachments* (pp. 25–60). New York: Plenum Press.

Melzak, R., & Scott, T. H. (1957). The effects of early experience on response to pain. *Journal of Comparative and Physiological Psychology, 50,* 155–161.

Moore, L., Crawford, F., & Lester, J. (1994, June). *Security of attachment at 30 months: Maternal, infant, and family variables.* Paper presented at the symposium "Quality of attachment in the Preschool Years," P. M. Crittenden, chair, International Conference on Infant Studies, Paris, France.

Mowrer, R. R. (1988). A cuing treatment reestablishes the US pre-exposure effect following context change. *American Journal of Psychology, 101,* 539–548.

Mowrer, R. R., & Gordon, W. C. (1983). Effects of cuing in an "irrelevant" context. *Animal Learning and Behavior, 11,* 401–406.

Neisser, U. (1991). Two perceptually given aspects of the self and their development. *Developmental Review, 11,* 197–209.

Ornstein, R., & Thompson, R. F. (1984). *The amazing brain.* New York: Houghton Mifflin.

Plutchik, R. (1980). *Emotion: A psychoevolutionary synthesis.* New York: Harper & Row.

Pulkkinen, L., & Ronka, A. (1994). Personal control over development, identity formation, and future orientation as components of life orientation: A developmental approach. *Developmental Psychology, 30,* 260–271.

Putnam, F. (1995). Development of dissociative disorders. In D. Cicchetti & D. Cohen (Eds.), *Developmental Psychopathology: Vol. 2. Risk, disorder, and adaptation* (pp. 581–608). New York: Wiley.

Radke-Yarrow, M., Cummings, E. M., Kuczynski, L., & Chapman, M. (1985). Patterns of attachment in two- and three-year-olds in normal families and families with parental depression. *Child Development, 56,* 884–893.

Renken, B., Egeland, B., Marvinney, D., Mangelsdorf, S., & Sroufe, A. (1989).

Early childhood antecedents of aggression and passive-withdrawal in early elementary school. *Journal of Personality, 57,* 257–282.

Roland, A. (1988). *In search of self in India and Japan.* Princeton, NJ: Princeton University Press.

Rosaldo, M. (1984). Toward an anthropology of self and feeling. In R. Schweder & R. LeVine (Eds.), *Culture theory: Essays on mind, self, and emotion* (pp. 137–157). New York: Cambridge University Press.

Seligman, M. E. P. (1975). *Helplessness: On depression, development, and death.* San Francisco: Freeman.

Seligman, M. (1971). Preparedness and phobias. *Behavior Therapy, 2,* 307–320.

Selye, H. (1976). *The stress of life.* New York: McGraw-Hill.

Stern, D. (1985). *The interpersonal world of the infant.* New York: Basic Books.

Teti, D. M., Gelfand, D. M., Messinger, D. S., & Isabella, R. (1995). Correlates of preschool attachment security in a sample of depressed and non-depressed mothers. *Developmental Psychology, 31,* 364–376.

Tooby, J., & Cosmides, L. (1990). On the universality of human nature and the uniqueness of the individual: The role of genetics and adaptation. *Journal of Personality, 58,* 17–67.

Tulving, E. (1972). Episodic and semantic memory. In E. Tulving & W. Donaldson (Eds.), *Organization of memory.* New York: Academic Press.

Tulving, E. (1985). How many memory systems are there? *American Psychologist, 40,* 385–398.

Tulving, E. (1995). Introduction. In M. Gazzaniga (Ed.), *The cognitive neurosciences* (pp. 751–753). Boston: MIT Press.

U.S. Department of Health and Human Services, National Center on Child Abuse and Neglect. (1994). *Child maltreatment 1992: Reports from the states to the National Center on Child Abuse and Neglect.* Washington, DC: U.S. Government Printing Office.

Vygotsky, L. S. (1987). *The collected works of L. S. Vygotsky* (R. W. Rieber & A. S. Carlton, Eds.; N. Minick, Trans.). New York: Plenum Press.

Winnicott, D. W. (1958). Psychoses and childcare. In *Collected papers: From pediatrics to psychoanalysis* (pp. 219–228). London: Tavistock.

Youniss, J. (1992). Parent and peer relations in the emergence of cultural competence. In H. McGurk (Ed.), *Childhood social development* (pp. 131–147). Hove, England: Erlbaum.

Zillmann, D. (1984). *Connections between sex and aggression.* Hillsdale, NJ: Erlbaum.

SECTION II

RISK AND PREDICTION

4

Attachment Networks in Postdivorce Families: The Maternal Perspective

INGE BRETHERTON
REGHAN WALSH
MOLLY LEPENDORF
HEATHER GEORGESON

Surprisingly few researchers have studied divorce-related family processes and outcomes from an attachment-theoretic perspective. Yet attachment theory is especially well suited for helping us untangle the complexities of children's and parents' postdivorce experiences, complexities that are not well captured by labeling such families "single-parent."

Increasingly, children in postdivorce families retain contact with both parents (Maccoby & Mnookin, 1992). More frequently than in the past, joint custody arrangements provide for children to shuttle regularly between parental homes, even when their primary physical placement is with the mother. The resulting increase in interparental contact poses new challenges to the postdivorce coparental relationship and is likely to impact children's sense of security with both parents. In addition, many fathers and mothers build relationships with new partners who, irrespective of whether they are cohabiting, may play important—if sometimes tempo-rary—quasi-parental roles in the child's life. The child or the other parent may see even temporary partners as competitors or intruders or, more positively, as additional parental figures. If the partner has children from a previous marriage, they too may be seen as friends or as potential rivals for the father's or mother's affections.

97

In addition, ex-spouses' extended families, especially the mothers' parents, often serve as supportive figures to their adult children during and after a divorce and may act also as quasi-parental figures for grandchildren. If this support relationship functions smoothly, a mother's ability to serve as secure base for her child may be bolstered. If a mother's parents are critical of her parenting or ex-spousal and partner relationships, or if they form alliances with the former spouse, relationships within the whole attachment network may be adversely affected.

The complexity of attachment networks in postdivorce families requires that we go beyond the traditional assessments of child–mother and –father attachment quality and address issues of separation, loss, loyalty conflict, jealousy, anger, and resolution of mourning. Though the latter topics are discussed in Volumes 2 and 3 of Bowlby's attachment trilogy (Bowlby, 1973, 1980) and appear to have influenced clinical work with divorced families, they have inspired few research efforts. However, writings on loss and marital separation by Colin Murray Parkes (1971) and Robert Weiss (1974), both of whom were guided by Bowlby's theorizing, are relevant to the postdivorce situation.

Parkes's (1971) influential article on psychosocial transitions extends loss phenomena to situations other than bereavement. Parkes construes any redefinition of an important interpersonal relationship as a loss calling forth the grief and anger responses of normal and pathological mourning, even in the case of divorce, when the termination of a relationship is deliberately sought as the solution to an unbearable situation.

In a subsequent qualitative study of marital separation, Weiss (1974) observed that many separating and divorcing couples experienced difficulties in renegotiating the postdivorce relationship. Many continued to harbor strong though ambivalent attachment feelings toward a former wife or husband. Some ex-spouses even felt compelled to drive down the street where the former husband or wife lived, or to call the ex-spouse on the telephone when feeling lonely (i.e., to engage in proximity seeking), though the overt purpose of contact—when it was achieved—was to harass the former spouse. Few ex-spouses were able to be mutually considerate. The majority engaged in open hostility. Murderous fantasies were not rare, and ex-spouses found it especially difficult to mourn the loss of a marital attachment and its future potential while at the same time continuing to coparent their children (see also Wallerstein & Blakeslee, 1989). For these reasons, parents and children in many postdivorce families continue to face attachment-related adjustments long after the divorce decree, a point also made by Kalter, Pickar, and Lesowitz (1984).

The popular and clinical literature on divorce (e.g., Ahrons, 1994; Ahrons & Wallish, 1987, Cummings & Davies, 1994; Tschann, Johnston, Kline, & Wallerstein, 1989; Whitehead, 1993) calls on former spouses to respond with sensitivity to their children's love for the other parent, their fear of being caught in the middle or being abandoned, and their hope for parental reconciliation. The literature also tells divorced parents that if they can abstain from blaming each other for their children's distress or misbehavior and refrain from competing for their children's affections, they are more likely to be successful in supporting the children's sense of security and well-being (Wallerstein & Kelly, 1980). Additional justification for such recommendations comes from Amato and Keith's (1991) meta-analyses of divorce outcomes, which revealed consistent negative effects of postdivorce parental conflict on children (see also Emery, 1988).

However, in our view, the challenges faced by divorcing and postdivorce parents in trying to resolve grief and anger over their failed marriage while at the same time renegotiating the task of coparenting often have not been acknowledged sufficiently. Nor has enough consideration been given to the fact that such renegotiations are not limited to the immediate postdivorce period but arise anew each time the postdivorce family is faced with developmental and relationship issues. These include one or both ex-spouses' exploration of new partner relationships or the responses of the extended family to the divorce. In this chapter we examine some of these issues as they are discussed by preschoolers' mothers who have been divorced for at least 2 years, focusing on positive and negative aspects of postdivorce coparenting, maternal evaluation of the father–child relationship, and the roles of new partners and the mothers' own parents.

METHOD

Participating Families

Fifty divorced mothers participated in the study. Most families were identified through public court records, but 8 of the 50 families were recruited through local preschools. Only mothers who were employed outside of the home or pursuing a degree (or both) and who had been legally separated or divorced for at least 2 years were eligible for the study. We wanted to study postdivorce families' adjustment without the added stress of dire poverty and after the initial turmoil of the divorce process had been surmounted (see Hetherington, 1989). Overall, 44% of the mothers identified through court records and who fulfilled study criteria agreed to participate. Some of the mothers who had unlisted phone numbers and did not respond to our letter of invitation may have been ineligible rather than reluctant to participate. Hence, the percentage of eligible but nonparticipating mothers may have been lower than 56%.

Mothers

The mothers' ages ranged from 23 to 41 years, with a mean of 32 years. All mothers had graduated from high school, 34% had also attended college, and 20% had obtained bachelor or higher degrees. Their average income (including child support) was about $24,000. Fifteen mothers had one child, 26 had two children, and 9 had more than two children. In all cases one of the children was a preschooler aged 4.5 to 5.0 years.

Fathers

Fathers' educational and occupational levels (Hollingshead, 1978) were highly correlated with the mothers', $r(49) = .53$, $p < .0001$, and $r(49) = .30$, $p < .05$, respectively. All but two of the fathers were employed at the time of the study.

Custody-Related Information

The children's primary physical placement was with the mother in 45 cases and was shared equally with the father in 5 cases. Mothers had sole legal custody in 15 cases; for the other 35 cases legal custody was joint.

The fathers of 90% of the children lived within easy reach (less than 10 miles away). Seventy-five percent of the children in the study saw their fathers at least every 2 weeks (usually over the weekend). Out-of-state fathers received or made visits a few times per year. Two fathers with drug/alcohol problems were restricted to supervised visits, and 11 fathers were reported by the mothers to have serious drinking or drug problems. Some of these were the fathers who did not have regular contact with their children. One child had not seen his father since the age of 6 months although there was telephone contact between the two parents.

Procedure

The findings reported in this chapter come from a larger study of attachment organization in postdivorce families which included family observations, child assessments, maternal interviews, and a series of questionnaires. This chapter focuses on the mothers' perceptions of their families' attachment networks, though many of the instruments on which our data are based are not traditional attachment measures.

Mothers evaluated the members of their attachment networks as well as interrelationships among network members through open-ended interviews and a number of questionnaires. Their responses yielded descriptions and ratings of the ex-spousal and coparental relationships and relationships with other social network members, including new partners, parents, relatives, and friends. Information about members of the formal network (church/temple, child's teacher, doctors, mental health professionals, and books/media) also was collected but is not considered here because the main emphasis of this chapter is on attachment issues. In addition, we asked the mothers to rate retrospectively the spousal attachment relationship at the time of permanent separation.

Instruments

Qualitative information about the mother's relationships with the child's father, new partners, and her own parents was obtained through the Social Network Interview and the Parent Attachment Interview. Some of the information obtained through these two interviews was later quantified for use in statistical analyses.

Social Network Interview

This structured interview provided detailed information about the members of the mother's and the child's social networks. It was adapted from a similar interview by Cochran, Larner, Riley, Gunnarsson, and Henderson (1990) and was administered to the mothers by a female researcher at a place of her choice (work, home, or university). It took about 2 hours, and was audiotaped.

Initially, the mother was asked to name all the people who were part of her broader social network (relatives, neighbors, friends, workmates, organizational contacts, and professionals). Systematic information about types of help, proximity, and frequency of contact was obtained for each of the persons named, but this information is not reported in this chapter. The next step was to identify the primary network members, that is, those members of the overall network whom mothers regarded as *most* important. Mothers were then asked to list reasons why these primary network members were important and to discuss network members whom they experienced as stressful. Finally they were asked to list and discuss members of the child's social network and to describe how the child responded to parental dating or involvement with a new partner. Because mothers did not use identical categories to describe all of their network members' supportive and problematic behavior, distinct descriptive categories were developed for the various types of network members. This task was undertaken by a coder who had no knowledge of other data from the study. This coder's work was subsequently checked by two additional coders. Disagreements (mostly omissions) were resolved by discussion.

The categorized positive and negative descriptions from the Social Network Interview (SNI) were used in two ways: (1) qualitatively, to present a more vivid picture of how postdivorce mothers experience their social network; and (2) quantitatively, to compare the SNI data with other measures. Quantitative SNI measures of support and stress were generated by summing across the number of different positive and negative categories generated from each mother's statements about the child's father, her parents, and new partners (boyfriends and fiances).

Parent Attachment Interview

Additional information about the child's father was extracted from the Parent Attachment Interview (PAI; Bretherton, Biringen, Ridgeway, Maslin, & Sherman, 1989). The interview was administered and audio-taped during a laboratory session. The interview takes between 1 and 2 hours. It was transcribed verbatim.

The primary purpose of the PAI was to assess the mother's perception of the mother–child attachment relationship through 25 structured, open-ended questions. Questions focus on mother–child emotional communication, autonomy negotiations, and attachment situations (bedtime, separations). Although only one of these questions concerned the father–child relationship directly, mothers spontaneously provided a substantial amount of information about coparenting issues and the child's relationship with the father in the course of responding to other PAI questions. To analyze this information more closely, all interview segments pertaining to father-related information were extracted verbatim from the PAI transcripts.

Careful and repeated reading of these transcripts revealed that mothers addressed five general father-related topics during the PAI: (1) coparenting issues related to transitions between parental residences, (2) issues related to the child's stay at the father's home, (3) the child's relationship with the father, (4) quality of fathering, and (5) mother–child conversations about divorce-related topics. Assignment of statements to major categories and subcategories by the first coder were checked by two subsequent coders who had no or very limited knowledge of other data about the families. Disagreements (mostly omissions rather than conflicts over interpretation) were resolved by discussion.

Some of the information from the PAI was quantified using the method developed for analyzing the SNI. Aggregate scores relevant to quality of fathering were derived from the number of different positive and negative descriptive categories mothers used to discuss their former spouses as fathers. These scores were used in subsequent correlational analyses.

Sources of Help Questionnaire

The Sources of Help Questionnaire (SOHQ), developed by Wan, Jaccard, and Ramey (1996), was given to mothers for completion at home after the SNI, and was collected during a subsequent lab session when mothers were administered the PAI.

The SOHQ uses a 5-point scale to rate the helpfulness of various sources of help, in this case the helpfulness of the mothers' parents (the child's maternal grandparents), other relatives, close friends, coworkers, church or temple, doctors, counselors/therapists, and books (from 1 = "is not helpful," to 5 = "extremely helpful"). Each source of help is rated separately for the provision of (1) informational support (specifically, parenting advice), (2) emotional support, (3) tangible help, and (4) companionship. The frequency of contact with each source also is rated on a 5-point scale (from 1 = "not at all," to 5 = "once a week or more"). Overall satisfaction with help from each source was evaluated by an 11-point scale (ranging from –5 = "extremely dissatisfied," to +5 = "extremely satisfied"). Mothers were asked not to rate network members who were unavailable (i.e., if their parents had died, or they were not in contact with their former husbands or with relatives, they were to indicate this rather than give a low rating).

The introduction to the questionnaire read as follows:

> "When parents have problems or need perspectives on raising their children or managing their family, they frequently turn to other people for advice, help, and support. We would like to find out whom you contact for help and advice related to your family, how often you contact them, and how satisfied you are with the help that they provide. We will ask you to do separate ratings for each of four types of help."

For the purposes of this questionnaire, types of support were defined as follows: (1) informational support as advice about parenting; (2) emotional support as listening, reassuring, and showing care; (3) tangible help as running errands, babysitting, financial assistance, or other forms of material help; and (4) companionship as sharing time in leisure and recreational activities, offering a sense of friendship, and participating in shared activities.

Based on a factor analysis of data from their initial validation study of the SOHQ, Wan et al. (1996) concluded that separate assessments of the four different forms of help were useful. Although ratings for different forms of help tend to be significantly correlated, in their study, some social network members specialized in particular types of help.

Marital Autonomy and Relatedness Inventory

After the lab session during which the PAI took place, the mothers were given a second packet of questionnaires, including the Marital Autonomy and Relatedness Inventory (MARI). The MARI (Schaefer & Edgerton, 1979) has scales for love, rejection, autonomy, and controllingness, as well as for agreement/disagreement about childrearing. Respondents rate their partners. Hence, the love and rejection scales pertain to the mothers' ratings of the fathers' loving and rejecting behavior toward them. Mothers were asked to fill out the MARI retrospectively, that is, in terms of how they perceived spousal behavior at the time of permanent separation (i.e., the rejection scale assessed how rejected the mother remembered herself to feel by the child's father at that time). The MARI was chosen for this study because of its compatibility with attachment theory (it assesses relatedness, autonomy, rejection, and controllingness in the marital relationship), and because its parental scales allowed us to evaluate former spouses' agreement/disagreement about childrearing issues. MARI items are rated from 1 = "not at all like him/her," to 5 = "very much like him/her."

RESULTS

We begin by reporting qualitative analyses concerning the mother's perspective on the child's father, new maternal partners, and the mother's parents, based on the SNI and PAI. Next we consider maternal ratings based on the SOHQ concerning the child's father, the mother's parents, and other close relatives and friends. For each source, we report mean helpfulness ratings for the four separate types of support and for frequency of contact (5-point scales) as well as ratings of satisfaction with overall support (11-point scale). In addition, we show intercorrelations among ratings for the overall satisfaction scores. Finally we report correlations that represent the overall functioning of the family's attachment network based on the quantified SNI and PAI data and the SOHQ ratings. In addition, we discuss correlations of mother's MARI ratings with her responses to the SOHQ, SNI, and PAI.

Social Network Interview

Who Was Mentioned

Eighty-four percent of the mothers listed the child's father as a member of their extended social network (in many cases exclusively as a source of stress). Only 24% of the 50 mothers placed the child's father in their primary network. Mothers also discussed the fathers as members of the child's network.

Ninety-two percent of the mothers nominated one or both of their own parents as members of their overall social network and 82% included one or both parents in their primary network (14% of the mothers had divorced parents). In addition, 70% of the mothers named relatives other than parents as additional members of their primary network. The vast majority of these were siblings. Mothers identified 40 sisters and 18 brothers as primary network members, but nominated only three of their grandmothers, two aunts, two uncles, and one sister-in-law in this category.

Ninety-four percent of the mothers named friends (including neighbors and coworkers who had become friends) as members of their primary networks and 64% of the mothers included a partner in their overall social network. Of these 32 men, 84% were also listed on the mothers' primary network though only 22% were cohabiting. Because the focus of this chapter is on attachment issues, we limit our further discussions to the child's father (as attachment figure for the child to whom the mother may or may not have an unresolved marital attachment), the mother's new partner (who may function as an attachment figure for the mother as well as for the child), and the mother's parents, who may serve as subsidiary attachment figures for the children.

Relationship with the Child's Father

Mothers provided considerably more different reasons why they considered the child's father as stress-inducing than why they considered him supportive, $M = 3.2$ versus $M = .9$, respectively, $t(49) = 5.07$, $p < .0001$.

Mothers' positive statements about the child's father centered on communication quality and emotional support. Twenty-eight percent of mothers noted that both parents were working on improving communication for the sake of the child or children, and 16% emphasized that they tried to be polite or get along with the child's father:

> "We're both committed to working to provide the best thing for the children."

> "We don't expect it to be perfect, so we get along."

Twelve percent mentioned that they could ask the child's father for both tangible help and/or emotional support:

> "I wouldn't hesitate if I was broken down somewhere to call and ask him to pick me up."

> " . . . when I can't handle it anymore and [I] vent all the frustrations on him and he listens."

Mothers' negative statements focused on the father's lack of interest in and attention given to the children, problems with child support and with the child's transitions between parental residences, lack of trust between the parents, and emotionally hurtful statements that fathers addressed to mothers and/or their children.

The most common source of stress (36%) was the father's perceived lack of interest in the children even while they were staying with him, such as "He just plops them down in front of the TV." Along the same lines, 30% of the mothers judged that the father's time with the children was insufficient in order to develop a close relationship:

> "I wish that he would see her more often. He only takes her when he's supposed to—he never plans for anything more, like on a vacation or going camping."

> "His dad really hangs out with the adults. If he has something planned, it doesn't matter if the kids are there or not."

Thirty percent of the mothers voiced their upset about problems related to the father's payment of child support:

> "When I took him back to family court and I told him I wanted his support reviewed, he immediately quit his two part-time jobs."

Mothers also reported difficulties with the transition between maternal and paternal residences, and were irked by fathers' negative comments about the mother, either to the children or directly to the mother herself:

> "At the beginning of the divorce he was calling me 'Mommy Dearest,' telling the children I'm Mommy Dearest and a bad person."

Inability to trust the father and fathers' lack of respect for the mother were additional stresses.

Thus, in terms of attachment quality, many mothers saw fathers as less than adequate attachment figures who also frequently undermined the mother's ability to serve as secure base by criticizing her or calling her names directly or via the children. However, in a minority of families a fairly amicable, even supportive coparental relationship had emerged.

The Mother's Parents

Mothers generated far more positive than negative statements about their own parents, $M = 3.5$ versus $M = 1.6$, $t(47) = 4.27$, $p < .0001$. The two most common reasons for considering their parents important were the provision of child care (52%) and of emotional support (46%). In addition, 32% of the mothers made strong statements about the degree to which they could rely on their parents as attachment figures:

> "She would do anything for me."

> "He is always there for me."

> "My mom would bend over backwards for me."

> "I can always count on my mom."

> "Whatever I need, they're there."

Other mothers considered their parents important because of the special bond or close relationship between them (36%), because they felt comfortable calling on parents when needed (32%), or because of parents' financial help (28%), instrumental help (22%), supportiveness regarding the divorce (16%), fondness for the grandchildren (16%), or serving as role models for their grandchildren or the mother (14%). Six percent of the mothers mentioned that they provided important reciprocal support to their parents.

Mothers felt unsupported and stressed, on the other hand, when their parents were judgmental about the divorce (24%):

> "You made your bed, now lie in it."

> "My mother would say things like: 'It's not like he ever hit you.' "

> "This is totally against anything that they believe in. . . . People don't get divorced."

Twenty-four percent of the mothers felt stressed by their parents' behavior toward themselves or their children, and 16% reported parental put-downs:

> "I'm not what my mother wanted."

> "He will not approve of my discipline."

> "If I did lose my job my mother would probably curl up and die."

Other mothers mentioned past problems, such as a parent's alcoholism, which still caused conflict in the current relationship (16%) .

In addition, several mothers (12%) commented that accepting help carried obligations or was conditional, and 12% mentioned that one or both parents were overly controlling:

> " . . . they would expect things in return . . . they would expect to be able to give advice."

> "The obligation stress. . . . "

> "She makes me feel like I can't say or be critical at all."

> "You kind of feel like you reverted back in a way to having to listen to what Mom and Dad say all of a sudden."

A few mothers commented that their parents provided less help or emotional support than expected (12%), that they felt stressed because of current problems in the parents' lives (12%), that parents were not helping with child care (4%) or finances (2%), or that they had problems contacting the parents (4%). One mother even felt that her efforts to seek help from her parents were rejected outright.

In summary, the mothers' parents, especially the mothers' mothers, served frequently as secure havens and bases for adult daughters and/or the grandchildren. However, when parents were controlling or judgmental of their adult daughter, their support (whether emotional or material) was perceived as less helpful. Serving as an attachment figure to an adult child requires much tact on both sides because it may reinstitute the asymmetry of attachment relations in childhood.

The Mother's New Partner

Sixty-four percent of the mothers mentioned a boyfriend or fiance. In contrast to their statements about the child's father, mothers were very positive about their new partners and mentioned few stresses, $M = 4.4$ versus $M = 1.1$, $t(31) = 6.3$, $p < .0001$. Of the 32 mothers who discussed partners as members of their social network, slightly more than half ($N = 17$) also commented that the child liked, loved, or felt positively toward the partner:

> "They [children] are fond of [partner]; once in a while they call him Daddy."

> "[Child] has got him wrapped around her little finger."

> "[Child] wants to have him as part of the family."

And 37% commented that the partner was interacting well with the children:

> "He is so good with the kids."

> " . . . a lot of effort to try and accommodate with the children."

Mothers also mentioned that partners helped with child care and children's activities (50%):

> "Roughhousing, watch cartoons, go a lot of places, the zoo."

> "Plays with [child] and took care of her."

> "[Partner] fixes [child's] bike if it needs fixing."

> "Wrestles around on the floor, reads to them, go for walks together."

"He built a tree-house for the boys, and [child] loves to play in that."

"They play catch in the backyard . . . and helping him ride the bike . . . trying to get [child] to try new things."

Overall, mothers made positive statements about 75% of the 32 partners in one or more of the three child-related categories. Many mothers stated that they were less interested in partners who had no commitment to children.

As regards the partner's relationship with the mother herself, 97% of the 32 mothers with partners made one or more positive statements. Forty-four percent of the mothers noted that the partners provided emotional support:

"My own needs, my own time, my own support."

" . . . boosting my ego."

" . . . takes up all the slack."

Forty-one percent of the mothers with partners mentioned positive personality characteristics, an indirect way of talking about the partner's style of relating:

"Very honest and hardworking, very caring."

"I didn't know a man could have so much compassion."

"He has a great sense of humor, and I didn't know how much I would value that."

Having similar interests or values was mentioned by several mothers (25%), as was having a positive relationship (21%):

"We click on every level."

"Real close to him, we get along well."

Being a good listener, open communication, and support with divorce and postdivorce issues were mentioned by 16% of mothers. Fewer mothers reported the following qualities or behaviors: understanding the mother's situation," someone to do things with," offering good advice, "always there" to provide support, and helping with chores. Only one mother mentioned financial support.

Fifty-nine percent of the 32 mothers with partners discussed one or more stressful aspects of their partner relationships, but the statements were quite varied. Nine percent of the mothers mentioned difficulties in trusting the partner and a few mothers each made one of the following negative comments about their relationship with him: doubts about continuing the relationship; the partner living too far away, having a problematic ex-spouse or girlfriend; not being a positive influence in the mother's life; and having a problem with alcohol. A few mothers also commented on child-related problems with the partner: not interacting well with the child, not being a good role model for the child, interfering in the mother–child relationship, and disagreeing about childrearing and daily routines. One mother reported that she "got rid" of a boyfriend whom she regarded as detrimental to the children and most mothers mentioned that they did not expose their children to the men they were dating unless a close relationship had developed.

Partners, in summary, were appreciated because they were friends—even budding attachment figures—for the children, and because they offered emotional support and communication to the mothers. For many of the mothers the partners seemed to serve as emerging marital attachment figures. Negative statements about the partners were not numerous and were extremely varied.

Additional Information about the Child's Father from the Parent Attachment Interview

In the course of answering questions posed during the PAI, many mothers spontaneously provided extensive additional information about the child's father even though only one question pertained specifically to him. As previously noted, mothers' comments covered five broad topics: (1) the child's transition between parental residences, (2) the child's stay at the father's house, (3) the father–child relationship, (4) the quality of fathering, and (5) mother–child conversations about the divorce and/or the child's father.

Transitions: Comings and Goings

Given that the children's parents had been divorced for at least 2 years and, in most cases, permanently separated for much longer, it was noteworthy that transitions between the mother's and father's homes still presented problems for many, though not all, families.

Positive Responses to Transitions. On the positive side, 16% of the 50 mothers explicitly stated that transitions from mother to father or vice versa were now going well or better:

> "At first he always cried and he told his daddy that he wanted to come home, but . . . his dad is starting to do things like bow, you know, shooting bows and arrows and things like that, so now he is starting to enjoy being there."

> "It's been at least a year since she had a problem with it [going to father] . . . and it's like when they're ready to leave [their dad], they're anxious to come back to my house and vice versa, so. But it's never really, like I said, a big production or a big (*pause*), I mean either way, their dropping off or coming back. They're pretty flexible, I guess."

> "He handles it real well, he looks forward to going to his dad's."

Transition Difficulties. Stressful transitions were more commonly reported than were smooth ones. Remember that 7 of the 50 children had little or no contact with their fathers. With respect to the remaining 43 families, 81% of the mothers reported at least one transition-related difficulty, though we must stress that these problems did not necessarily occur during every transition.

Fewer than half of the mothers reporting transition difficulties mentioned the child's transition to the father's residence, whereas almost three-quarters described problems related to the child's return to the mother's house. Some of the children merely offered resistance during departure to the father's house, some also had tantrums, and others cried:

> "So I took him over there and handed him to [father] and he just screamed, he didn't want to go and screamed and screamed . . . he did not want to be with him, he did not want to be with him."

> "A lot of times he will say: 'Mommy, don't go, I need you,' and he'll start crying when I leave when I drop him off at his [father's], but once I'm gone he's fine. It's that initial leaving."

> "She'll get sad or upset on transition days, going from one house to the next. Um, and I know it's hard for her, but I think that's normally when I think of her being sad."

Regarding returns to the maternal home, three types of negative responses were described. Some children did not to want leave the father's house:

> "And then he can even, I come back to pick him up, and he can even change his mind and say: 'No, I want to stay at [father's] now,' so he can change his mind."

> "And it's not just [being sad] leaving my house. It's like when she leaves her dad's to come to my house. . . . Just you know, once she's been in one place for a little while and now she's going to the other."

A few children were reported to be clingy when they returned home to mother:

> "So he wants to sit on my lap, so I know he missed me."

More common and more troublesome for the mothers were behavior problems associated with returning:

> "I get everything all clean and all perfect and, you know, then they come and start fighting right away and throwing things around."

> "Her worst behavior is when I pick her up from her [father's] house. She'll hit me, scream at me at that point. . . . I just let her go through the stage, even though it rips me up inside."

Staying at the Father's Residence: Mothers' and Children's Positive and Negative Responses

Positive Responses. Fifty-one percent of the 43 mothers whose children had regular father contact reported that their children enjoyed their stay at the father's house, despite the fact that transition problems occurred in over half of these families:

> "Both kids really, and especially [child] really enjoys the time at her dad's."

> " . . . he really likes being with his dad, and his dad has a fiancee now, and he likes being with her."

Some mothers (14%) reported that they were able to communicate with their children while at the father's residence:

> "And on Sunday nights we usually talk to each other, I'll call over to his dad's or he will call and talk to me, and it's just: 'What are you doing, Mom?' Or I'll call: 'What are you doing, [child]?' 'Oh, eating supper.' And I'll say: 'Are you having fun?' "

A few mothers reported feeling relieved or relaxed when the children were at the father's:

> "It's nice to have the freedom every two weeks or so."

> "When they're with their dad I worry less, and, you know, I actually feel I can relax and enjoy myself a bit."

Negative Responses. On the other hand, 70% of the mothers whose children had regular father contact commented on their own or the child's negative feelings during father visits. Fifty-six percent of the 43 mothers said they worried about their children's physical or psychological well being:

> "And some of the things she comes back with after there, basically when she is with him, that is my most difficult time, and just things she is allowed to see and hear. I lose my input, my ability to protect her from things that she doesn't need to deal with yet."

Twenty-eight percent of the mothers reported that their children became upset during visits to their father's house. A few mothers were chagrined that the father did not let the children call their mothers on the telephone while they were staying with the father or that the father prevented the mother from talking to the children:

> "His dad doesn't let him call me on the weekends, so they have no contact with me over the weekend."

> "I think the hardest is when they are on vacation and there was no phone, so I couldn't even talk to them on the phone. That's tough because then I worry, you know, and I mean I know their dad is competent, but he's still their dad (*laugh*). . . . [When I haven't] heard anything for a week, that's when it's hard."

Finally, 46% of the mothers of children with regular father contact reported that their children asked to be with their fathers while they were staying at their mother's, or wanted to know why their fathers did not come or call. A few of the mothers also expressed disappointment that the father never called the child at the mother's house, or requested to speak to the child when he was calling the mother.

Quality of Fathering

Positive Statements. In contrast to the many negative statements during the SNI, whose emphasis was on the coparental relationship, the percentage of mothers making positive statements about the child's father was higher during the PAI, presumably because this interview was focused more on the parent–child rather than on the ex-spousal relationship. Eighty-six percent of the 50 mothers made one of more positive statements about the child's father. Eighteen percent of the mothers volunteered that their ex-spouses had actually become better parents after the divorce:

> "[Father] would take him in the beginning and bring him back by 11:30 on Sunday, so he could watch a Packer game without having to fuss with [child], and that's just the way he was. . . . Now their relationship is changing, he's had a couple of different boats since we divorced and he takes [child] out in those and [child] really looks forward to that."

An additional 18% of the mothers believed their ex-spouses to be good fathers, and 34% commented favorably on the fathers' activities with their children:

> "[Child's father] is good for them and good to them, he does a lot of things with them . . . it's all fun time, so I get a little frustrated that way, but that's OK."

Most common (46%) were positive statements about the child's affection for the father or the father's affection for the child:

> "She talks very highly of him. She loves him, misses him. So I'm assuming she's the same with him [Note: very affectionate]."

> "We're just both really affectionate with her. She's just a really easy kid to want to hug."

"He [child's father] loves his kids more than anything and nothing
will take their place."

In addition (as already noted), many mothers reported that their children
enjoyed visiting their fathers, despite the fact that in some of these cases
mothers were not particularly satisfied with the quality of fathering the
children received:

"He really looks forward to that [visiting father at work] and gets
all excited because his dad works at a warehouse and drives a forklift
around, and he will put him in his lap and take off. The things that
[child] does with his dad are kind of fun."

A substantial minority of mothers (30%) reported that they were able
to communicate reasonably well or very well with the child's father about
coparenting issues or gave an example of good coparental communication:

"His dad and I have become pretty good friends."

"One thing I'm really glad we do, even though we are divorced, is
neither of us makes a major decision about the kids without consulting
the other. . . . I mean even the other day, when she had such a rough
day at school, I called [child's father] and said: 'Well, this is what
happened, and this is how they handled it. What do you think, what
is your opinion on how I should handle it?' Because we try and be
consistent. . . . I think we both have the kid's best interest in mind."

In addition, many mothers stressed that they refrained from making
negative comments about the father to the child (as noted later under
mother–child talk). Finally, 28% of the mothers reported that fathers were
willing to take care of the children while they were out of town on business
or vacations:

"Even when I go [on a trip] by myself [father] and the kids take me
to the airport, so they know I haven't just disappeared . . . so they
stay there the whole time until they see me off . . . it doesn't seem to
bother them, they have such a good relationship with their dad."

In 24% percent of the families, fathers looked after the children for longer
stays, including summer vacations.

"Since the divorce, they have been with their father in the summer
for a whole week at a time . . . and they're going on a vacation with

him just this next week, too . . . I know that he is well taken care of, no matter who has him [meaning the grandparents or other relatives], even his father."

Negative Statements. All 50 mothers made one or more negative statements about the father's coparenting or parenting. Their statements fell into seven general categories: (1) unreliability in keeping appointments, (2) dangerous situations during the visit, (3) lack of paternal sensitivity, (4) lack of involvement during visits, (5) disagreements about discipline, (6) fathers spoiling the children or letting themselves be manipulated, and (7) interparental communication difficulties.

Thirty-two percent of the 43 mothers whose children had regular father contact reported that the father was not reliable in terms of visiting or keeping visitation appointments, for example cancelling a visit because the father was not "emotionally up to it . . . " or because the children had a cold. Thirty-nine percent of the mothers described serious risk issues such as the father using alcohol or drugs while the children were with him, leaving the child or children alone in the house, or matters related to sexual activities with partners. Sixty-five percent of the mothers criticized the father for being selfish or insensitive with respect to the child. Another common complaint was that the father was not involved enough with the child during visits (let them watch too much TV, did not do much with them), an issue that had already come up during the SNI. In addition, 37% of the mothers reported that fathers criticized them directly in front of the child or to the child.

> "When we first separated, he told them that Daddy could have girlfriends, but Mommy couldn't have any boyfriends. . . . He's done some other things that I find disturbing."

> "I'm trying to deflate it and telling him: 'No, I'm not a bad person,' and it really screwed him up, you know, he would come home and say: 'Daddy says you are a bad person.' "

> "A particular time when (*pause*) his dad brought him home and his dad just laid into me like crazy, and at that time I was depressed and didn't know it yet, I just started bawling and he [child] came over and gave me a hug."

Concerning discipline issues, 74% of the 43 mothers whose children had regular father contact reported that their strategies differed from the fathers'. In most of the families with childrearing disagreements, fathers were said to be more lax than the mothers:

"In playing we're a lot alike. When it comes to discipline, he [father] doesn't discipline like he should, so when [child] comes back, it's hard. . . . He lets [child] get away with almost anything."

"I'm a lot more strict than he is. Of course, I have to live with them a lot more than he does, so I expect them to respect me and do what I ask them to do. Of course, that takes a lot of work too . . . I think basically he is not strict, he basically lets them do a lot more of what they want to do and when they want to do it, like stay up late."

In the remaining families (about 26% of those with disagreements), fathers were said to be more controlling. Moreover, in 42% of the families with regular father contact, mothers believed that fathers spoiled the children or let themselves be manipulated by the them (by buying whatever they wanted, letting them drink pop and eat junk food whenever they asked, etc.):

"Like chewing gum. I haven't wanted her to chew gum 'cause I . . . didn't want her choking on it and swallowing and chomping on it. Her dad lets her chew gum, and has since she was 2. Well, she didn't understand that [Note: the mother had said the child had to wait until she was 5]. . . . 'Well how come Daddy lets me chew gum?' "

" . . . and 'Daddy bought me this, and Daddy lets me have candy, Daddy took me there.' I don't know what he is feeling, but it's almost like he is trying to buy back time he doesn't have with her."

A minority of mothers (21%) commented that coparental communication about the child was either extremely negative or nonexistent.

Mother–Child Talk about Divorce Issues

Many mothers provided examples of their children's questions and statements about divorce and coparenting topics. Many also discussed their answers.

Children. Altogether, 76% of the 50 mothers in the study mentioned that their children talked to them about divorce and parenting issues. A few reported that their child idealized the father as superhero or fantasized about activities with him (such as going fishing) that had never occurred. In three of these families the father had no contact with the child.

Forty-six percent of the 50 mothers reported that their children asked or talked about the parents' feelings for each other. Thirty-six percent asked questions about parental reunions or affection between the parents. For example, one child told the mother that she had tried to get her father to buy a Mother's Day card, but the father refused. Another mother said:

> "Lately she has been focusing on the fact that we should be together, and um, out of the blue one day at dinner table she turned to me and said: 'Mommy, do you love Daddy?' "

Twelve percent of the mothers mentioned that their children wanted to know why the parents had divorced, 24% of the children wondered why the parents did not live together, and 6%, wondered why they could not get along or argued:

> "[She] can't understand why we are not married anymore (*child looking at parents' wedding photos*)."

> "The most pain that [child] seems to have right now is why his mother and father are not married, and he wants us to be married again, because he sees us, we get along real well now, and he sees us get along and he wants us to be married and like his friend, he says he wants Daddy in the house."

In addition, 26% of the mothers reported that their children talked to them about the father's behavior, his extended family, or his girlfriend. For example, a boy whose father had a girlfriend commented that he now had two mothers, and a girl invited her mother to attend the father's remarriage ceremony. A third mother said:

> "Now if we drive past his dad's fiancee's house and his dad's car is there, if we have time [child] will ask if we can stop, and so I do that now, so that's been real difficult for me."

Most mothers experience a child's expressed wish to live with the father as very threatening. Sixteen percent of the mothers reported that their child had done so:

> "And sometimes she'll tell me separate from having been over there, that she wishes she could go live with him. 'Why?' "Cause I miss him.' "

> "And there's been times when he said [to his father: 'I want to live with you,' and it's been a weekend when he's been there, and [father]

said: 'You're too young now, maybe some day you can come and live with me,' but I'm hoping he will stay with me and yet I hope that [child's father] and I will always live close enough so it won't be a problem."

As mentioned in an earlier section, a number of mothers mentioned that their children wanted to know why they could not see the father whenever they wanted to or why he did not come to see them. Also painful or frustrating for most mothers, 16% of the children were said to use statements like "Dad lets us do that," to get their own way with the mother.

Mothers. Whereas many mothers reported that their children asked questions about the divorce or divorce-related issues, they also explained that they tried to shield the children from information they (the children) were not ready to hear or comprehend. In fact, 66% of the mothers said they refrained or tried to refrain from sharing negative feelings and/or information about the father. Thirty percent of the mothers said they would not discuss reasons for the divorce, and 50% decided not to divulge their negative feelings about the current situation:

"When I talk about his dad, you know, I was told by everyone that I should leave my feelings for my ex away when I talk to the kids and, you know, have a (*pause*) neutral ground and don't say bad things about him, so I try and do that."

"Only if I would be angry about her father, that would be the only time [not to share feelings]. I mean, we keep that as sunny between us as, you know, we do get along real well, but there are times when I am real frustrated with him or there's problems and that I would not [share]."

Thirty-eight percent of the mothers explicitly stated that they were trying to protect the child's feelings by withholding information that, in their view, should not be shared with a child:

"I don't tell him too much because I think he should be a child and not to have to worry about his mother."

"I don't share my feelings about not liking the fact that [father's girlfriend] is becoming more like a mother to them, you know, because I don't want to put her [child] in the position like feeling she has got to choose between the two of us, so you know—there is . . . if I'm going to be putting her in an awkward position by sharing my feelings, making her feel guilty about her (*pause*), then

I feel I shouldn't share what I'm feeling with her. As far as her and any of the other kids know, I like [father's girlfriend]."

"I don't want him hurt, and to explain, I have to lie about his dad yet because it would hurt him too much."

Some of these mothers told children (untruthfully) that the father was busy rather than unwilling when he called to cancel a visit. A few (8% of the 50 mothers) expressed the hope that the children would form their own independent opinion of the father. Another 8% described their attempts to engender positive feelings about the visit, despite the negative feelings they harbored.

Whereas many mothers described attempts to cover up their own negative feelings about the child's father or about divorce issues, a minority (28%) discussed their attempts to be open in response to the child's questions:

"She's asked some pretty tough questions, and I've been pretty honest with her. I haven't sugar-coated a lot and I'm sure it hurts her. 'Do you love my dad?' and I've had to tell her, 'No.' If I said yes, then, 'Why aren't you living with him?' So, no, I don't. She started crying, she wanted me to tell her, 'I do love him,' and she got the honest answer, she cried. I didn't put her down, 'That's just the way it is, honey. You still love him, but I don't.' "

"He doesn't understand why I don't want to live with his dad anymore. And I was trying to explain to him that sometimes people could care about each other, but they really couldn't live together. And I think I overdid it, because he said, 'Mom, now I really want to tell you something.' And I thought, 'Oh, no. Here it comes. He's going to tell me I'm a bad mom.' And he said, 'I really want to go to Wal-Mart.' "

Some mothers tried to provide answers regarding more difficult issues such as the father's alcoholism:

"We have had to have this conversation around the alcohol and how it can be dangerous to drive and, or if they go to the hotel and his dad wants him to swim and that maybe sometimes when you drink he can't be as attentive and he can't watch the kids as well."

"I just tell him that Daddy is sick [drunk] and Daddy can't always take care of you, so when Daddy is sick, Grandma has to be there, and so, just in case Daddy is sick while you're with him, Grandma needs to be there to help take care of Daddy."

Another mother talked to her child about the father's behavior at the time of permanent separation:

> "I strive for honesty, no matter what. . . . His daddy is the something we talk about quite a bit . . . his daddy was very cruel, very, very cruel and [child] has to sort that out . . . I'm telling him the truth, I'm telling him that Daddy didn't want to live with us anymore, that Daddy told us we had to leave, and people don't agree with that. Unfortunately, I have made a very firm decision that I want my son to know that what Daddy did, Daddy did not do right . . . I don't want him to grow up and think that's OK."

When this mother's parents divorced while she was a child, her mother had painted a positive picture of her father. She had felt confused and wanted to prevent her son from experiencing similar confusion.

Three mothers mentioned that they had told their children to communicate directly with their father about issues that bothered them:

> "I've tried to be positive when he says he doesn't want to go there. I just tell him that I think it's important that he talk to Daddy about that and 'tell him how you feel.' "

In one case this had disastrous consequences, because the father blamed the child for breaking up the relationship between him and his girlfriend after he had complained to his father in the girlfriend's presence.

Mothers' and Fathers' New Partners as Described in the Parent Attachment Interview

Some additional, though less extensive, information about new partners also emerged during the PAI. Mothers tended to compare their boyfriends and fiances favorably with the child's father, though these new relationships were not always without problems. Some mothers discussed problems that arose with how the father and boyfriend were to be addressed. In a few cases, the children called both the father and the fiance "Daddy" (adding the first name when they refer to either father, i.e., Daddy Bob). Several mothers reported that children became attached to their partners and asked for them after a breakup: "Where is John?" "Why can't we see Rick anymore?" One child consoled her mother about the loss of her boyfriend: "If he won't be your friend anymore, then I'll be your friend." On the other hand, a few children became very upset at seeing someone else close to their mothers.

Regarding the fathers' new partners, altogether 58% of the fathers were reported to have new partners (3 were remarried). Some mothers expressed gratitude at the presence of these women because they believed that, as a result, their children received better care at the fathers' house, and, as already noted, one mother reported that a father accused the child of breaking up the relationship with his girlfriend (the child complained about her to the father in her presence). A few mothers described their efforts at fostering good relationships with their former husbands' partners. For example, one mother reluctantly invited the girlfriend to her house for the child's birthday because they had a tradition of the father coming to celebrate birthdays. Other mothers felt pained when they heard that the father tells the children to call his new partner "Mommy."

It appears that many children have both intense positive and negative feelings about their parents' partners. In the past, such feelings have been studied in the context of remarriage, but they also play an important role whenever there is significant contact with a parent's partner, whether or not that partner is cohabiting.

Questionnaire Data

Findings Obtained with the Sources of Help Questionnaire

Means and standard deviations of mothers' SOHQ ratings of perceived helpfulness concerning the child's father, the mothers' parents, other relatives, and close friends are shown in Table 4.1. The ratings of relatives

TABLE 4.1. Means and Standard Deviations of Perceived Helpfulness Ratings by Source, Type of Support, Frequency of Contacting the Source, and Overall Satisfaction with Support (from SOHQ)

Sources of help	Mean (SD) helpfulness ratings (5-point scale)				Frequency of support	Total satisfaction (−5 to +5)
	Parenting advice	Emotional support	Tangible support	Compan-ionship		
Child's father (48)	$1.9^a(1.1)$	$1.6^b(1.0)$	$1.9^a(1.1)$	$1.4^b(1.0)$	3.3(1.5)	−2.0(3.2)
Mothers' parents (48)	$3.6^b(1.2)$	$3.6^b(1.3)$	$3.7^b(1.5)$	$4.0^a(1.3)$	3.6(1.6)	2.7(2.8)
Relatives (48)	$3.1^b(1.2)$	3.4 (1.2)	$3.0^b(1.4)$	$3.5^a(1.4)$	3.1(2.4)	2.2(2.4)
Close friends (50)	$3.6^b(1.0)$	$4.2^a(1.0)$	$3.3^c(1.3)$	$3.9^b(3.9)$	4.0(1.1)	2.9(2.0)

Note. Numbers in parentheses after each source of help refer to the number of mothers who provided ratings for the particular source. Helpfulness ratings range from 1, "is not helpful," to 5, "extremely helpful." SOHQ, Sources of Help Questionnaire.

$^{a, b, c}$ Within sources of help, means labeled *a* are greater than means labeled *b*; means labeled *b* are greater than means labeled *c* (significance tested with Tukey's HSD post hoc test, $p < .05$).

and friends are included to provide contextual information, although these relationships are not a focus of this chapter. The number of mothers who rated a particular network member is shown in parentheses. These numbers vary because mothers had been asked not to rate the helpfulness of an individual who was unavailable (e.g., her parents if they had died, or a former spouse who was not in contact with her at all).

In line with the information gleaned from the SNI, mothers rated the support received from children's fathers as very substantially lower than that of all other sources of help. None of the mean ratings for the different types of helpfulness were greater than 2 on a 5-point scale. The lowest mean was, understandably, for companionship. In addition, the mean overall satisfaction rating for the father (on a scale from −5 to +5) was negative, that is, expressing dissatisfaction. For the child's maternal grandparents (the mother's parents), on the other hand, all mean helpfulness ratings were above 3. The ratings for relatives and friends were in the same range.

The low ratings of father support (the four separate categories of support and the overall rating) were especially interesting in light of the fact that ratings of contact frequency for fathers and the mothers' parents were similar. A within-subjects analysis of variance (ANOVA) for frequency of contact with the child's father, the mother's parents, relatives, and close friends was significant, $F(4,40) = 3.8, p < .005$, because relatives and friends were rated significantly higher than were other network members. However, the frequency ratings for the child's father and the mother's parents were not significantly different (using Tukey's HSD test). On the other hand, the ANOVA for overall satisfaction ratings was not only highly significant, $F(4,40) = 34.4, p < .0001$, but also subsequent HSD tests showed that ratings for the child's father were significantly lower than were ratings for the mother's parents, relatives, and close friends. The low ratings of maternal satisfaction with the child's father are especially interesting when contrasted with Wan et al.'s (1996) standardization sample of married families, in which spouses received the highest helpfulness ratings (with means in the range of 4.5 for the different types of helpfulness).

Because we had not expected that mothers' boyfriends and fiances would be involved in children's lives in very significant numbers, we failed to ask the mothers to rate them separately on the SOHQ. However, for those six mothers who rated their boyfriends or fiances under the category "other," helpfulness ratings were very high ($M = 4.6$ for the overall satisfaction ratings). Note that, of these rated partners, only three lived with the mother. Overall, 7 of the 32 partners, or 23%, lived with the child's mother.

Intercorrelations among Sources of Help. Given that maternal SOHQ ratings were correlated with a number of demographic variables, maternal age and education were controlled in all subsequent computations (interestingly, income was not consistently related to variables of interest). The correlations among mothers' overall support satisfaction scores for the child's father, the mother's parents, other relatives, and close friends are displayed in Table 4.2 (the intercorrelations among the four scales assessing types of support are similar). The number of ratings on which the separate correlation coefficients are based varies somewhat as a function of the number of mothers who provided a response for the particular source of help. Interestingly, mothers' ratings of satisfaction with support from their children's fathers were not correlated with corresponding ratings of the maternal grandparents, relatives, and friends. The variations in father ratings can, hence, not be ascribed to a mother's general ease or difficulty in getting along with other figures in her primary network.

Correlations of the Sources of Help Questionnaire Ratings with Aggregated Scores from the Social Network Interview and Parent Attachment Interview

As described in the methods section, we derived quantitative aggregate scores from the SNI and PAI information and correlated these with the overall satisfaction scores from the SOHQ. From the SNI we developed support and stress scores for the child's father, the mother's parents, and the mother's partner. From the PAI we derived aggregate scores pertaining to low quality of fathering, father involvement with the child during visits, and father–child affection.

Mothers' SOHQ ratings of satisfaction with support from the child's

TABLE 4.2. Correlations among SOHQ Ratings of Overall Satisfaction with Various Sources of Support (Controlling for Mother's Age and Education)

Support source	Child's father	Mother's parents	Relatives
Child's father (48)			
Mothers's parents (48)	−.14		
Other relatives (48)	.12	.51***	
Close friends (50)	.00	.28*	.55***

Note. Numbers in parentheses after each source represent the number of mothers making this rating. For example, the maternal grandparents are not rated by mothers whose parents have died. SOHQ, Sources of Help Questionnaire.

$^†p < .10;$ $^*p < .05;$ $^{**}p .< 01;$ $^{***}p .< 001.$

father were positively correlated with SNI scores of father support and negatively correlated with SNI scores of father stressfulness, as reported in Table 4.3. That is, SOHQ father ratings appear to be attenuated by stresses in the ex-spousal and coparental relationships. This finding is further supported by the correlations of the SOHQ father ratings with aggregate measures from the PAI. Paternal affection and involvement scores from the PAI were correlated positively with SOHQ father ratings. By contrast, low quality fathering scores from the PAI were negatively correlated with SOHQ father ratings.

The findings for the mother's parents revealed similar effects. When the mother made more positive statements about her parents during the SNI, she also rated them as more helpful on the SOHQ. Conversely, problems and stresses in the mother's relationship with her own parents as reported during the SNI were negatively correlated with corresponding SOHQ ratings. Here too, we observe the attenuation of satisfaction with a support figure's assistance when aspects of the relationship are stressful (see Table 4.3).

The SNI support and stress/problem scores for the child's father were, however, not correlated with the SOHQ scores for the mother's parents. Nor were SNI support and problem scores for the mother's parents correlated with the SOHQ scores for the child's father. This parallels results reported already for within SOHQ correlations and suggests that the mother's negative or positive relations with the child's father cannot be attributed to a personality trait (general ability to get along).

TABLE 4.3. Partial Correlations of Helpfulness and Satisfaction Ratings from the SOHQ, Problem and Support Summary Scores from the SNI, and Fathering Variables from the PAI (Controlling for Mother's Age and Education)

SNI and PAI variables	SOHQ satisfaction with father's support	SOHQ satisfaction with mother's parents' support
Child's father supportive (SNI)	.49***	
Child's father stressful (SNI)	−.45***	
Father–child affection (PAI)	.42**	
Father involved with child (PAI)	.56***	−.40**
Low-quality fathering (PAI)	−.49***	
Mother's parents supportive (SNI)		.43**
Mother's parents stressful (SNI)		−.26*
Mother's partner supportive (SNI)	−.34*	
Mother's partner stressful (SNI)		.26†

Note. Only coefficients with $p < .10$ are shown. PAI, Parent Attachment Interview; SNI, Social Network Interview; SOHQ, Sources of Help Questionnaire.
†$p < .10$; *$p < .05$; **$p < .01$; ***$p < .001$.

Instead, we discovered some "trade-off" effects in the correlational patterns. When mothers reported the father to be more involved with the child (PAI), the SOHQ ratings for mothers' parents tended to be lower. Likewise, when boyfriends and fiances presented more problems, mothers' parents were rated as more supportive (though this correlation was significant only at the $p < .10$ level and must be treated as suggestive only). We also noticed trade-off effects with respect to fathers and partners. When mothers viewed their boyfriends/fiances as more supportive, they tended to rate themselves as less satisfied with support from the child's father. Although these correlations apply only to the subset of mothers with partners ($N = 32$), there also was a significant negative correlation between having or not having a partner and satisfaction with helpfulness of the child's father, $r = -.27, p < .05$, controlling for mothers' age and education.

These trade-off effects as indexed by correlations between positive and negative assessments of the child's father, the mother's parents, and her new partner could be explained in a variety of ways: (1) when a father is more involved with the child, support from the mother's parents may be less crucial, or (2) when a boyfriend or fiance is problematic, the mother's parents may become more important. It could be that daughters seek help from parents less when another support source is more immediately available or that the mother's parents withdraw when they perceive that their daughter has such support, or both. Parents as attachment figures to their adult children, in other words, may make themselves available according to their daughters' expressed need or their own perceptions of their daughters' and grandchildrens' needs.

Correlations between the Marital Autonomy and Relatedness Inventory and Aggregate Scores Derived from the Social Network Interview and Parent Attachment Interview

Both SNI and the PAI data suggest that about one-quarter to one-third of the mothers were able to communicate very well or reasonably well about joint parenting issues with the child's father. However, a majority of mothers expressed varying degrees of anger and disappointment at the quantity and quality of their former husbands' coparenting efforts, although many tried not to communicate these negative feelings to their children ("I don't tell them I'd like to shoot him.").

Interestingly, the aggregated SNI and PAI scores of father support and stress (SNI) and fathering quality, father involvement, and father–child affection (PAI) were correlated meaningfully with the MARI (see Table 4.4). The MARI was used in preference to other well-known marital questionnaires because of its compatibility with attachment theory. It was

TABLE 4.4. Partial Correlations between Father Support and Problem Measures and the MARI (Controlling for Mother's Age and Education)

Maternal perceptions of child's father	MARI scales (mother's perception of father's feelings and behaviors)						
	Loves mother	Rejects mother	Grants autonomy to mother	Controlling of mother	Parenting agreement	Father more lenient	Father stricter
Satisfaction with support (SOHQ)	.36**	−.48***			.51***		−.24†
Father supportive (SNI)	.57***	−.47***	.30*	−.21†	.47***	−.39**	
Father stressful (SNI)		.26*	.30*	.30*	−.37**		
Father–child affection (PAI)	.34**	−.36**			.30*		
Father involved with child (PAI)	.39**	−.51***			.42***	−.23†	−.38***
Low-quality fathering (PAI)	−.35**	.50***		.23†	−.37		−.32*

Note. Only coefficients with *p* < .10 are shown. MARI, Marital Autonomy and Relatedness Inventory; PAI, Parent Attachment Interview; SNI, Social Network Interview; SOHQ, Sources of Help Questionnaire.

†*p* < .10; *p* < .05; **p* < .01; ***p* < .001.

designed to evaluate the balance between how loved, rejected, controlled, and autonomous a spouse feels in the relationship. Furthermore, unlike other instruments, the MARI contains scales assessing parental agreement and disagreement about childrearing issues. Given that it was used retrospectively, we cannot, of course, assume that mothers' MARI ratings were uninfluenced by their present feelings about the ex-spouse. The ratings are hence best viewed as current appraisals of the past.

It is not surprising that the MARI scales of agreement/disagreement with the child's father were related to the PAI aggregate scores representing the father's parenting quality, his involvement with the child, and the assessment of father–child affection. It is intriguing, however, that the PAI-derived postdivorce assessments of fathering quality, father involvement, and father–child affection also were related strongly to the love and rejection scales of the MARI, because these scales evaluated maternal perceptions of the former spousal rather than the former coparenting relationship. Our findings indicate that a mother's feelings about the child's father as a former spouse are related closely to how she now judges him as a parent. It is also noteworthy that these correlations emerged despite the fact that the mean ratings on the love scale were quite low, whereas those for rejection and controllingness scales were quite high, in contrast to responses by married parents participating in previous studies, for whom exactly the opposite was the case (Bretherton, Winn, Page, MacFie, & Walsh, 1993).

Our findings could be interpreted in two (not mutually exclusive) ways: (1) there is continuity between ex-spousal and coparental relationships as experienced at the time of divorce and the present, or (2) the perception of the current relationship is influencing the ratings of the past relationship. Whichever interpretation one accepts, the father's supportiveness, fathering quality, and affection for the child are closely linked in the mother's mind to her evaluations of the spousal and ex-spousal relationship. This suggests that, for postdivorce parents to function as secure bases for their children, the resolution of their marital attachment relationship (i.e., emotional divorce) is of the highest importance.

CONCLUDING REMARKS

The findings reported in this chapter call on researchers to acknowledge more explicitly and gain a greater understanding of attachment-related problems inherent in coparenting with an ex-spouse. In particular, we need a deeper exploration of the lengthy process of adult attachment dissolutions/resolutions and the compensatory roles of new partner relationships and adult child–parent attachments. Weiss (1974) suggested that the continuing powerful feelings of postdivorce parents toward their former spouses derive from (1) unresolved attachment, (2) the effect of this on coparental communication and the ability to trust the coparent, (3) the effect of this on supporting rather than undermining the ex-spouse's parental role, and (4) the effect of unfavorable comparisons of ex-spouse vis-à-vis a new partner.

These conflicting feelings may motivate a variety of counterproductive behaviors, from stalking to attacking the coparent and drawing the child into coparental power struggles and other conflicts. Some of these feelings may be exacerbated by blame and criticism from other important supportive figures, in particular the mother's parents, or they may be eased when parents help the mother to resolve her feelings about the ex-spouse by providing emotional and material support.

Our qualitative analyses corroborate much that was reported in Weiss's (1974) book on marital separations, though Weiss's study did not provide frequency or correlational data. Furthermore, participants in Weiss's study were for the most part more recently separated or divorced than were the mothers in our study, who had been divorced or legally separated for at least 2 years. The average age of the now-4.5-year-old children at the time of permanent separation was 16 months, but despite the passage of time the postdivorce relationship continued to be problematic for many families in our study.

The reasons mothers gave for this state of affairs during the SNI and PAI were not primarily linked to the quality of the predivorce marital relationship, but rather they centered on ongoing problems with managing communication and coparenting: low levels of trust, respect, and sense of control; competition for the child's love; and low regard for the father's parenting, tempered by many mothers' acknowledgment that there was father–child affection. However, even though mothers' comments during the SNI and PAI focused primarily on the present situation, the quantified SNI and PAI scores of supportive and problematic behaviors by the child's father were meaningfully and significantly correlated with mothers' retrospective ratings of the marital relationship. Whereas this demonstrates a close link between mothers' current perceptions of the former marriage and their current perceptions of coparental and father–child relationships, only longitudinal studies beginning during the divorce process will be able to document the extent to which predivorce ratings of the marriage predict postdivorce coparenting quality.

Our study also highlights the need to explore how postdivorce families' attachment networks change during parental courtship and commitment to new (not necessarily permanent) partners who assume a parenting role. Our data suggest that such changes affect all family relationships and reverberate into the extended family. We were especially intrigued by the suggestion of trade-off effects wherein the perceived helpfulness of support from the mothers' own parents is negatively related to father or partner helpfulness. Other related research topics suggested by our study are children's longing for departed parental partners; jealousy of parental partners, problems with postdivorce kinship names (calling the new partners "Mommy" or "Daddy"), children's adaptation to repeated separations; parents' worries about their children's well-being associated with lack of knowledge and control while the children are staying with the other parent; and children's distress over not being able to access an attachment figure when they wish to. Because our findings are limited to the maternal perspective on postdivorce attachment networks in a relatively small sample, larger-scale longitudinal studies investigating both parents' perspectives on attachment issues in divorced families are badly needed.

Finally, although there is ample evidence that postdivorce parental conflict affects children adversely, we need further studies on how children perceive these postdivorce parental relations (see the review by Grych & Fincham, 1992). We know that children become concerned when their parents argue (Cummings & Davies, 1994; Peterson & Zill, 1986). They may be afraid of being caught in the middle or of being abandoned, and may blame themselves for their parent's divorce because a parent threatened, in the past or present, to leave if a child misbehaved (Bowlby, 1973). We are beginning to learn, however, which types of interparental conflict lead to less damaging attributions by children. For example, Jouriles et al. (1991) reported that consequences for children are less adverse when the parental conflict concerns nonchild issues than when the parents argue about the child. Furthermore, Grych and Fincham's review (1992) revealed that openly expressed conflict has more deleterious effects on children's adjustment than does concealed conflict. Moreover, whereas exposure to interparental conflict tends to sensitize children and hence leads to more intense reactions (Cummings, Zahn-Waxler, & Radke-Yarrow, 1981), children's awareness of conflict resolution seems highly beneficial (though these findings were based on witnessing nonparental interadult anger), even when only the outcome of the resolution, not the resolution itself, was directly observed (Cummings, Ballard, El-Sheikh, & Lake, 1991; Cummings, Simpson, & Wilson, 1993).

Given these findings, parents in the process of divorce might benefit from learning not only about the potentially adverse effects of conflict, but also about the conditions under which children are less affected by interparental conflict (see Cummings & Davies, 1994). Just as important, however, are attempts to gain a better understanding of why a substantial minority in our study and other studies were able to negotiate fairly friendly coparental relations. Better predivorce relations may have contributed to more positive postdivorce coparenting in these families, but other postdivorce factors may also be important, as suggested by a few mothers' comments that their ex-husbands had become better fathers after the divorce.

Furstenberg and Cherlin (1991) point out that to aim for and expect an at-most businesslike postdivorce relationship may be more realistic than to expect amicable interactions. In some cases, even a businesslike relationship may be unrealistic, and avoiding direct communication between parents may be the best solution (Johnston & Campbell, 1988). However, a greater acknowledgment and awareness of the diverse and intense emotional challenges posed by the interrelated attachment processes operating in divorcing and postdivorce families is as important as the many current attempts to ameliorate postdivorce coparenting by substituting mediation for the adversarial climate of the legal divorce process (Kelly, Gigy, & Hausman, 1988). To discover what factors enable some postdivorce families to resolve old attachment issues and to negotiate new attachment issues more successfully should be a high priority, in view of the percentage of parents and children currently involved in marital breakups.

ACKNOWLEDGMENTS

This study was funded by Grant No. R01 HD267766-01 from the National Institutes of Health and by support from the Graduate School Research Committee and the Waisman Center of the University of Wisconsin–Madison to the first author. We would like to express our deepest thanks to the mothers who shared their experiences with us. We are also grateful to Barbara Golby and Chris Halvorsen for assistance with data collection and to Margaret Peterson, Charmaine Harbort, and Julia North for transcribing the interviews.

REFERENCES

Ahrons, C. R. (1994). *The good divorce.* New York: HarperCollins.
Ahrons, C. R., & Wallish, L. S. (1987). The relationship between former spouses. In D. Perlman & S. Duck (Eds.), *Intimate relationships: Development, dynamics and deterioration* (pp. 269–296). Newbury Park, CA: Sage.
Amato, P. R., & Keith, B. (1991). Parental divorce and the well-being of children. *Psychological Bulletin, 110,* 26–46.
Bowlby, J. (1973). *Attachment and loss: Vol. 2. Separation.* New York: Basic Books.
Bowlby, J. (1980). *Attachment and loss: Vol. 3. Loss.* New York: Basic Books.
Bretherton, I., Biringen, Z., Ridgeway, D., Maslin, C., & Sherman, M. (1989). Attachment: The parental perspective. *Infant Mental Health Journal, 10,* 203–220.
Bretherton, I., Winn, L., Page, T., MacFie, J., & Walsh, R. O. (1993, March). *Concordance of preschoolers' family stories with parental reports of family*

climate, family stress and child temperament. Paper presented at the biennial meeting of the Society for Research in Child Development, New Orleans, LA.

Cochran, M., Larner, M., Riley, D., Gunnarsson, L., & Henderson, C. R. (1990). *Extending families.* New York: Cambridge University Press.

Cummings, E. M., & Davies, P. T. (1994). *Children and marital conflict.* New York: Guilford Press.

Cummings, E. M., Ballard, M., El-Sheikh, M., & Lake, M. (1991). Resolution and children's responses to interadult anger. *Developmental Psychology, 27,* 462–470.

Cummings, E. M., Simpson, K. S., & Wilson, A. (1991). Children's responses to interadult anger as a function of information about resolution. *Developmental Psychology, 19,* 978–985.

Cummings, E. M., Zahn-Waxler, C., & Radke-Yarrow, M. (1981). Young children's responses to expressions of anger and affection by others in the family. *Child Development, 52,* 1274–1282.

Emery, R. E. (1988). *Marriage, divorce and children's adjustment.* Newbury Park, CA: Sage.

Furstenberg, F., & Cherlin, A. J. (1991). *Divided families.* Cambridge, MA: Harvard University Press.

Grych, J. H., & Fincham, F. D. (1992). Interventions for children of divorce: Toward greater integration of research and action. *Psychological Bulletin, 111,* 434–454.

Hetherington, E. M. (1989). Coping with family transitions: Winners, losers, and survivors. *Child Development, 60,* 1–14.

Hollingshead, A. B. (1978). *The four-factor index of social status.* Unpublished manuscript, Yale University, New Haven, CT.

Johnston, J., & Campbell, L. E. G. (1988). *Impasses of divorce.* New York: Free Press.

Jouriles, E. N., Murphy, C. M., Farris, A. M., Smith, D. A., Richters, J. E., & Waters, E. (1991). Marital adjustment, parental disagreements about child rearing, and behavior problems in boys: Increasing the specificity of the marital assessment. *Child Development, 62,* 1424–1433.

Kalter, N., Pickar, J., & Lesowitz, M. (1984). School-based developmental facilitation groups for children of divorce: A preventive intervention. *American Journal of Orthopsychiatry, 54,* 612–623.

Kelly, J. B., Gigy, L., & Hausman, S. (1988). Mediated and adversarial divorce: Initial findings from a longitudinal study. In J. Folberg & A. Milne (Eds.), *Divorce mediation: Theory and practice* (pp. 453–473). New York: Guilford Press.

Maccoby, E. E., & Mnookin, R. H. (1992). *Dividing the child: Social and legal dilemmas of custody.* Cambridge, MA: Harvard University Press.

Parkes, C. M. (1971). Psycho-social transitions: A field for study. *Social Science and Medicine, 5,* 101–115.

Peterson, J. L., & Zill, N. (1986). Marital disruption, parent–child relationship, and behavior problems in children. *Journal of Marriage and the Family, 49,* 295–307.

Schaefer, E. S., & Edgerton, M. (1979). *Short report on the marital relatedness and autonomy inventory (MARI)*. Unpublished manuscript, University of North Carolina.

Tschann, J. M., Johnston, J. R., Kline, M., & Wallerstein, J. S. (1989). Family process and children's functioning during divorce. *Journal of Marriage and the Family, 51*, 431–444.

Wallerstein, J. S., & Blakeslee, A. (1989). *Second chances: Men, women, and children a decade after divorce*. New York: Ticknor & Fields.

Wallerstein, J. S., & Kelly, J. B. (1980). *Surviving the breakup*. New York: Basic Books.

Wan, C. K., Jaccard, J., & Ramey, S. L. (1996). The relationships between social support and life satisfaction as a function of family structure. *Journal of Marriage and the Family, 58*, 502–513.

Weiss, R. S. (1974). *Marital separation*. New York : Basic Books.

Whitehead, B. (1993, April). Dan Quayle was right. *Atlantic Monthly*, pp. 47–84.

5

Intergenerational Transmission of Attachment: A Move to the Contextual Level

MARINUS H. VAN IJZENDOORN
MARIAN J. BAKERMANS-KRANENBURG

Attachment theory has been presented by John Bowlby (1907–1990) in the three volumes of *Attachment and Loss* (Bowlby, 1969/1984, 1973/1980, 1980/1981). During the last decade it has become so widely known that a brief overview will be sufficient here. Bowlby postulated that for children, the contact with their parent or caregiver is very important, especially when under stress. By nature, children seek proximity and contact and show behavior that brings about such contact (e.g., crying or crawling) or that is meant to maintain contact (e.g., smiling). For toddlers it is the parent's psychological availability rather than his or her physical presence that is supposed to be essential. Children who are securely attached to their caregivers are confident of the caregivers' availability; they know that they can rely on them when distressed (Bowlby, 1969/1984). Children who are securely attached are prone to grow up as socially competent preschoolers (Arend, Gove, & Sroufe, 1979; Waters, Wippman, & Sroufe, 1979).

Infant–parent attachment relationships can, however, develop less favorably as well. Bowlby (1969/1984) already formulated criteria for observing differences in patterns of attachment, but it is Mary Ainsworth (born 1913) who devised a laboratory observation procedure that enabled researchers to discriminate systematically attachment patterns among

1-year-old infants: the Strange Situation (Ainsworth, Blehar, Waters, & Wall, 1978). In this procedure infants are confronted with three stressful components: a strange environment, interaction with a stranger, and two short separations from the caregiver. This stressful situation elicits attachment behavior and on the basis of infants' reactions to the procedure, three patterns of attachment can be distinguished. Infants who actively seek proximity to their caregivers upon reunion, communicate their feelings of stress and distress openly, and then readily return to exploration are classified as *secure* (B) in their attachment to that caregiver. Infants who seem undistressed and ignore or avoid the caregiver after reunion (although physiological research shows that their arousal during separation is similar to other infants'; Spangler & Grossmann, 1994), are classified as *insecure–avoidant* (A). Infants who combine strong proximity seeking and contact maintaining with contact resistance or who remain unsoothable, without being able to return to play and explore the environment, are classified as *insecure–ambivalent* (C). In the balance between attachment and exploration, ambivalent infants maximize attachment behaviors. Avoidant infants minimize or deactivate attachment behaviors and try to hide their upset emotions. Secure infants strike a balance between activating attachment behaviors upon reunion and returning to exploration after some time. An overview of all American studies with nonclinical samples (21 samples with a total of 1,584 infants, studies conducted in the years 1977 to 1990) shows that about 67% of the infants are classified as secure, 21% are classified as insecure–avoidant, and 12% are classified as insecure–ambivalent (van IJzendoorn, Goldberg, Kroonenberg, & Frenkel, 1992).

Recently, Main and Solomon (1990) identified a fourth category: Some children showed *disorganized/disoriented* behavior during the Strange Situation, for instance, contradictory or undirected behavior or indices of apprehension regarding the parent. It turned out that parents of infants who show these signs of disorganization often either suffer from unresolved mourning due to loss or other potentially traumatic experiences (Ainsworth & Eichberg, 1991; Main & Hesse, 1990), or abuse or neglect their children (Carlson, Cicchetti, Barnett, & Braunwald, 1989; Crittenden, 1985; Lyons-Ruth, Repacholi, McLeod, & Silva, 1991). In nonclinical samples about 15% of the infants are classified as disorganized (van IJzendoorn et al., 1992). A second classification of secure, insecure–avoidant or insecure–ambivalent, is assigned to indicate the child's attachment strategy apart from the moments of disorganization.

It is hypothesized that infants' behaviors in the Strange Situation reflect their current *working model of attachment,* generated in the first year of life. The infant's attachment working model contains a representation of the caregiver and the caregiver's behavior toward him together with a complementary representation of himself in the interaction. The attachment working model is rooted in the infant's experiences during interactions with the caregiver. Several studies show that mothers of securely attached infants respond sensitively to their children's signals; that mothers of avoidant infants are unresponsive or rejecting to their children's signals and are, in particular, distant and not inclined to physical contact; and that ambivalent infants have mothers who are inconsistently responsive to their signals (Ainsworth et al., 1978; Belsky, Rovine, & Taylor, 1984; Grossmann, Grossmann, Spangler, Suess, & Unzner, 1985; Isabella, 1993; Maslin & Bates, 1983).

THE ADULT ATTACHMENT INTERVIEW

The influence of childhood attachment experiences on attachment relationships in adulthood is an intriguing but complex issue. Clinical and retrospective data seem to suggest that abused children are likely to become abusive parents, and that in general troubled parents look back on a troublesome childhood (although the estimates of intergenerational transmission of abuse vary widely, see Belsky, 1993; Malinosky-Rummell & Hansen, 1993; and Kaufman & Zigler, 1987). The basic model to describe the intergenerational transmission of attachment is simply the following:

Parent's early attachment experiences
↓
Parenting behavior
↓
Infant's attachment experiences

This model emphasizes heavily the continuity of development across the lifespan and does not take into account discontinuities caused by contextual or experiential discontinuities. However, the link between early attachment experiences and later parenting behavior can be broken because of later attachment experiences with parents, intimate friends, spouses, or therapists. Bowlby (1988) emphasized that positive experiences in a partner relationship can bring about the reconstruction of an originally insecure attachment working model; a partner or therapist can provide a "secure base" for exploring and dealing with early attachment experiences. Therefore, to acquire insight into continuity and change of intergenerational transmission of attachment, it is crucial to pay attention to the working model (or mental representation) of attachment experiences of parents. For decades, adequate measures to assess adult attachment representations were lacking. In fundamental as well as in clinical research, self-report measures like the Parental Bonding Instrument (PBI; Parker, Tupling, & Brown, 1979) and the Mother–Father–Peer Scale (Epstein, 1983) dominated the field, but they had at least two shortcomings: first, these self-report measures about childhood experiences with parents are based on an unwarranted optimistic view on respondents' autobiographical memory capacities, and second, they do not take into account phenomena such as repression or idealization of past experiences.

The introduction of the Adult Attachment Interview (AAI; George, Kaplan, & Main, 1985) was a simple but revolutionary shift in attention from the "objective" description of childhood experiences to the current representation of these experiences, and from the content of autobiographical memories to the form in which this autobiography is presented. The AAI is based on two assumptions: (1) autobiographical memory is the ongoing reconstruction of one's own past in the light of new experiences; and (2) repression, dissociation, and idealization of the past—especially of negative childhood experiences—exist and can be traced by studying form and content of the autobiographical narrative separately. Taking these considerations into account, the first model can be extended as follows:

Parent's early attachment experiences
↓
Parent's attachment representation
↓
Parenting behavior
↓
Infant's attachment experiences

According to attachment theory, there is no direct link between parents' early attachment experiences and their parenting behavior. Past attachment experiences are always filtered through the current mental representation of attachment in influencing parenting behavior and the construction of new attachment relationships. The current attachment representation is formed not only on the basis of the early attachment experiences, but also is influenced by later relationships. A good friend, spouse, or therapist can provide a "secure base" for exploring and working through adverse childhood experiences. In addition, parenting behavior is influenced by the social context. A supporting social network might moderate the effects of otherwise unfavorable circumstances (Belsky, 1984), and specific childrearing conditions may affect infants' attachment experiences negatively (Sagi et al., in press). Furthermore, some children may make it difficult for parents to respond sensitively to their attachment signals, because the infants' severe physical handicaps or highly irritable temperament impair the communication (van IJzendoorn et al., 1992). We can add these factors to our model as following:

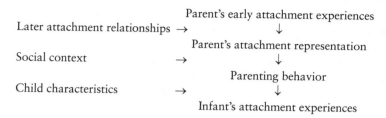

Our contextual model is, of course, simplified, but it makes clear that in attachment theory intergenerational transmission of attachment is interpreted in a quite specific way; in fact, almost all AAI studies available today start their search for the roots of current attachment relationships in parents' minds—and not in their pasts. In this respect, AAI research shows some affinity to recent studies on parental belief systems and their influence on parenting behavior (Goodnow & Collins, 1990; see also Lieberman, Chapter 9, this volume).

What is the structure of the AAI? The AAI is a semistructured interview which probes alternately for general descriptions of past relationships with parents, specific supportive or contradictory memories, and descriptions of current relationships with parents. After a warming-up question about the composition of the family of origin, the subjects are asked to present five adjectives that describe their childhood relationship to each parent and they also are asked the following: (1) why they chose these adjectives; (2) to which parent they felt the closest; (3) what they did when—as a child—they were upset, hurt, or ill; (4) what they remember about separations from their parents; and (5) whether they have ever felt rejected by their parents. In addition to these questions about experiences in childhood, subjects are asked how they think their adult personalities are affected by these experiences; why, in their view, their parents behaved as they did; and how the relationship with their parents has changed over time. In addition, some questions are asked about the subject's experiences of loss through death of important figures, both as a child and as an adult. In total, it takes about an hour to complete the interview (George et al., 1985).

Interviews are transcribed verbatim and coded with the complex AAI coding system. An important criterion for the classification is the interview's coherence. Coherence is defined in terms of Grice's (1975) maxims of quality, quantity, relevance, and manner. In adequate discourse subjects provide evidence for what they say and avoid contradictions (*quality*), subjects are succinct, and yet complete (*quantity*), subjects keep to the point (*relevance*), and they present the information in a clear and orderly way (*manner*).

Coding leads to three classifications, indicating three types of attachment representations: dismissing, autonomous, and preoccupied. *Dismissing* (Ds) subjects emphasize their independence; when they acknowledge negative aspects of their childhood they insist on their not being influenced negatively by those experiences. More often, however, they offer a very positive evaluation of their attachment experiences, without being able to illustrate their positive evaluations with concrete events demonstrating secure interaction. They often appeal to a lack of memory of childhood experiences. In particular because of internal contradictions between general evaluations and specific illustrations, the narrative of dismissing subjects is incoherent. *Autonomous* (F; derived from "Free") subjects tend to value attachment relationships and to consider them important for their own personality. They are able to describe attachment-related experiences coherently, whether these experiences were negative (e.g., parental rejection or over involvement) or positive. They present a coherent and balanced picture without contradictions or other major violations of Grice's rules for adequate discourse. *Preoccupied* (E; derived from "Enmeshed") adults are still very much involved and preoccupied with their past attachment experiences and are therefore not able to describe them coherently. Passivity and vagueness may characterize their biography, or they may express anger when they discuss the present relationship with their parents. Dismissing and preoccupied subjects both are considered to be insecure. Some autonomous, dismissing, or preoccupied subjects indicate through their incoherent discussion of trauma (usually involving loss) that they have not yet completed the process of mourning. These subjects receive the additional classification *Unresolved* (U), which is superimposed on their main classification (Main & Goldwyn, 1991).

In this section three questions concerning the AAI will be addressed: (1) the instrument's reliability, (2) the instrument's discriminant validity, and (3) the distribution of classifications in studies with the AAI conducted so far. Furthermore, we will briefly describe instruments that are available as alternatives for the time-consuming AAI. In the next section we will describe research on the intergenerational transmission of attachment. Addressing these questions, we will rely on the increasing number of studies in which the AAI has been applied since its development about 10 years ago and on some meta-analyses based on these studies (van IJzendoorn, 1995a; van IJzendoorn & Bakermans-Kranenburg, 1996).

Reliability: Interviewer Effect, Intercoder Reliability, and Test–Retest Reliability

As the AAI resembles a natural dialogue about personal issues rather than an objective, impersonal interview, it is possible that the conversation is influenced in a certain direction by the interviewer's personality or interviewing style. Thus far two studies of a potential interviewer effect have been conducted. In The Netherlands, 83 mothers were interviewed twice, by two out of five interviewers, in counterbalanced order (Bakermans-Kranenburg & van IJzendoorn, 1993). The interviewers did not provoke systematically different AAI classification distributions. Furthermore, each pair of interviewers showed about the same stability of AAI classifications over time. In a replication and extension of this study, 59 Israeli college students were interviewed by interviewers who also served as coders (Sagi, van IJzendoorn, Scharf, et al., 1994). The interview outcome was not influenced by the interviewer, whether that interviewer also coded the interview or not. The roles of interviewer and coder of the same interview do not seem to be incompatible. Provided that interviewers are adequately trained, we may conclude that AAI classifications are robust against potential interviewer effects.

It is not the audiotape but rather the verbatim transcription that is coded. Although the reliability of the transcription is, therefore, essential, this fact hardly ever is underscored. The intercoder reliability, however, is established and reported in almost every AAI study. On the basis of 18 studies, we found an average intercoder reliability of about 80%, a reasonable but not perfect reliability.

It is important that the test–retest reliability of the AAI be examined. Although Bowlby chose the term "attachment working model" to emphasize that it is an open, dynamic model that can be restructured on the basis of new experiences (Bowlby, 1988), the model itself stimulates continuity more than change, as internal working models become more rigid over the years (Sroufe, 1988). For adults, stability of the attachment representation may be expected, especially when no major life events take place. Therefore, it is crucial for a measure of adult attachment representations to be stable over time. Thus far, four studies considered the test–retest reliability of the AAI (Bakermans-Kranenburg & van IJzendoorn, 1993; Benoit & Parker, 1994; Sagi, van IJzendoorn, Scharf, et al., 1994; Steele & Steele, 1994). Test–retest reliabilities between 77% and 90% were reported, with an intervening period that varied from 1 to 15 months. Note that the test–retest reliability cannot be 100%, due to imperfect intercoder reliability. After all, it is improbable that all interviews that were coded incorrectly on the first occasion were coded incorrectly again on the second occasion—and in the same (wrong) direction. On the basis of these findings it can be concluded that the instrument seems suitable to examine the *stability* of the attachment working model after changes in life circumstances, major life events, or therapeutic intervention. Note, however—with an eye to the high stability reported by Benoit and Parker (1994), who conducted the interview some weeks before and a year after the delivery—that the birth of the first child is not yet so far reaching that it brings about changes in the parents' attachment representations.

Discriminant Validity: Intelligence, Memory, Social Desirability, and Temperament and Adaptation

Intelligence

The AAI relies on subjects' speech production. The classification is based on the verbatim text of the discourse and the coding system heavily emphasizes coherence in the sense of Grice (1975): The discourse should embody the maxims of quality, quantity, relevance, and manner. Therefore, the coherence of AAI transcripts could be determined by subjects' logical reasoning abilities. In three studies, associations between AAI classifications on the one hand and verbal fluency and logical reasoning on the other hand have been explored. Bakermans-Kranenburg and van IJzendoorn (1993) found that a verbal IQ test (Groningen Intelligence Test; Luteijn & van der Ploeg, 1982) and a logical reasoning test (Raven's Standard Progressive Matrices; Raven, 1958) were not related to the AAI classifications. Sagi, van IJzendoorn, Scharf, et al. (1994) replicated this result with a college admission battery test in a group of Israeli students. If anything, the dismissing students tended to perform somewhat better on this test than did the other students. Crowell et al. (1993), however, found a difference between preoccupied and autonomous mothers: Autonomous mothers scored better on the Henmon–Nelson Test of Mental Ability. Therefore, they propose that in studies with the AAI, an IQ measure should be used as a covariate. Taking into account that two other studies did not confirm this result (Rosenstein & Horowitz, 1996; Ward, Botyanski, Plunket, & Carlson, 1991), it is questionable whether this conclusion is justified.

Memory

Several questions of the AAI consider experiences in the subject's childhood. Although these experiences do not play a major role in the subject's classification, it is nevertheless indicated by the coding system that a lack of memory of childhood events might be interpreted as characteristic of an insecure attachment working model. It is supposed that dismissing subjects are not open to negative aspects of their early attachment relationships and fall back on a lack of memory to avoid reflecting on or discussing those aspects. However, an alternative interpretation would be that dismissing subjects are just not able to remember as many childhood experiences in as much detail as are the other subjects. In the latter case, dismissing subjects would be unable to provide the interviewer with enough material to back up idealized descriptions, but the lack of supporting evidence would be the result of a cognitive rather than a emotional factor. It is therefore important to examine whether the AAI assesses subjects' attachment representations or general cognitive differences in subjects' autobiographical memory abilities.

The two studies that addressed this issue are the aforementioned studies of Bakermans-Kranenburg and van IJzendoorn (1993) in Leiden, The Netherlands, and of Sagi, van IJzendoorn, Scharf, et al. (1994) in Israel. The 83 mothers in the Dutch study evaluated their own long-term and autobiographical memory abilities on a self-report memory questionnaire and completed a memory test with questions about common issues in childhood not related to family attachment experiences. The dismissing mothers did not indicate that they perceived their autobiographical memory abilities as less developed than the other subjects', and they performed even somewhat better on the memory test. In the Israeli study, subjects were asked in a remote memory test to choose among four titles of TV programs, out of which three were fake and only one actually ran during their childhood. Furthermore, subjects completed a paired associate test for relatively short-term memory (3 months). Finally, using Galton's method of Semantic Cuing (Crovitz & Quine-Holland, 1976), subjects were asked to think of memories from their childhood associated with each of 12 cue words and to indicate the age when the event took place. No significant differences among the attachment categories were found; dismissing subjects, however, tended to recall the information on the Semantic Cuing task from a somewhat later age (average age for recall was 8 years for the dismissing subjects and 7 years for the other subjects). This difference is small; it seems justified to conclude that the classification of the AAI is not influenced by differences in autobiographical memory. Without further evidence, dismissing subjects' appeals to a lack of memory for attachment experiences cannot be attributed to general memory deficits.

Social Desirability

In an open, semistructured interview like the AAI, in which subject and interviewer communicate in an intensive way about sensitive issues of childhood and daily life, subjects may be inclined to present their answers in a socially desirable way. Dismissing subjects might, therefore, not be idealizing their childhood to avoid facing negative experiences, but rather to create a pleasant atmosphere and to impress the interviewer favorably.

In that case, AAI classifications do not indicate subjects' representation of attachment, but instead their tendency to give socially desirable answers. In two studies with the AAI, a measure of social desirability (the Marlowe–Crowne scale; Crowne & Marlowe, 1960) was included (Bakermans-Kranenburg & van IJzendoorn, 1993; Crowell et al., 1993). Neither of these studies showed an association between social desirability and attachment classification.

Temperament and Adaptation

The AAI aims at internal working models of attachment, assessing mental representations and behavior within the context of intimate relationships. Although some association with temperament and social adjustment may be expected, the measure pretends to be more specific, not overlapping too much with measures of general personality traits or mental and physical health. Relations with variables within the attachment domain (e.g., infant attachment, parental responsiveness) should be dominant. If this were not the case, the AAI would lack specificity and a firm foundation in attachment theory (Crowell et al., 1993). Two studies focused on relationships between AAI classifications and personality traits.

De Haas, Bakermans-Kranenburg, and van IJzendoorn (1994) examined the association between the EAS (Emotionality, Activity, Sociability scale; Buss & Plomin, 1984) and the attachment categories. No significant relationships between temperament and adult attachment were found. Neither were the AAI classifications related to subjects' mental and physical health (assessed by the General Health Questionnaire; Goldberg, 1972, 1978). In the second study, Crowell et al. (1993) detected a significant relation between the AAI classifications and an instrument for social adjustment (the Social Adjustment Scale; Weissman & Paykel, 1974). Secure mothers were better adjusted than were dismissing mothers; preoccupied mothers yielded the lowest scores. Crowell et al. (1993), however, found also that this association disappeared when they controlled for differences in IQ between the subjects. In sum, the conclusion that the psychometric characteristics of the AAI are excellent seems warranted.

Distributions of Classifications in Normal and Clinical Samples

Standard Distribution

Normative data about the distribution of interview classifications can be found by means of a meta-analytic combination of the separate primary studies. More than 2,000 AAIs have been classified and reported, and such an impressive number of classifications provides a basis for analyses of the reported distributions. In Table 5.1, these data are presented briefly. Compared with the combined samples of "normal" infant–mother dyads observed in the Strange Situation (21% avoidant, 67% secure, and 12% ambivalent; van IJzendoorn et al., 1992), the overall AAI distribution of nonclinical mothers shows an underrepresentation of autonomous mothers (58%) and an overrepresentation of preoccupied mothers (18%). As a result, the percentage of insecure mothers is relatively high. When the classification of unresolved is taken into account as a separate category, 19% of the nonclinical mothers are classified as such for unresolved loss or trauma of other kinds. The majority of these unresolved mothers are from the insecure categories, so that the percentage of autonomous mothers does not decrease drastically (from 58% to 55%; see van IJzendoorn & Bakermans-Kranenburg, 1996, for details). Mothers' nationality or socioeconomic status appeared not to influence the distribution. The distribution of fathers is remarkably similar to the standard distribution of mothers. Although it could be imagined that men tend to be more dismissing than are women (Gilligan, 1982), this idea is not confirmed by the data. The distribution of adolescents' AAI classifications corresponded to the distribution of classifications of adults. Finishing school, getting married, and having children do not seem to affect the attachment representations, at least on the level of the global distribution of classifications. The question of whether this applies to individuals as well can be answered only by longitudinal studies.

In five studies, both partners of, in total, 226 couples were interviewed (Cohn, Silver, Cowan, & Pearson, 1992; Crittenden, Partridge, & Claussen, 1991; Miehls, 1989; Steele, Steele, & Fonagy, 1993; van IJzendoorn, Kranenburg, Zwart-Woudstra, van Busschbach, & Lambermon, 1991). Autonomous wives appeared to be most often married to autono-

TABLE 5.1. Distributions of AAI Classifications in Normal and Clinical Samples

Population	N	Distribution (%)		
		Dismissing	Autonomous	Preoccupied
Mothers (normal)	584	24	58	18
Fathers (normal)	286	22	62	16
Low SES	254	28	57	15
Adolescents	237	26	56	19
Parents of clinical children	148	41	14	45
Clinical adults	291	41	12	47

Note. Derived from van IJzendoorn and Bakermans-Kranenburg (1996). SES, socioeconomic status.

mous husbands, although one-third of the autonomous wives were married to a dismissing or a preoccupied husband. The same was true of autonomous husbands. About one-third of them were married to insecure wives (van IJzendoorn & Bakermans-Kranenburg, 1996). That means that there seems to be a tendency toward stabilization of security or insecurity by the choice of a partner, but that there also are many exceptions to the rule that husbands and wives share the same working model of attachment. Therefore, many chances for breaking the intergenerational cycle of insecurity exist (Rutter, Quinton, & Hill, 1990).

Clinical Groups

The AAI has become increasingly popular in clinical psychology, developmental psychopathology, and child psychiatry. The attraction of the measure for diagnostics and evaluation of therapeutic processes may stem from the theoretical roots of the instrument, in which knowledge of normal development is combined with psychopathological insights. The application of the AAI in clinical samples—that is, adults with psychiatric problems and parents of children with problem behavior—has led to two hypotheses. First, it is supposed that clinical groups show an overrepresentation of insecure attachment representations compared with the standard distribution in nonclinical samples. Secondly, it is hypothesized that externalizing problems such as oppositional behavior are rooted in a dismissing representation of attachment, whereas internalizing problems such as depressive symptoms are associated with a preoccupied representation of attachment (Rosenstein & Horowitz, 1996; see also Goldberg, Chapter 6, this volume).

The AAI has been administered in a variety of clinical groups (for details, see van IJzendoorn & Bakermans-Kranenburg, 1996). The combined clinical groups indeed show a strong overrepresentation of insecure subjects. The dismissing as well as the preoccupied category are well represented (see Table 5.1). Whether the clinical problems are located primarily in the adults or in the children does not make a difference for the overall distributions. Thus, we found confirming evidence for the first hypothesis. The second hypothesis, however, concerning the relation of a specific kind of psychiatric disturbance—externalizing or internalizing—to a specific type of adult attachment representation could not be confirmed on the basis of our data (see also van IJzendoorn & Bakermans-Kranenburg, 1996). Although some studies showed a clear link between externalizing problems and dismissing attachment on the one hand, and internalizing problems and preoccupied attachment on the other hand (e.g., Rosenstein & Horowitz, 1996), other studies did not present such an unambiguous picture (e.g., Patrick, Hobson, Castle, Howard, & Maughan, 1992; see Goldberg, Chapter 6, this volume, for similar discussion with reference to the Strange Situation).

An example of the complicated associations between psychiatric diagnosis and AAI classifications is provided by the study of mentally disturbed criminal offenders that we carried out in cooperation with two Dutch forensic mental hospitals (van IJzendoorn et al., in press). The sample consisted of 40 forensic psychiatric inpatients of Dutch ethnicity who were sentenced for (attempted) murder, rape, or similar sexual crimes, and other major crimes, but who were found to be mentally ill at the time of their crime. The criminal offenders were subjected to a special juridical measure that imposes on criminal offenders with psychiatric disturbances a psychotherapeutic treatment of potentially unlimited duration in a maximum-security forensic hospital to protect society against repetition of their crimes. The subjects were interviewed with the AAI before entering the forensic hospital. After about 6 months they were interviewed with the Structured Interview for Disorders of Personality—Revised (SIDP-R; Pfohl, 1989), and therapists completed staff–patient interaction inventories to assess the quality of the patients interactions with the staff. Background information about crime characteristics and childrearing history was derived from court files.

We found that only 5% of the subjects were autonomous according to the AAI. The remaining subjects were distributed about equally among the dismissing, preoccupied, unresolved, and cannot classify (CC) categories. In particular, the high percentage of CC subjects is remarkable. The CC classification is used when subjects display contradictory attachment strategies, for example, highly dismissing toward their father as well as highly preoccupied with their mother (Hesse, 1996; see Fonagy et al., Chapter 8, this volume, for discussion of mismatched attachment strategies). Although we had expected to find more dismissing subjects diagnosed with an antisocial personality disorder, this was not the case. In fact, the dismissing subjects seemed to be less disturbed than were subjects in the other insecure categories. Eight out of 11 CC subjects were diagnosed with a personality disorder, whereas in total only 22 of 40 criminals reached the DSM-III-R (American Psychiatric Association, 1987) criteria for personality disorders. The preoccupied subjects showed elevated externalizing as well as internalizing problems (Goldberg, Chapter 6, this volume, reports the same findings with a sample of preschool children). Constructing a continuous AAI scale on which the autonomous subjects receive the lowest score, the unresolved and CC subjects the highest score, and plain dismissing and preoccupied subjects a score in the middle, we found that the more insecure the subjects were, the more personality disorders they had. It is interesting to note that 90% of the CC subjects were raised in institutional care, compared with 45% of the remaining subjects in the other AAI categories. Lastly, attachment security appeared to be related to the quality of patients' interactions with the staff: the autonomous and dismissing subjects did function better than did subjects in the other categories; the CC subjects performed worst (van IJzendoorn et al., in press). In a study on nonclinical subjects, Crowell et al. (1993) also found that subjects in the F (autonomous) and Ds (dismissing) categories seemed to be better socially adjusted. In sum, we did not find clear-cut associations between the AAI and type of personality disorder, although we found that more insecure delinquents were more disturbed. Furthermore, the AAI classifications were related to early childhood experiences, and to staff–patient interactions. Note that the AAI classifications were not based on the early childhood experiences per se.

To summarize the results on attachment in clinical groups, we displayed graphically the information in Figure 5.1. In Figure 5.1, the centers of gravity of the distributions of the clinical samples (with problems located in the adults and in the children, respectively) are projected against the background of the standard distribution of AAI classifications of nonclinical mothers. Figure 5.1 shows that the distributions of both types of clinical groups and the distribution of mentally disturbed criminal offenders diverge strongly from the standard distribution, which is located at the crossing of the three axes. Note also how close to the origin, that is the standard distribution, the distributions of the fathers and of the adolescents are situated. The centers of gravity for the clinical samples, however, are located far away from this origin, and indicate overrepresentations of dismissing as well as preoccupied subjects. Conclusions about the relation between specific clinical groups and attachment representation, however, are not yet warranted; the data base for systematic inferences about this issue is still rather small.

Alternative Measures

The AAI is a laborious instrument; administering, transcribing, and coding an interview require training and an impressive amount of time. Therefore, several researchers have been motivated to devise a questionnaire concerning the same issues of childrearing and attachment experiences. Hazan and Shaver (1987) developed a self-report questionnaire in which subjects choose which of three short descriptions of attachment styles fits their ideas best. Other questionnaires, such as Epstein's Mother–Father–Peer Scale (Epstein, 1983), the Egna Minnen Beträffende Uppfostran (EMBU; Perris, Jacobsson, Lindström, von Knorring, & Perris, 1980), the Inventory of Parent and Peer Attachment (Armsden & Greenberg, 1987), and the Adult

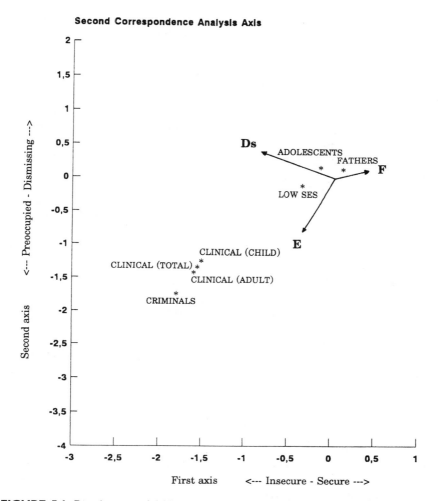

FIGURE 5.1. Distributions of AAI classifications in specific groups projected against the background of the standard AAI distribution.

Attachment Questionnaire (AAQ; Lichtenstein, 1991) focus on a description of the past and present relationship with subjects' parents. The Berkeley–Leiden Adult Attachment Questionnaire for Unresolved Loss and Other Trauma (BLAAQ-U; Main, van IJzendoorn, & Hesse, 1993) aims at identifying subjects who probably will be classified as unresolved on the basis of their AAI. The most obvious problem of these instruments is their validity. The questionnaires developed thus far lack satisfying

convergent validity and cannot be used as an alternative for the AAI despite
the advantages of questionnaires in large samples (van IJzendoorn et al.,
1991; De Haas et al., 1994). The BLAAQ-U seems to be rather successful
in identifying subjects with unresolved loss or other trauma, but does not
provide information about the other classifications. Taking stock of the
alternatives for the AAI, we must conclude that a good alternative is as yet
not available; that reliable self-classification may remain problematic; and
that—at least for the time being—we have to rely on the time-consuming
AAI. Attachment questionnaires bring insecure subjects into the paradoxical position of having to present a balanced self-diagnosis of their mental
representation of attachment, whereas they are insecure because they are
not able to reflect on their attachment experiences in a balanced way. One
of the consequences of this self-report paradox is that with the regular
questionnaire format, dismissive idealization and veridical description of
positive attachment experiences cannot be differentiated.

INTERGENERATIONAL TRANSMISSION OF ATTACHMENT

Infant's Attachment Classification

The development of the AAI was embedded in research on the question of
why some children are securely and others are insecurely attached to their
parents. Investigators examined whether the answer could be found in
parents' attachment representations; the coding system of the AAI classifications reflects the infants' attachment classifications in the Strange
Situation. The Strange Situation procedure and the classifications that can
be assigned have been described above (see also Goldberg, Chapter 6, this
volume; see Rutter, Chapter 2, this volume for a critique of the Strange
Situation). In the balance between exploration and attachment behavior,
children who are attached avoidantly to their parents minimize or deactivate attachment behavior, whereas ambivalently attached children maximize attachment behavior at the expense of exploration (Main, 1990).
Securely attached children strike the balance between attachment behavior
(asking for comfort) immediately after the reunion and return to exploration after some time. In the same vein, the AAI classifications are based on
the communication about emotions in attachment relations. Autonomous
subjects are characterized by an open and unbiased reflection on their
attachment experiences, dismissing subjects minimize the influence of early
attachment experiences on their adult personalities, and preoccupied
subjects are still preoccupied by their childhood experiences or the present
relationship with their parents. Thus a potential association between adult
and infant attachment goes further than Belsky's (1984) process model,

which states that the child is influenced by specific characteristics of the parent's personality that result from the parent's own upbringing. The intergenerational transmission of attachment suggests an analogy of adult and infant strategies, showing, as it were, two sides of the same coin: the manifestation of the strategy in the parent (at the level of verbal representation) on the one hand, and that of the infant (at the level of attachment behavior) on the other hand. In Figure 5.2 the corresponding attachment categories are presented. It is hypothesized that autonomous parents stimulate a secure relationship with their children by their openness to their children's attachment signals (Main, 1991), whereas the insecure parents' pasts interfere with the required open communication.

The correspondence between parental attachment and infant attachment has been examined in a number of studies during the past decade. Eighteen studies have been published or are in an advanced stage of publication thus far. (Due to the frequent use of the AAI in the field of attachment research, this collection of studies should be considered the current reflection of a growing number of AAI studies.) The correspondence between parents' unresolved loss and infants' disorganization in the Strange Situation has been addressed in a small minority of these studies. Therefore, we pay little attention to this issue. A short presentation of the 18 studies and details about the method of the meta-analysis can be found in van IJzendoorn (1995a). In most studies, the AAI was administered with mothers; four studies, however, concerned fathers (Main & Goldwyn, in press; Radojevic, 1992; Steele et al., 1993; and van IJzendoorn et al., 1991).

On these 18 studies (with a combined sample of 854 parent–child dyads) we performed three meta-analyses. First, we combined effect sizes for the correspondence between autonomous parents and secure infants. The combined effect size was $d = 1.06$, which is comparable to a correlation coefficient of $r = .47$. This effect size is quite strong; it would take 1,087

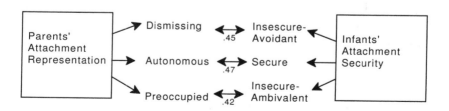

FIGURE 5.2. Intergenerational transmission of attachment: Correspondences between parents' and children's attachment representations. *Note:* Effect sizes are based on 18 studies with 854 parent–child dyads in total (van IJzendoorn, 1995a).

studies with null results to diminish the combined probability level to insignificance (Rosenthal, 1991). Studies with mothers showed a stronger relationship between parental attachment and infant's attachment than did studies with fathers; for mothers, the combined effect size was $r = .50$, whereas for fathers it was $r = .37$.[1] The four studies that assessed the attachment representations of the parents before the birth of their (first) child (Benoit & Parker, 1994; Fonagy, Steele, & Steele, 1991; Radojevic, 1992; Ward & Carlson, 1995) did not yield effect sizes different from studies that administered the AAI simultaneously with the Strange Situation, or even years after the assessment of the infant's attachment. The benefit of studies with a prospective design is that they can shed light on the direction of the causal link between parents' and infants' attachment classifications; these studies indicate that parents' prenatal attachment representations, which are of course uninfluenced by their unborn children, can predict the quality of the parent–child attachment relationship about 1 year later. The causal direction of the relation between parental and infant attachment thus goes from parent to child. Alternative explanations involving a third factor determining both the parent's and the infant's attachment do not seem very plausible; studies of the discriminant validity of the AAI show that parental IQ and temperament are not associated with the AAI classifications. Therefore, hereditary IQ or temperament may not be involved in establishing the association between AAI and Strange Situation classifications.

The second meta-analysis aimed at the correspondence between parents' dismissing attachment representation and infant's avoidant attachment. A comparable effect size was found ($r = .45$). Again, the correspondence was stronger for mothers ($r = .50$) than for fathers ($r = .32$). The third meta-analysis, concerning the relationship between the preoccupied AAI classification of the parent and the infant's ambivalent classification, yielded a combined effect size of $r = .42$ for fathers as well as for mothers. The effect sizes are presented in Figure 5.2. Although beyond the scope of this chapter, note that the studies in which the unresolved classification was assigned as well showed a combined effect size of $r = .31$ for this category. In that case, however, the association between the preoccupied and the ambivalent classification decreased to $r = .19$ (see van IJzendoorn, 1995a).

Parental Responsiveness

Responsiveness has been defined as the "ability to perceive and to interpret accurately the signals and communications implicit in the infant's behavior, and given this understanding, to respond to them appropriately and promptly" (Ainsworth, Bell, & Stayton, 1974, p.127). Parental responsiveness fosters a secure parent–infant attachment relationship. For that reason, responsiveness is supposed to be a mediating factor in the relationship between parents' attachment representations and their children's attachment working models. Parental attachment representations determine the way the parents are inclined to communicate about emotions in intimate relationships, in particular in the attachment relationship with their children. Parents who tend to dismiss their negative feelings about their own childhood experiences may also be inclined to be less open to their infants' feelings of anxiety and distress. For parents who still are strongly preoccupied with their own attachment experiences as children, these past experiences may be in the way of an open and balanced communication about their children's feelings in stressful situations. These parents also might feel threatened by the negative and ambivalent emotions of their children, as they remind them of their own past. Parents with autonomous attachment representations, however, can be expected to be open for communication about their children's anxiety and distress.

In 10 studies, with a total of 389 parent–child dyads, AAI classifications have been related to measures for sensitive responsiveness. Within studies, often more than one scale for sensitive responsiveness was used. Therefore, these measures were combined through separate meta-analyses (van IJzendoorn, 1995a). The combined effect size for the ten studies was $r = .34$. At least 156 studies with null results would have to be conducted to diminish the probability level to insignificance. Unfortunately, this effect size describes only the association between a secure or insecure attachment representation and sensitive responsiveness; it would be interesting to distinguish between dismissing and preoccupied representations as well. In that case, we could examine whether these different types of insecurity are related systematically to quality of responsiveness, for example, over- and understimulation. The available studies, however, lack relevant data to perform meta-analyses exploring this issue.

The Transmission Gap

The rather modest effect size for the relation between AAI classifications and sensitive responsiveness indicates the existence of an uncharted territory in the field of transmission of attachment, referred to as a "transmission gap" (van IJzendoorn, 1995a). After all, only a limited part of the correspondence between parents' attachment representations and children's attachment classifications can be ascribed to the mediating force of sensitive responsiveness, and the complete process of intergenerational transmission of attachment still remains unexplained.

This unexplained part can be quantified as follows (see van IJzendoorn, 1995a). The effect size for the association between AAI classifications and sensitive responsiveness was $r = .34$. Goldsmith and Alansky's (1987) meta-analysis of the relation between responsiveness (assessed with Ainsworth's measure for sensitivity at home) and children's attachment classifications in a selected set of studies yielded a combined effect size of $r = .32$. As the effect size of the correspondence between parental attachment representations and infants' attachment classifications amounts to .47, the unexplained part must be equal to .36 (i.e., .47–[.34 × .32]). Differences in responsiveness between parents with different attachment representations play a part in the explanation of transmission of attachment across generations, but this part is, as we saw, only modest. Alternative explanations can be found in correlated errors of measurement (but the measures involved may not share much systematic error variance because they are so different), genetic factors (but Suomi, 1995, discussed an ethological study in which the substantial intergenerational transmission of parenting between biologically related primates and their offspring did not differ from the transmission in adoptive "families"), and/or the hypothesis that the current measures of responsiveness may not capture all relevant aspects of the parent–child interaction (e.g., that we do not pay enough attention to the interchange between parents' and children's facial expressions of emotions). The issue of the transmission gap is discussed more extensively in the debate between Fox (1995) and van IJzendoorn (1995b).

Environmental Influences

Is intergenerational transmission of attachment restricted to specific childrearing conditions? This question is raised in the first place because the correspondence of $r = .50$ implies that there also are autonomous parents with insecure children, and that the children of some insecure parents are nevertheless securely attached to them. In fact, in about 25% of the families, there is no correspondence between parental and infant attachment security (van IJzendoorn, 1996). These exceptions to the general rule seem important for generating knowledge about the process of intergenerational transmission of attachment on the case level (see Lieberman, Chapter 9, this volume). Secondly, the social context of the parent–child relationship should be taken into account. Most studies with the AAI have occurred in Western, industrialized countries with similar and relatively stable family constellations. Therefore, the issue of the ecological context might fade into the background. In a very discrepant ecological context, however, the general rule of intergenerational transmission may lose strength. In other words, the conclusion that a universal law of intergenerational transmission of attachment exists is not justified until the contextual limits of the transmission phenomenon are tested.

The Israeli kibbutzim appear to provide an opportunity to test the universality of intergenerational transmission of attachment. Although still a Western cultural setting, the childrearing context in kibbutzim, in particular in kibbutzim with communal sleeping arrangements, deviates strongly from the "normal" Western patterns of childrearing and family life (Aviezer, van IJzendoorn, Sagi, & Schuengel, 1994). In all kibbutzim children spend a large part of the day in special "infant houses" under the care of professional caregivers. Some kibbutzim, however, kept until recently to the practice of communal sleeping as well. In the communal sleeping arrangement, children spend only 3 to 4 hours in the afternoon at home; during the rest of the day and at night they are under the care of professional caregivers or watchwomen. Whereas the former kibbutzim appear to provide a situation similar to that of dual-earner families with full-time daycare, kibbutzim with communal sleeping arrangements deviate from this pattern. The care at night is provided by watchwomen who have to supervise many infants and children through intercoms. Sensitive responsiveness to infants' signals of anxiety and distress at night is, therefore, almost impossible.

In a quasi-experimental design, 20 mother–infant dyads from kibbutzim with communal sleeping arrangements and 25 mother–infant dyads from other kibbutzim (where the children slept at home) completed the AAI and the Strange Situation. The parents and children were comparable on potentially intervening variables, with the sleeping arrangement being the only difference (Sagi et al., in press). The distributions of mothers' attachment representations were quite similar; 65% of the mothers from communal sleeping kibbutzim were autonomous, and 72% of the mothers from other kibbutzim were classified as autonomous. These percentages are not significantly different. However, a significant difference between the children's attachment classifications appeared; whereas the distribu-

TABLE 5.2. Mothers' and Infants' Attachment Classifications in Two Types of Kibbutzim

Infant's attachment security	Mother's attachment representation			
	Communal sleeping		Home sleeping	
	Secure (*n*)	Insecure (*n*)	Secure (*n*)	Insecure (*n*)
Secure	6	5	16	4
Insecure	7	2	2	3
Correspondence	$\frac{8}{20} = 40\%$		$\frac{19}{25} = 76\%$	

Note. Derived from Sagi et al. (in press).

tion of the children who slept at home was comparable to the distribution of attachment classifications in normal, Western families (80% secure), only 55% of the children from kibbutzim with communal sleeping arrangements were securely attached (Sagi, van IJzendoorn, Aviezer, Donnell, & Mayseless, 1994). Relating type of kibbutz, maternal attachment, and infant attachment, a significant three-way interaction was found between type of kibbutz, infant attachment classification, and maternal attachment classification. Depending upon the sleeping arrangement, which thus seems to be an important aspect of the childrearing context, the intergenerational transmission of attachment was present or absent. In the kibbutzim where the children slept at home, the normal correspondence between mothers' and infants' attachment was found (76%). In kibbutzim with communal sleeping arrangement the correspondence between mothers' and infants' classifications was only 40%, with intergenerational transmission of attachment as the exception rather than the rule (see Table 5.2).

This remarkable result points at the limits of the hypothesis of intergenerational transmission. A closer look at the mismatches makes clear that, in particular, autonomous mothers with insecure infants are responsible for the low percentage of agreement. It is supposed that because of the inconsistent childrearing pattern in the communal sleeping arrangement, the transmission process is blocked, that the influence of a secure maternal attachment representation is overruled by the insensitive context. Two factors seem important. First, the infants spend only a few hours per day with the mother. The lower correspondence could be due to that factor, comparable to the lower effect size we found for fathers than for mothers. It may also be true of fathers that they do not spend enough hours per day with their children to be the deciding factor in their children's attachment. Secondly, infants in kibbutzim with communal sleeping arrangements might feel deserted by their attachment figures at night. Although they experience sensitive care during the afternoon, during the night their attachment signals and behaviors remain unanswered. The recurrent and prolonged separations might induce feelings of insecurity—notwithstanding the positive attachment experiences with the mother during parts of the day. We must conclude that intergenerational transmission of attachment is not context-free, and that cultural childrearing practices may block the transmission of security.

Attachment from Infancy to Adulthood

In coding the AAI the subjects' self-reports about their early years are not taken for granted. On the contrary, the form of the discourse about past and present attachment experiences, rather than the content of their autobiographies, is decisive for the classification. Nevertheless, early attachment experiences may play a role empirically in the formation of adult attachment representations. How strongly is the current mental representation of attachment expected to be rooted in early childhood (van IJzendoorn, 1995b)? And what data are available to address this issue empirically?

More than two decades ago, Bowlby (1973/1980, p. 411 ff.) wrote about the traditional model of lifespan personality development as resembling a railway system with a single main line along which are set a series of stations. Personality development was supposed to be fixed from the very beginning, and only temporary stops, regressions, or accelerations were allowed to exist. In contrast, Bowlby compared his alternative model to a railway system that starts with a single main route which leaves the city in a certain direction but soon forks into a range of distinct routes, some of which diverge from the main route, and others take a convergent course. At any point, critical junctions may show up at which the lines fork; once a train is on any particular line, homeorhesis (Waddington, 1957) tends to keep it on that line.

The development of attachment is not considered to be fixed during the first year of life, but should be regarded as "environmentally labile," in particular in the early years of life (Bowlby, 1973/1980, p. 414). More specifically, Bowlby (1973/1980) always contended that attachment is environmentally labile during the first 5 years, and that even during the decade after the fifth birthday the development of attachment is sensitive to environmental changes, albeit in steadily diminishing degrees. At any stage during the years of immaturity—infancy, childhood, and adolescence—changes in childrearing arrangements and life events such as rejections, separations, and losses (Egeland & Farber, 1984), but also positive experiences such as parents getting a job, adolescents finding a supportive partner (Rutter et al., 1990), or being in therapy (Bowlby, 1988) may provoke a change in the course of attachment development. Almost two decades ago, Sroufe (1978) wrote about his expectations for the longitudinal studies he was embarking upon: "We would not expect a child to be permanently scarred by early experiences or permanently protected from environmental assaults. Early experience cannot be more important than later experience, and life in a changing environment should alter the qualities of a child's adaptation" (p. 50).

There are four studies on attachment available now that cover the first 18 to 20 years of life, and more studies are in progress. The first study is the Bielefeld study of Zimmermann (1994), working with Klaus and Karin Grossmann. Forty-nine families from northern Germany participated in a study starting with home observations of parental sensitivity during the first year of life. Infants between 12 and 18 months of age were observed with their parents in the Strange Situation procedure. At 6 years of age, AAIs of the parents were collected. At 10 years of age, the children were interviewed to assess their mental representation of parental support. At 16 years of age, AAI data of 44 adolescents who were seen as babies became available. Life events such as divorce, life-threatening illness of the parents, and loss through death of parents or other family members were assessed. Zimmermann (1994) did not find a simple, bivariate correspondence between attachment security in infancy and security of attachment representation in adolescence. In particular, divorce and life-threatening illness of parents appeared to be associated with insecure adolescent attachment representation. In a multivariate hierarchical regression analysis, almost 70% of the variance of adolescent attachment security could be explained by life events, maternal attachment representations, and children's representation of parental support at 10 years of age.

Hamilton's (1994) study of 30 adolescents who as 1-year-olds were observed in the Strange Situation procedure showed that attachment may be amazingly stable across a 17-year period. She found that 77% of her subjects were classified similarly as secure or insecure at 1 year and at 17.5 years of age, when they completed the AAI. The subjects were recruited from a larger California sample in which children from families with alternative lifestyles such as communal living were overrepresented. Review of the case notes for each family, gathered over the full course of the study, suggested that the continuity of attachment was associated with certain family circumstances (Hamilton, 1994). Adolescents who retained a secure attachment classification grew up in families that experienced few stressful circumstances. In contrast, adolescents who were classified insecure at both assessments came from families characterized by marital dissolution in early childhood, often accompanied by family violence, persistent parental substance abuse, and financial stress (Hamilton, 1994). In other words, the stability of secure and insecure attachments was supported by stable positive or stable negative circumstances.

The third study has been carried out by Beckwith, Cohen, and Hamilton (1995) at UCLA. They followed 86 preterm children from the first months until 18 years of age. The sample covered a wide range of socioeconomic statuses and a diversity of ethnic groups and contained subjects with at least 28 weeks gestational age. Assessments of parent–infant interaction were derived from naturalistic home observations when the infants were 1, 8, and 24 months of age. A maternal responsiveness score for each age was computed, but—unfortunately—the Strange Situation procedure was not included. When subjects were 18 years of age, the AAI was administered. Results showed that dismissing subjects received lower mother–infant responsiveness scores than did the other two attachment groups, which did not differ from each other. Furthermore, mothers of dismissing subjects did not change their unresponsive behavior; they were equally less engaged at all three observations during infancy, whereas mothers of autonomous or preoccupied subjects changed their patterns over time. In particular, in the subgroup of boys, mothers of autonomous subjects became more sensitive across the three assessments, whereas the mothers of preoccupied subjects showed a steady decrease of responsiveness (Beckwith et al., 1995). The authors note also that 73% of the preoccupied adolescents had experienced a family breakup before 8 years of age, whereas only 28% of the autonomous and 20% of the dismissing subjects had experienced a divorce of their parents.

Waters, Merrick, Albersheim, and Treboux (1995) studied the attachment security of 50 white, middle-class subjects in infancy (using the Strange Situation procedure) and in young adulthood (using the AAI). The attachment security of the original sample of 60 infants and their mothers was highly stable from 12 to 18 months of age (Waters, 1978), and the sample may consist of very stable families. For example, 78% of the parents remained married during this 20-year period. Information about major life events was derived from the AAIs. The continuity of attachment across 20 years was remarkable: 70% of the subjects were classified in the same secure versus insecure category. Across the three categories (avoidant/dismissing; secure/autonomous; and ambivalent/preoccupied) the correspondence was 64%. In the group of subjects who did not experience major negative life events the percentage of correspondence amounted to 78%. Discontinuity of attachment appeared to be related to negative life events such as loss of a parent, parental divorce, life-threatening illness of parent or child, parental psychiatric disorder, or physical or sexual abuse.

Waters et al. (1995) consider the outcome of their longitudinal study as important support for the prototype hypothesis. This hypothesis states that the primary infant–mother attachment relationship serves as a prototype for later love relationships, and that mental representations of real attachment experiences constructed early in life—in fact, during the first year of life—account for the continuity (Waters et al., 1995). An alternative hypothesis is the idea that continuity of attachment is dependent on the stability of the environment in which the child is raised. If the childrearing environment provides enough sensitive care to stimulate the development of a secure attachment in the first year of life, it may continue to be optimal in later stages as well and therefore scaffold secure attachment throughout the first two decades of life. In fact, the four longitudinal studies illustrate how disruptions of caregiving arrangements may be responsible for discontinuities in the development of attachment. This seems to provide some support for the idea that the prototype is only effective under optimally stable conditions.

We may conclude that the studies show some continuity of attachment over the first 20 years of life. At the same time—and more interestingly—discontinuity of attachment can be explained by attachment-relevant life events such as loss or divorce. Lawful continuity as well as lawful discontinuity (Sroufe, 1988) are dependent on family circumstances and life events that threaten the equilibrium of the subjects' attachment representations. These pioneering studies can provide only a first impression of what is to be expected of attachment across the lifespan, and they seem to illustrate nicely Bowlby's (1973/1980) emphasis on the environmental lability of internal working models of attachment in the early years. What these studies do not support is a simplistic model of a critical period of attachment development. The development of attachment does not become fixed during the first year of life, but may remain open to external influences well into adolescence (see also Rutter, Chapter 2, this volume). How strong the environmental pressures have to be to cause a discontinuity in attachment development is still unclear. In general, the development of the childrearing environment has been studied somewhat less intensively than has the development of attachment across the lifespan. For example, the assessment of changes in childrearing circumstances has often been restricted to major negative life events. Smaller fluctuations in the sensitivity of the environment to the attachment signals of a developing individual have not been included in the longitudinal studies published so far. To test the prototype and the stable environment hypotheses more thoroughly, however, we need adequate measures for both dimensions (in van IJzendoorn, 1996, this line of reasoning has been detailed).

Breaking the Intergenerational Cycle of Insecure Attachment

Insecure attachment in infancy is associated with a higher risk of malfunctioning in the socioemotional domain during the preschool years (Sroufe, 1988). Although insecure attachment cannot be considered "pathological" per se, its status as a risk factor has urged researchers and clinicians to reflect on potentially preventive and corrective measures (Belsky & Nezworski, 1988). In recent years, several intervention studies aiming at the prevention or correction of insecure attachment have been performed. The studies take two, sometimes complementary, approaches. First, interventions may be directed at parental sensitivity, that is, at the behavioral level. Second, interventions may also focus on the parents' mental representation of attachment, that is, on the representational level, to pave the way for subsequent behavioral changes. The behaviorally oriented interventions are often short-term and focused, whereas the representational interventions often are long-term and broad-band therapeutic interventions. A good example of the first type of studies is the Anisfeld, Casper, Nozyce, and Cunningham (1990) study in which the effectiveness of a soft baby carrier was tested. A good example of the second type of interventions is the seminal study of Lieberman, Weston, and Pawl (1991), who modeled their approach after Fraiberg's ideas about mother–infant psychotherapy, in which the "ghosts" of the past are discussed.

Intervention studies may show different outcomes. Some interventions may be effective in changing parental sensitivity but not infant attachment; other interventions may change only parental attachment representations, but not infant attachment or parental sensitivity; and, of course, there may be studies that are successful in every domain: parents' attachment representation, infant attachment, and parental sensitivity. Unfortunately, most intervention studies do not report on changes in attachment representations. One of the most intriguing issues in this area is, however, the issue of generalizability: If the parent's insensitivity for infant's attachment signals has been changed and, as a consequence, also the infant's attachment insecurity, how firmly is this change rooted in the parent's personality and how long will its influence last?

We found four case studies and 12 experimental studies that aimed at changing at least the infant's attachment ($N = 869$; data derived from van IJzendoorn, Juffer, & Duyvesteyn, 1995). Eleven of 12 experimental studies also presented data on the effectiveness of the intervention in changing parental insensitivity. The combined effect size of these 11 studies was $d = .58$, an effect size of medium strength (Cohen, 1988). The combined effect size of the 12 studies on attachment security was much lower: $d = .17$. Some interventions even showed negative effects. These interventions used long-term and intensive approaches. In fact, the combined effect size for the long-term, broad-band interventions ($n = 7$) was $d = .00$, whereas the combined effect size for the short-term, behaviorally oriented interventions was $d = .48$. Of course, several explanations may be provided for this intriguing difference in effectiveness, for example, differential attrition (see van IJzendoorn et al., 1995, for elaboration).

A crucial issue is how effective the short-term interventions are in the long run. From the perspective of attachment theory, the generalizability of the interventions seems guaranteed only if the interventions not only change parental behavior or infant attachment, but also attachment representations. It may not be too difficult to teach a mother to be more responsive to the baby's crying, and this may be one of the factors changing the infant's attachment behavior in the Strange Situation procedure, but how deeply rooted is this change in the parent's personality, or more specifically, in his or her mental representation of attachment? In a case study we tried to address this issue in an exploratory and preliminary way (Juffer, van IJzendoorn, & Bakermans-Kranenburg, in press). An insecure–dismissing mother and her 5-month-old daughter participated in this study. The AAI and Ainsworth's 9-point sensitivity rating scale were used as pre- and posttests, and the Strange Situation was included in the posttest. The intervention was implemented between the 6th and 9th month after the birth of this firstborn baby. In four intervention sessions the mother received written information about sensitive interaction with infants and video home training with feedback on videotaped mother–infant interactions, and the intervenor involved the mother in discussions about her childhood attachment experiences in relation to the current interaction with the baby. At the pretest the mother appeared to be insecure–dismissing, and her sensitivity rating was rather low. At the posttest the mother again had to be classified as insecure–dismissing, but her sensitivity rating was almost two scale points higher. This change on the behavioral level was reflected in the Strange Situation. At 14 months of age the child was classified as securely attached to her mother (B3/B2). It is remarkable that only four intervention sessions were effective in changing the mother's insensitive behavior, and in changing the child's attachment insecurity (assuming that the girl was insecurely attached to her mother before the intervention). This is an illustration of the remarkable effectiveness of several short-term intervention studies (e.g., van den Boom, 1988). At the same time, the mother's representation of attachment remained insecure. If parents only acquire new behavioral strategies to interact with their infant, they may not be able to find sensitive ways to deal with the attachment needs of the developing child. Because they are still dismissing or preoccupied they might be less creative and flexible, and more defensive in the communication about emotions with their child. The generalizability of the intervention effects may therefore be restricted. In the long run, the discrepancy between the representational and the behavioral levels may even be counterproductive because the child may experience several shifts in sensitivity of the parent across the years. Another interpretation would be more optimistic. The change at the behavioral level may, after some time, induce a change at the representational level. A securely attached child may provoke positive interactions with the parent, and may reinforce the mother's sensitive behavior, even at a later stage of development. In this way, the child may help to break the intergenerational cycle of insecure attachment. Until more data from experimental longitudinal studies, including data on parental representations, become available, we have no empirical evidence to support one or the other alternative (van IJzendoorn et al., 1995; Juffer et al., in press).

CONCLUSION

In sum, we may conclude that, according to a growing number of studies, intergenerational transmission of attachment should be considered an established fact. The AAI as the assessment of parental attachment representations plays a central part in these studies. We see not the specific events in parents' childhoods per se, but rather the representation of attachment experiences to be of overriding importance. Results on the reliability and discriminant validity of the AAI yielded satisfactory results. The AAI is a psychometrically sound instrument. Alternatives for the time-consuming AAI are not yet available; most questionnaires lack convergent validity. On the basis of a meta-analytic combination of the separate primary studies, a normative standard distribution of interview classifications in normal samples could be derived. The distributions of clinical groups diverge strongly from this standard distribution; irrespective of the location of the problems (in the children or in the parents), the insecure attachment categories are overrepresented. It seems impossible, however, to show systematic associations between type of attachment insecurity and type of psychiatric disturbance.

Responsiveness appears to be a mediating factor in the intergenerational transmission of attachment, but the rather modest effect sizes of the relations between parental responsiveness and parental attachment representations on the one hand, and between parental responsiveness and children's attachment on the other hand suggest a "transmission gap" of attachment. The limits of the intergenerational transmission have been explored on the basis of a quasi-experimental study with two types of Israeli kibbutzim. Apparently, intergenerational transmission of attachment can be blocked by culture-specific childrearing conditions. Intergenerational transmission of attachment may also be discontinued by major life events such as loss of attachment figures or a breakup of the family. Furthermore, interventions aiming at changing attachment insecurity are successful on the behavioral level, but it is still unclear under which conditions the intergenerational transmission of insecure attachment can be changed permanently.

The AAI enabled us to make substantial progress in addressing the issue of intergenerational transmission of attachment in normal as well as in clinical groups, and in different cultural contexts. The AAI also provoked numerous precise questions and hypotheses about the transmission of attachment across generations that deserve our attention in the years to come.

ACKNOWLEDGMENTS

This study was supported by a PIONEER award from the Netherlands Organization for Scientific Research (NWO, Grant No. PGS 59-256) to Marinus van IJzendoorn. Parts of this chapter were presented by the first author at the PAOS/RUL symposium on "Personality, Developmental Psychology, and Psychopathology" (P. D. Treffers, Chair), Leiden, The Netherlands, June 10–11, 1993.

NOTE

1. Effect sizes are presented as correlation coefficients, as this statistic is well known and can easily be interpreted.

REFERENCES

Ainsworth, M. D. S., Bell, S. M., & Stayton, D. J. (1974). Infant–mother attachment and social development: "Socialization" as a product of reciprocal responsiveness to signals. In M. P. M. Richards (Ed.), *The integration of a child into a social world* (pp. 173–225). Cambridge, England: Cambridge University Press.

Ainsworth, M. D., Blehar, M. C., Waters, E., & Wall, S. (1978). *Patterns of attachment: A psychological study of the Strange Situation.* Hillsdale, NJ: Erlbaum.

Ainsworth, M. D. S., & Eichberg, C. (1991). Effects on infant–mother attachment of mother's unresolved loss of an attachment figure, or other traumatic experience. In C. M. Parkes, J. Stevenson-Hinde, & P. Marris (Eds.), *Attachment across the life cycle* (pp. 160–183). London: Routledge.

American Psychiatric Association. (1987). *Diagnostic and statistical manual of mental disorders* (3rd ed., rev.). Washington, DC: Author.

Anisfeld, E., Casper, V., Nozyce, M., & Cunningham, N. (1990). Does infant carrying promote attachment? An experimental study of the effects of increased physical contact on the development of attachment. *Child Development, 61,* 1617–1627.

Arend, R., Gove, F., & Sroufe, L. A. (1979). Continuity of individual adaptation from infancy to kindergarten: A predictive study of ego-resiliency and curiosity in preschoolers. *Child Development, 50,* 950–959.

Armsden, G. L., & Greenberg, M. T. (1987). The inventory of parent and peer attachment: Individual differences and their relationship to psychological well-being in adolescence. *Journal of Youth and Adolescence, 16,* 427–454.

Aviezer, O., van IJzendoorn, M. H., Sagi, A., & Schuengel, C. (1994). "Children of the Dream" revisited: 70 years of collective early child care in Israeli kibbutzim. *Psychological Bulletin, 116,* 99–116.

Bakermans-Kranenburg, M. J., & van IJzendoorn, M. H. (1993). A psychometric study of the Adult Attachment Interview: Reliability and discriminant validity. *Developmental Psychology, 29,* 870–879.

Beckwith, L., Cohen, S. E., & Hamilton, C. E. (1995, March). *Mother–infant interaction and parental divorce predict attachment representation of late adolescence.* Paper presented at the biennial meeting of the Society for Research in Child Development, Indianapolis.

Belsky, J. (1984). The determinants of parenting: A process model. *Child Development, 55,* 83–96.

Belsky, J. (1993). Etiology of child maltreatment: A developmental–ecological analysis. *Psychological Bulletin, 114,* 413–434.

Belsky, J., & Nezworski, T. (Eds.). (1988). *Clinical implications of attachment.* Hillsdale, NJ: Erlbaum.

Belsky, J., Rovine, M., & Taylor, D. (1984). The Pennsylvania infant and family development project II: Origins of individual differences in infant–mother attachment: Maternal and infant contributions. *Child Development, 55,* 706–717.

Benoit, D., & Parker, K. C. H. (1994). Stability and transmission of attachment across three generations. *Child Development, 65,* 1444–1457.

Bowlby, J. (1984). *Attachment and loss: Vol. 1. Attachment* (2nd ed.). Harmondsworth: Penguin. (First edition published 1969)

Bowlby, J. (1980). *Attachment and loss: Vol. 2. Separation: Anxiety and anger.* Harmondsworth: Penguin. (Original work published 1973)

Bowlby, J. (1981). *Attachment and loss: Vol. 3. Loss: Sadness and depression.* Harmondsworth: Penguin. (Original work published 1980)

Bowlby, J. (1988). *A secure base: Clinical applications of attachment theory.* London: Routledge.

Buss, A. H., & Plomin, R. (1984). *Temperament: Early developing personality traits.* Hillsdale, NJ: Erlbaum.

Carlson, V., Cicchetti, D., Barnett, D., & Braunwald, K. (1989). Disorganized/disoriented attachment relationships in maltreated infants. *Developmental Pschology, 25,* 525–531.

Cohen, J. (1988). *Statistical power analysis for the social sciences.* New York: Academic Press.

Cohn, D. A., Silver, D. H., Cowan, P. A., & Pearson, J. (1992). Working models of childhood attachment and couple relationships. *Journal of Family Isues, 13,* 432–449.

Crittenden, P. M. (1985). Maltreated infants: Vulnerability and resilience. *Journal of Child Psychology and Psychiatry and Allied Disciplines, 26,* 85–96.

Crittenden, P. M., Partridge, M. F., & Claussen, A. H. (1991). Family patterns of relationships in normative and dysfunctional families. *Development and Psychopathology, 3,* 491–512.

Crovitz, H. F., & Quine-Holland, K. (1976). Proportion of episodic memories from early childhood by years of age. *Bulletin of the Psychonomics Society, 7,* 61–62.

Crowell, J. A., Waters, E., Treboux, D., Posada, G., O'Connor, E., Colon-Downs, C., Feider, O., Fleischman, M., Gao, Y., Golby, B., Lay, K. -L., & Pan, H. (1993, April). *Validity of the Adult Attachment Interview: Does it measure what it should?* Poster presented at the biennial meeting of the Society for Research in Child Development, New Orleans.

Crowne, D. P., & Marlowe, D. (1960). A new scale of social desirability independent of psychopathology. *Journal of Consulting Psychology, 24,* 349–354.

De Haas, M. A., Bakermans-Kranenburg, M. J., & van IJzendoorn, M. H. (1994). The Adult Attachment Interview and questionnaires for attachment style, temperament, and memories of parental behavior. *Journal of Genetic Psychology, 155,* 471–486.

Egeland, B., & Farber, E. A. (1984). infant–mother attachment: Factors related to its development and changes over time. *Child Development, 55,* 753–771.

Epstein, S. (1983). *The Mother–Father–Peer scale.* Unpublished manuscript, University of Massachusetts at Amherst.

Fonagy, P., Steele, H., & Steele, M. (1991). Maternal representations of attachment during pregnancy predict the organization of infant–mother attachment at one year of age. *Child Development, 62,* 891–905.

Fox, N. A. (1995). Of the way we were: Adult memories about attachment experiences and their role in determining infant–parent relationships: A commentary on van IJzendoorn (1995). *Psychological Bulletin, 117,* 404–410.

George, C., Kaplan, N., & Main, M. (1985). *Adult Attachment Interview.* Unpublished manuscript, University of California at Berkeley.

Gilligan, C. (1982). *In a different voice.* Cambridge, MA: Harvard University Press.

Goldberg, D. (1972). *The detection of general illness by questionnaire* (Maudsley monograph No. 21). London: Oxford University Press.

Goldberg, D. (1978). *Manual of the General Health Questionnaire.* Windsor, Berks: NFER–Nelson Publishing Company.

Goldsmith, H. H., & Alansky, J. A. (1987). Maternal and infant temperamental predictors of attachment: A meta-analytic review. *Journal of Consulting and Clinical Psychology, 55,* 805–816.

Goodnow, J. J., & Collins, W. A. (1990). *Development according to parents: The nature, sources and consequences of parents' ideas.* London/Hillsdale, NJ: Erlbaum.

Grice, H. P. (1975). Logic and conversation. In P. Cole & J. L. Moran (Eds.), *Syntax and semantics III: Speech acts* (pp. 41–58). New York: Academic.

Grossmann, K., Grossmann, K. E., Spangler, G., Suess, G., & Unzner, L. (1985). Maternal sensitivity and newborns' orientation responses as related to quality of attachment in northern Germany. In I. Bretherton & E. Waters (Eds.), Growing points in attachment theory and research. *Monographs of the Society for Research in Child Development, 50*(1–2, Serial No. 209), 233–278.

Hamilton, C. E. (1994). *Continuity and discontinuity of attachment from infancy through adolescence.* Unpublished doctoral dissertation, University of California at Los Angeles.

Hazan, C., & Shaver, P. (1987). Romantic love conceptualized as an attachment process. *Journal of Personality and Social Psychology, 52,* 511–524.

Hesse, E. (1996). Discourse, memory, and the Adult Attachment Interview: A note with emphasis on the emerging Cannot Classify category. *Infant Mental Health Journal, 17,* 4–11.

Isabella, R. A. (1993). Origins of attachment: Maternal interactive behavior across the first year. *Child Development, 64,* 605–621.

Juffer, F., van IJzendoorn, M. H., & Bakermans-Kranenburg, M. J. (in press). Intervention in transmission of attachment: A case study. *Psychological Reports.*

Kaufman, J., & Zigler, E. (1987). Do abused children become abusive parents? *American Journal of Orthopsychiatry, 57,* 186–192.

Lichtenstein, J. (1991, April). *The adult attachment questionnaire (AAQ): Validation of a new measure.* Poster presented at the biennial meeting of the Society for Research in Child Development, Seattle.

Lieberman, A. F., Weston, D. R., & Pawl, J. H. (1991). Preventive intervention and outcome with anxiously attached dyads. *Child Development, 62,* 199–209.

Luteijn, F., & van der Ploeg, F. A. E. (1982). *Groninger Intelligentie Test. Handleiding* [*Groningen Intelligence Test. Manual*]. Lisse, The Netherlands: Swets & Zeitlinger.

Lyons-Ruth, K., Repacholi, B., McLeod, S., & Silva, E. (1991). Disorganized attachment behavior in infancy: Short-term stability, maternal and infant correlates, and risk-related subtypes. *Development and Psychopathology, 3,* 397–412.

Main, M. (1990). Cross-cultural studies of attachment organization: Recent studies, changing methodologies, and the concept of conditional strategies. *Human Development, 33,* 48–61.

Main, M. (1991). Metacognitive knowledge, metacognitive monitoring, and singular (coherent) vs. multiple (incoherent) model of attachment. Findings and directions for future research. In C. M. Parkes, J. Stevenson-Hinde, & P. Marris (Eds.), *Attachment across the life cycle* (pp. 127–159). London/New York: Tavistock/Routledge.

Main, M., & Goldwyn, R. (1991). *Adult Attachment Classification System: Version 5.0.* Unpublished manuscript, University of California at Berkeley.

Main, M., & Goldwyn, R. (in press). Interview-based adult attachment classifications: Related to infant–mother and infant–father attachment. *Developmental Psychology.*

Main, M., & Hesse, E. (1990). Parents' unresolved traumatic experiences are related to infant disorganized attachment status: Is frightened and/or frightening parental behavior the linking mechanism? In M. T. Greenberg, D. Cicchetti, & E. M. Cummings (Eds.), *Attachment in the preschool years* (pp. 161–182). Chicago/London: University of Chicago Press.

Main, M., & Solomon, J. (1990). Procedures for identifying infants as disorganized/disoriented during the Ainsworth Strange Situation. In M. T. Greenberg, D. Cicchetti, & E. M. Cummings (Eds.), *Attachment in the preschool years* (pp. 121–160). Chicago/London: University of Chicago Press.

Main, M., van IJzendoorn, M. H., & Hesse, E. (1993, March). *Unresolved/Unclassifiable responses to the Adult Attachment Interview: Predictable from unresolved states and anomalous beliefs in the Berkeley–Leiden Adult Attachment Questionnaire (BLAAQ-U).* Paper presented at the biennial meeting of the Society for Research in Child Development, New Orleans.

Malinosky-Rummell, R., & Hansen, D. (1993). Long-term consequences of childhood physical abuse. *Psychological Bulletin, 114,* 68–79.

Maslin, C. A., & Bates, J. E. (1983, April). *Precursors of anxious and secure attachments: A multivariate model at age 6 months.* Paper presented at the biennial meeting of the Society for Research in Child Development, Detroit.

Miehls, D. A. (1989). *Marital attachment patterns and change in one's mental representations.* Unpublished dissertation, Smith College School for Social Work, London, Ontario, Canada.

Parker, G., Tupling, H., & Brown, L. B. (1979). A parental bonding instrument. *British Journal of Medical Psychology, 52,* 1–11.

Patrick, M., Hobson, R. P., Castle, P., Howard, R., & Maughan, B. (1992). *Personality disorder and the mental representation of early social experience.* Unpublished manuscript, Tavistock Institute, London.

Perris, C., Jacobsson, L., Lindström, H., von Knorring, L., & Perris, H. (1980). Development of a new inventory for assessing memories of parental rearing behaviour. *Acta Psychiatrica Scandinavica, 61,* 265–274.

Pfohl, B. (1989). *Structured Interview for the DSM-III-R Personality Disorders (SIDP-R).* Iowa City: University of Iowa Hospitals and Clinics.

Radojevic, M. (1992, July). *Predicting quality of infant attachment to father at 15 months from prenatal paternal representations of attachment: An Australian contribution.* Paper presented at the 25th International Congress of Psychology, Brussels.

Raven, J. C. (1958). *Standard progresssive matrices: Sets A, B, C, D, and E.* London: Lewis.

Rosenstein, D. S., & Horowitz, H. A. (1996). Adolescent attachment and psychopathology. *Journal of Consulting and Clinical Psychology, 64,* 244–253.

Rosenthal, R. (1991). *Meta-analytic procedures for social research.* Beverly Hills, CA: Sage.

Rutter, M., Quinton, D., & Hill, J. (1990). Adult outcome of institution-reared children: Males and females compared. In L. N. Robins & M. Rutter (Eds.), *Straight and devious pathways from childhood to adulthood* (pp. 135–157). Cambridge, England: Cambridge University Press.

Sagi, A., van IJzendoorn, M. H., Aviezer, O., Donnell, F., & Mayseless, O. (1994). Sleeping away from home in a kibbutz communal arrangement: It makes a difference for infant–mother attachment. *Child Development, 65,* 992–1004.

Sagi, A., van IJzendoorn, M. H., Scharf, M., Joëls, T., Koren-Karie, N., Mayseless, O., & Aviezer, O. (in press). Ecological constraints for intergenerational transmission of attachment: In search of determinants of transmission failures. *International Journal of Behavioural Development.*

Sagi, A., van IJzendoorn, M. H., Scharf, M., Koren-Karie, N., Joëls, T., & Mayseless, O. (1994). Stability and discriminant validity of the Adult Attachment Interview: A psychometric study in young Israeli adults. *Developmental Psychology, 30,* 988–1000.

Spangler, G., & Grossmann, K. E. (1994). Biobehavioral organization in securely and insecurely attached infants. *Child Development, 64,* 1439–1450.

Sroufe, L. A. (1978). Attachment and the roots of competence. *Human Nature, 1,* 50–57.

Sroufe, L. A. (1988). The role of infant–caregiver attachment in development. In J. Belsky & T. Nezworski (Eds.), *Clinical implications of attachment* (pp. 18–38). Hillsdale, NJ: Erlbaum.

Steele, H., & Steele, M. (1994). Intergenerational patterns of attachment. In D. Perlman & K. Bartholomew (Eds.), *Advances in personal relationships* (Vol. 5, pp. 93–120). London: Kingsley.

Steele, M., Steele, H., & Fonagy, P. (1993, March). *Associations among attachment classifications of mothers, fathers, and their infants: Evidence for a relationship-specific perspective.* Paper presented at the biennial meeting of the Society for Research in Child Development, New Orleans.

Suomi, S. J. (1995). Influence of attachment theory on ethological studies of biobehavioral development in nonhuman primates. In S. Goldberg, R. Muir, & J. Kerr (Eds.), *Attachment theory: Social, developmental, and clinical perspectives* (pp. 185–202). Hillsdale, NJ: Analytic Press.

van den Boom, D. C. (1988). *Neonatal irritability and the development of attachment: Observation and intervention.* Unpublished doctoral dissertation, Leiden University, Leiden, The Netherlands.

van IJzendoorn, M. H. (1995a). Adult attachment representations, parental responsiveness, and infant attachment: A meta-analysis on the predictive validity of the Adult Attachment Interview. *Psychological Bulletin, 117,* 387–403.

van IJzendoorn, M. H. (1995b). Of the way we are: On temperament, attachment, and the transmission gap: A rejoinder to Fox (1995). *Psychological Bulletin, 117,* 411–415.

van IJzendoorn, M. H. (1996). Continuity of attachment across the lifespan: Early prototypes or stable environments. Commentary to Mayseless (1996). *Human Development, 39,* 224–231.

van IJzendoorn, M. H., & Bakermans-Kranenburg, M. J. (1996). Attachment representations in mothers, fathers, adolescents, and clinical groups: A meta-analytic search for normative data. *Journal of Consulting and Clinical Psychology, 64,* 8–21.

van IJzendoorn, M. H., Feldbrugge, J. T. M., Derks, F., De Ruiter, C., Verhagen, M., Philipse, M., Van der Staak, C. P. F., & Riksen-Walraven, M. (in press). Attachment, representations of personality disordered criminal offenders. *American Journal of Orthopsychiatry.*

van IJzendoorn, M. H., Goldberg, S., Kroonenberg, P. M., & Frenkel, O. J. (1992). The relative effects of maternal and child problems on the quality of attachment: A meta-analysis of attachment in clinical samples. *Child Development, 63,* 840–858.

van IJzendoorn, M. H., Juffer, F., & Duyvesteyn, M. G. C. (1995). Breaking the intergenerational cycle of insecure attachment: A review of the effects of attachment-based interventions on maternal sensitivity and infant security from a contextual perspective. *Journal of Child Psychology and Psychiatry, 36,* 225–248.

van IJzendoorn, M. H., Kranenburg, M. J., Zwart-Woudstra, H. A., van Busschbach, A. M., & Lambermon, M. W. E. (1991). Parental attachment and children's socio-emotional development: Some findings on the validity of the Adult Attachment Interview in the Netherlands. *International Journal of Behavioral Development, 14,* 375–394.

Waddington, C. H. (1957). *The strategy of genes.* London: Allen & Unwin.

Ward, M. J., Botyanski, N. C., Plunket, S. W., & Carlson, E. A. (1991, April). *Concurrent validity of the AAI for adolescent mothers.* Paper presented at the biennial meeting of the Society for Research in Child Development, Seattle.

Ward, M. J., & Carlson, E. A. (1995). Associations among adult attachment representations, maternal sensitivity, and infant–mother attachment in a sample of adolescent mothers. *Child Development, 66,* 69–79.

Waters, E. (1978). The reliability and stability of individual differences in infant–mother attachment. *Child Development, 39,* 483–494.

Waters, E., Wippman, J., & Sroufe, L. A. (1979). Attachment, positive affect, and competence in the peer group: Two studies in construct validation. *Child Development, 50,* 821–829.

Waters, E., Merrick, S. K., Albersheim, L. J., & Treboux, D. (1995, March). *Attachment security from infancy to early adulthood: A 20-year longitudinal study.* Paper presented at the biennial meeting of the Society for Research in Child Development, Indianapolis.

Weissman, M., & Paykel, E. (1974). *The depressed woman: A study of social relationships.* Chicago: University of Chicago Press.

Zimmermann, P. (1994). *Bindung im Jugendalter: Entwicklung und Umgang mit aktuellen Anforderungen [Attachment in adolescence: Development and interaction with present circumstances].* Unpublished doctoral dissertation, University of Regensburg, Regensburg, Germany.

6

Attachment and Childhood Behavior Problems in Normal, At-Risk, and Clinical Samples

SUSAN GOLDBERG

The notion that early parent–child relationships play an important role in the etiology of psychopathology is not unique to attachment theory (Bowlby, 1969). However, the development of Ainsworth's Strange Situation procedure (Ainsworth, Blehar, Waters, & Wall, 1978) for assessing the quality of infant–adult relationships provided an important tool for empirical tests of this proposition and gave rise to a substantial body of research on this topic. More recently, the development of tools for assessing attachment in other age periods has further broadened the opportunities to establish links between psychopathology and childhood experiences of parental care. As we have gained the technology to provide clear empirical tests of the relation between early experiences with parents and later psychopathology, we have also become more sophisticated in understanding that developmental outcomes, including psychopathology, are complexly determined and an established link between parent–child relationships and psychopathology can only be one element in a complex process.

Parent–child relationships are not the only or even the most important determinant of childhood behavior problems. Furthermore, parental behavior itself is complexly determined. Demonstrated links between parent–child relationships and behavior disorders do not necessitate "blaming parents" but rather assume that each parent does the best job of childrearing that he or she can do under the circumstances of his or her life.

171

ATTACHMENT CLASSIFICATIONS AND MEASUREMENT

Most measures of attachment are based on Ainsworth's observations of infants in the Strange Situation, during which she observed three basic patterns: one considered secure and two considered *insecure*. The latter have been descriptively called *avoidance* and *resistance* in infancy. Each of these is considered to represent a primary strategy for maintaining the attention (and therefore protection) of the attachment figure.

Secure infants are confident of the availability of their attachment figure and explore freely in his or her presence. They may or may not be overtly distressed by separations but will limit exploration in the caregiver's absence. Upon return they are positive in their greeting, make contact if distressed, and are quickly able to return to exploration. In normative samples, 65% of infants show this pattern (van IJzendoorn & Kroonenberg, 1988).

Avoidant infants have learned that the attachment figure is unlikely to be available for comfort in time of need. To avoid potential rejection, they avoid expressing their attachment needs. Thus they appear precociously independent; though seemingly preoccupied with exploration, they explore less freely than do secure children. They rarely show overt distress at separations and at reunions they ignore or avoid the caregiver for prolonged periods. About 20% of infants in normative samples show this pattern (van IJzendoorn & Kroonenberg, 1988).

Resistant infants have learned that the attachment figure is unpredictable; attention can be ensured only with a great deal of effort on their part and their exploration is limited by preoccupation with the caregiver. They are extremely distressed by separations and often refuse to be comforted upon reunions. The resistant pattern occurs in 10% to 14% of infants in normative samples (van IJzendoorn & Kroonenberg, 1988). Because most studies encounter only a few resistant infants, we know little about their history and development. In a recent review, Cassidy and Berlin (1994) summarized what is known about this group of infants. They noted that a pattern of low maternal availability coupled with maternal interference with infant exploration characterized mother–infant dyads with resistant infants.

In spite of the labels "secure" and "insecure," the avoidant and resistant patterns are envisioned not as pathological forms of attachment but rather as variations within the normal range. I particularly like Crittenden's (1995, and Chapter 3, this volume) notion that avoidance reflects reliance on cognition rather than affect, whereas resistance reflects reliance on affect in preference to cognition. Secure individuals are those who achieve a balance in which cognition and affect have equal weight and credibility.

As attachment research expanded to include risk and clinical samples, other types of insecurity were identified (e.g., Crittenden, 1985; Radke-Yarrow, Cummings, Kuczynski, & Chapman, 1985). The most important of these for this chapter is what Main and Solomon (1986, 1990) identified as *disorganized/disoriented* (which I will call *disorganized* for convenience). Unlike avoidance and resistance, disorganization is characterized by absence of a coherent attachment strategy, accompanied by odd behaviors which make sense only if one can assume that the child is confused or fearful with respect to the caregiver. If a child is given a primary classification of disorganized, he or she is also assigned the best fitting alternative from among the other three (avoidant, secure, or resistant).

Because this pattern is frequent in maltreated samples (e.g., Lyons-Ruth, Connell, Grunebaum, & Botein, 1990; Carlson, Cicchetti, Barnett, & Braunwald, 1989) and has subsequently been found to occur with high frequency in some clinical samples (see van IJzendoorn, Goldberg, Kroonenberg, & Frenkel, 1992), it may be a more likely candidate for pathology per se than are other forms of insecurity. Nevertheless, because it is a recent discovery and is less clearly linked with home observations than the others, it is appropriate to be cautious about such an assumption.

With the exception of the disorganized classification, schemes for assessing attachment have been based on observations of normally developing children with low risk for psychopathology. One key question concerning attachment and psychopathology is whether these systems adequately capture variations in attachment seen in clinical samples.

Another direction of expansion in attachment research has been the development of assessment procedures and schemes for age groups beyond infancy. Two of these are relevant to this chapter. Several studies utilized the preschool system developed by Cassidy and Marvin (1992). It relies on observation of reunions in the Strange Situation (or modifications thereof) and retains the same basic four categories. The main changes are that resistance is now called "dependence" (but remains very similar in pattern), and the disorganized pattern gives way to several forms of "controlling" behavior (patterns in which the child seems to take charge of the relationship in inappropriate ways). Whereas they do not resemble the disorganized pattern of infancy, there may be brief flurries of disorganized activity and this pattern seems to be the developmental outcome of disorganization in infancy (Main, Kaplan, & Cassidy, 1985). There is also an "insecure–other" category which includes children who clearly are insecure but do not fit any of the other patterns. This group is often combined with the "controlling" group for analyses.

Main's Adult Attachment Interview (AAI; George, Kaplan, & Main, 1984) identifies the parental *state of mind* consistent with having an infant in each of the four major attachment patterns. Parents of avoidant infants are most often identified as *dismissing* of attachment (individuals who remember little of the emotional quality of their childhood or who idealize their experiences and assert that these experiences have not influenced them). Parents of resistant infants are likely to be *preoccupied* (heavily invested in continuing struggles with parents with little perspective of themselves or their parents independent of these conflicts). Parents of secure infants are most often judged *autonomous* (individuals who value intimacy, appreciate its effect on them, and have a realistic perspective of childhood experiences). Parents of disorganized infants often have experienced a traumatic loss with respect to attachment with which they have been unable to come to terms and are therefore considered *unresolved*. Like disorganized infants, adults who are unresolved are also assigned the best-fitting alternative from the other three.

ATTACHMENT AND PSYCHOPATHOLOGY: THE THEORY

An obvious suggestion about the relation between early attachment and later behavior problems is that children are more likely to develop behavior problems if they are insecurely attached to their primary caregiver than if they are securely attached. Several studies are concordant with this supposition (Erickson, Sroufe, & Egeland, 1985; Lewis, Feiring, McGuffog, & Jaskir, 1984; Renken, Egeland, Marvinney, Mangelsdorf, & Sroufe, 1989) although the data are by no means clear cut. At least two studies, one of them mine (Bates & Bayles, 1988; Goldberg, Lojkasek, Minde, & Corter, 1990), failed to find such associations. Furthermore, those that find such associations often find them with qualifications, for example, that the association holds only for boys (e.g., Renken et al., 1989).

However, as long as we constrain ourselves to focus on the secure–insecure dichotomy, a key aspect of attachment theory is ignored. Virtually all theories of child development predict that optimal conditions at an early age lead to better subsequent outcomes than do early nonoptimal conditions. Attachment theory offers a typology of nonoptimal early relationships and it seems logical to expect that these are associated with different outcomes. In particular, I want to address the question of whether there is any evidence that different kinds of childhood behavior problems are associated with different types of insecurity.

Theoretical reasoning (e.g., Cassidy & Kobak, 1988; Renken et al., 1989) links avoidant attachment with externalizing behavior problems, that is, those in which child behavior causes disruption and inconvenience for others (e.g., aggression, conduct disorder). It is argued that children engaged in an early avoidant relationship learn through the caregiver's lack of response to distress that "you cannot count on or trust others." They assume that others are uncaring and act accordingly, in a manner that may imitate or exaggerate the way they perceive themselves to have been treated. In addition, the frustration of unmet attachment needs gives rise to anger which is not expressed toward the caregiver, but is displaced toward others.

My initial reaction to this formulation was that it was counterintuitive. After all, is it not avoidant infants who learn to "cover up" their feelings and needs? Physiological recordings during the Strange Situation show that avoidant infants are just as aroused as are secure infants, although they appear unperturbed and rarely cry (Donovan & Leavitt, 1985; Spangler & Grossmann, 1994; Sroufe & Waters, 1977). Why would this not lead to "internalizing" problems, those in which the child experiences pain and misery but rarely disturbs others (e.g., depression, social withdrawal)? Such a script also is more consistent with the more recent observations that avoidance is associated with a style of emotional expression that inhibits or restrains emotions, particularly negative emotions (Berlin, 1993; Blokland, 1993; Cassidy, 1994).

Traditional theorizing links resistant (or dependent) attachment with internalizing disorders (e.g., Erickson et al., 1985; Renken et al., 1989). Because the caregiver responds inconsistently, the child becomes preoccupied with maintaining the caregiver's attention at the expense of exploring the larger world. Consequently, the child is fearful of undertaking new endeavors and remains isolated and withdrawn.

However, observations of resistant babies and dependent preschoolers in the Strange Situation with their pouty or frankly tantrumming behavior seem more obviously associated with externalizing problems. Recent studies also suggest that resistant or dependent individuals are characterized by a style of emotional expression that exaggerates feelings, particularly negative feelings, which might be more consistent with externalizing disorders (Berlin, 1993; Blokland, 1993). Of course, the bottom line is the empirical evidence.

ATTACHMENT AND PSYCHOPATHOLOGY: THE EVIDENCE

There are two basic strategies for testing the proposition that early parent–child relationships play a role in the etiology of psychopathology, and this chapter reviews examples of each type. The first is to follow individuals longitudinally from infancy. While this allows us to have direct measures of parent–child relationships (whether in Ainsworth's Strange Situation or in other observational settings), only a small number of clinical cases will emerge. The study of populations at high risk for psychopathology can increase substantially the size of the clinical group, but this remains a strategy which invests a great deal of time and energy (not to mention dollars) studying individuals who for the most part do *not* develop behavior disorders. It is possible that variations in problematic behavior within the normal range are not informative for understanding frank psychopathology. Existing studies of children fall almost exclusively into this category, and I currently am engaged in such a study (see Study 1, below).

An alternative strategy is to study concurrent parent–child relationships of children within clinical samples. This approach ensures a substantial number of clinical cases, but we cannot necessarily infer the nature of earlier parent–child relationships. First, presenting psychopathology can alter or obscure the underlying nature of attachments. Second, although there is some evidence for short-term stability of attachment in infancy (e.g., Waters, 1978) and from infancy to early school age (Main et al., 1985; Wartner, Grossmann, Femmer-Bombik, & Suess, 1994), data on stability from infancy to preschool are less consistent. In our own longitudinal study, less than 50% of children maintained the same attachment pattern from infancy through 4 years of age (Goldberg, Washington, Birenbaum, & Simmons, 1994). In a second study (Beckwith & Rodning, 1991), 42% of children were stable from infancy to preschool. There are few published studies of concurrent attachment in clinical samples.

Longitudinal Studies

In this approach, a psychiatric diagnosis is rarely, if ever, the outcome variable. Because the majority of children in these studies are well adjusted, it is not cost effective to conduct a psychiatric assessment of each child. Investigators generally rely on standardized instruments for parent and teacher reports of behavior problems.

Previous longitudinal studies paint an equivocal picture of the relation between infant attachment and later behavior problems: several studies have found that secure infants fare better during preschool and early school age than do insecurely attached peers (Erickson et al., 1985; Lewis et al., 1984; Renken et al., 1989), but others failed to find such connections (Bates, Maslin, & Frankel, 1985; Goldberg et al., 1990). In most studies, however, the number of resistant infants was small and they were either dropped from the analysis or avoidant/resistant comparisons were not pursued. Thus, it is possible that reported secure/insecure differences really are accounted for by avoidance rather than by insecurity per se. Indeed, links between resistance and internalizing problems have been reported in only one study (Lewis et al., 1984). This absence of effects may reflect both the rarity of resistant attachment and the relative invisibility of internalizing disorders in children.

Predicted links between avoidance and externalizing problems have indeed been found (Erickson et al., 1985; Lewis et al., 1984; Renken et al., 1989). Most recently, Lyons-Ruth, Alpern, and Repacholi (1993) found that infant disorganized attachment was the best predictor of teacher ratings of hostile behavior in 5-year-olds. However, a high percentage of this group were also considered to have an underlying avoidant strategy.

Study I: Health and Illness

Since 1984 we have been conducting a prospective longitudinal study based on the premise that children with chronic medical conditions are more likely to develop behavior disorders than are their healthy peers. An epidemiological study of 4- to 16-year-olds in Ontario confirmed this, showing that children with a physical problem were 2.4 times as likely as healthy peers to have a diagnosable psychiatric disorder (Cadman, Boyle, Szatmari, & Offord, 1987). Furthermore, meta-analysis of in-depth studies of adjustment in children with chronic medical conditions suggests that these groups are particularly likely to have internalizing disorders (Lavigne & Faier-Routman, 1992). Because internalizing disorders rarely are detected in young children, pediatric samples may provide us with a unique opportunity to examine precursors of internalizing disorders. Our study included two such pediatric groups: children diagnosed in infancy with either cystic fibrosis or congenital heart disease. These medical groups were selected because they represent chronic health conditions with different natural histories.

Cystic fibrosis is a genetic disease characterized by excessive mucous secretions that interfere with many bodily functions, particularly digestion and respiration. Parents can be responsible for several hours of daily therapeutic treatments, including administration of enzymes and high caloric intake to ensure adequate nutrition, as well as inhalation masks and physiotherapy to keep the airways clear. With regular aggressive treatment young children with cystic fibrosis maintain good health, but the disease is progressive and life expectancy is shortened.

Congenital heart disease covers many different diagnoses. Our study included children with the four most common conditions with good prognosis (ventricular septal defect, tetralogy of Fallot, coarctation of the aorta, and transposition of the great arteries). All conditions were self-correcting or surgically correctible and most infants' hearts had been surgically corrected when they entered the study. Other than careful monitoring and some administration of medications, parents do not have daily therapeutic responsibilities. These children were expected to be on an improving course of health. We recruited also a comparison group of healthy infants (see Goldberg, Gotowiec, & Simmons, 1995, for details).

As part of the larger longitudinal study, each infant participated with his or her mother in a Strange Situation at 12 to 18 months of age and both parents completed the Child Behavior Checklist (CBCL; Achenbach, 1992) when their child was 2, 3, 4, and 7 years of age. The CBCL yields three summary scores for Total, Internalizing, and Externalizing problems. Because the predictions regarding different types of attachment focus on the internalizing/externalizing dichotomy, these three scores were the focus of analysis.

This section reports CBCL data linking early attachment and behavior problems at age 4. In most cases, it is similar to the published 2- to 3-year data (Goldberg et al., 1995). (The 7-year data are still incomplete.) The 4-year sample includes 40 healthy children, 43 with cystic fibrosis, and 43 with congenital heart disease. Mother and father reports on the CBCL were highly correlated (r's = .51–.67) and for purposes of analysis we averaged mother and father scores on each of the main CBCL scales: Total, Internalizing, and Externalizing.

First, there were differences in infant attachment between the three groups. The medically diagnosed groups include fewer children who were secure as infants and more who showed disorganized attachment than was the case in the healthy group (Figure 6.1), $\chi^2(6) = 15.26$, $p < .01$. This difference reflected primarily differences between the healthy group and each of the diagnosed groups, which did not differ from each other.

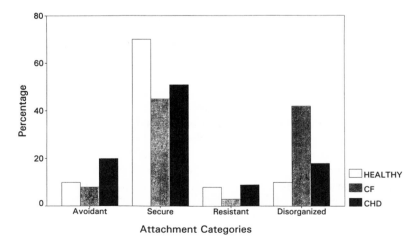

FIGURE 6.1. Distribution of infant attachment patterns by diagnostic group. CF, cystic fibrosis; CHD, congenital heart disease.

Furthermore, attachment was not related to family demographics or to child gender.

At age 4 years, average Total scores on the CBCL for each of the three groups were well within normal range, but the healthy children had the lowest scores, followed by the cystic fibrosis and then the congenital heart disease groups (Figure 6.2). These differences were not significant. In the sample as a whole, 32 children scored above the clinical cutoff on the CBCL by mother or father report (17% of the healthy group and 16% of the medically diagnosed groups).

A two-way analysis of variance (ANOVA) with attachment and diagnostic group as the factors yielded a main effect of attachment (Figure 6.3), $F(3, 114) = 4.11$, $p < .01$, only for Internalizing scores, for which there also was a marginally significant interaction, $F(6, 114) = 1.96$, $p < .07$. Because there was no main effect of diagnostic group and minimal evidence of attachment × medical group interactions, we collapsed across diagnostic groups for further analyses.

To test the specific prediction that those who were secure as infants should have fewer reported problems than those who were insecure, I conducted planned contrasts (B vs. ACD) for Total, Internalizing, and Externalizing CBCL scores. We also contrasted secure and avoidant infants (B vs. A) to test the possibility that avoidance, rather than insecurity, is the influential aspect of attachment. For Total scores, the secure–insecure contrast (B vs. ACD) was not significant, but the secure–avoidant contrast

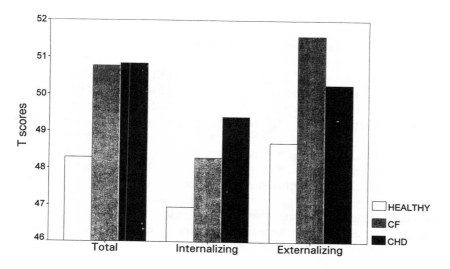

FIGURE 6.2. CBCL scores by diagnostic group. CF, cystic fibrosis; CHD, congenital heart disease.

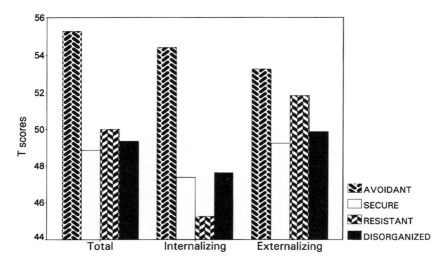

FIGURE 6.3. CBCL scores by infant attachment group.

was: $t(63) = 2.74$, $p < .01$. For Internalizing scores, the same pattern emerged: the secure–insecure contrast was not significant but the secure–avoidant contrast was: $t(50) = 2.74$, $p < .01$. There was a similar pattern for Externalizing scores: B versus ACD, ns; A versus B, $t(62) = 1.92$, $p < .06$. When we group these same children by (concurrent) attachment at 4 years of age, there are no statistically significant differences related to attachment status.

Thus, unlike most of the previous studies, our data show a link between avoidance and reports of internalizing problems rather than reports of externalizing problems. This may reflect the fact that we have a population that is biased toward internalizing problems. However, this pattern was evident in the healthy group as well as the two medically diagnosed groups.

To further examine this and to see what we could learn about predicted differences between children who had been avoidant and resistant as infants, we compared these groups directly, thus controlling for effects of security. Here our numbers are relatively small, so rather than use standard statistical techniques, we looked for consistency of patterns. We did this by conducting a mini-meta-analysis of our own data. Each diagnostic group in the study was considered a "replication" for which A–C difference effect sizes were calculated for averaged mother and father Internalizing and Externalizing scores.

On the Internalizing scale, the avoidant group consistently scored higher than did the resistant group. Effect sizes ranged from 0.33 to 1.44

(moderate to large; Cohen, 1992). When Rosenthal's method (Rosenthal, 1991) was used to combine the associated t values weighted by sample size, this was a highly significant effect, $z = 1.66$, $p < .005$ (two-tailed). For Externalizing scores, the avoidant group again scored higher than did the resistant group. Effect sizes ranged from 0.18 to 0.93 (small to large; Cohen, 1992) and the combined weighted t values indicated an effect of marginal significance, $z = 1.66$, $p < .10$ (two-tailed).

These data suggest that it is avoidance in infancy that is related to *both* internalizing and externalizing problems in childhood. Many researchers find high correlations and overlap between the Internalizing and Externalizing scales of the CBCL (Achenbach, 1991; $r = .59$; our study, $r = .60$). Thus, the problem in distinguishing internalizing and externalizing disorders may be a measurement problem. On the other hand, this overlap may also reflect reality; it is not uncommon for children to display both internalizing and externalizing symptoms. In the Ontario Child Health Study (Offord, Boyle, Fleming, Monroe-Blum, & Rae-Grant, 1989), 68% of children identified as having one psychiatric disorder met diagnostic criteria for at least one other disorder. Furthermore, some comorbid disorders "crossed" the internalizing–externalizing boundary. For example, one-third of children with conduct disorder also met criteria for emotional disorder and one-fourth of the conduct-disordered group also had a somaticizing disorder. Thus, while this is a conceptually appealing dichotomy, it is a difficult distinction to make in practice.

Another testable hypothesis about different kinds of insecure attachment is that early disorganized attachment places children at greater risk for subsequent psychopathology than does other forms of insecurity. To test this, we compared the disorganized group with the combined other insecure group (D vs. AC), again using the effect size strategy for Total CBCL scores. The disorganized group generally obtained lower scores than did the combined avoidant and resistant groups. Thus, there is no evidence that disorganization per se constitutes a special risk for psychopathology in our population. However, this also may reflect a sample bias. Lyons-Ruth et al. (1993) found disorganization highly predictive of hostile behavior in preschoolers, an externalizing problem. Because our sample was one predisposed to internalizing problems, there may not have been enough extreme Externalizing scores to reveal such an effect.

Cross-Sectional Studies

Previous cross-sectional studies of attachment in children with psychiatric diagnoses come from Greenberg and Speltz, who conducted two studies of children with externalizing disorders (Greenberg, DeKlyen, Speltz, & Endriga, Chapter 7, this volume; Greenberg, Speltz, DeKlyen, & Endriga, 1991; Speltz, Greenberg, & DeKlyen, 1990). The main finding from these studies was that a large majority of preschoolers with externalizing disorders were concurrently insecurely attached and a substantial majority of the insecure group showed a specific form of insecure attachment: controlling.

The following studies were conducted recently in Toronto. All have been or will be published independently, so they are presented here in brief form. The main purpose of reviewing them is to make comparisons across samples to see whether this informs us about links between specific attachment patterns and disorders. The populations can be grouped into three categories: "normal," "at risk," and "diagnosed with a disorder."

Study 2: Romanian Adoptees

The second study conducted in our laboratory included 56 children adopted into Canada from Romania, 19 with prolonged experiences of deprivation in institutional settings (institution group) and 37 being adopted directly from deprived homes or institutions in the first few months of life (home group). In this study attachment was assessed in the preschool years (ages 2 through 6 years). Because they had not had an opportunity for normal attachment-related experiences in infancy and because they had made a major adjustment to a change of home, it was predicted that many adoptees would not only be insecurely attached, but also would show unusual attachment patterns. An important question is whether these children retain the ability to form satisfactory attachments after early depriving experiences. Without knowing how long it should take a child to form a relationship with an adopting family, we arbitrarily decided not to assess attachment in any child until he or she had been with the adopting family for at least 6 months. Most had been with their families for considerably longer when we saw them. The range of time with adopted family ranged from 6 months to over 4 years.

The resulting distribution of attachment patterns (Figure 6.4) was unusual. As a convenient, potentially normative comparison sample, the figure includes attachment at 4 years of age for the healthy group from the previous study. This group of families was similar to adopting families in socioeconomic status, but parents were younger (mean age of the comparison mothers was 31.0 vs. 38.9 years in adopting families; fathers, 33.1 vs. 40.2 years). As far as we know, the effect of parent age on attachment has not been widely studied. However, this discrepancy between the two groups suggests caution in interpreting differences. The most striking feature of the distribution of attachment patterns was that not one adoptee was considered to be avoidant, which is the most common form of insecure

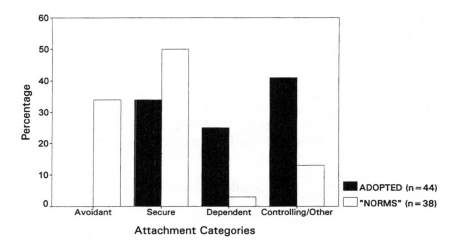

FIGURE 6.4. Distribution of preschool attachment patterns for adoptees and comparison ("norms") group.

attachment in normative samples. The proportion of controlling and insecure–other cases also is elevated relative to the comparison group, $\chi^2(3)$ = 28.9, $p < .00001$. There were no differences between home and institution groups.

We have considered several reasons for the absence of avoidant attachment:

1. In the deprived backgrounds of these children avoidance would not have been an adaptive strategy. Indeed, it is possible that children who did adopt such a strategy did not survive in severely depriving environments. Alternatively, because care was inconsistent children could quickly have become preoccupied with maintaining adult attention.
2. Parents who choose to adopt, particularly to adopt children at risk because of depriving environments, are unlikely to be sufficiently rejecting to raise avoidant children.
3. The formation of emotional bonds is a normal preoccupation in adopting families, so that avoidant attachment is unlikely.
4. The adopted child might also recognize avoidance as a relatively risky strategy in forming an alliance with new adoptive parents.

The lack of differences between home and institution groups is surprising. A possible explanation is suggested by a separate pilot study which included true controls for 18 of the present adoptees, case-matched for age, gender, and attachment classification (Sabbagh, 1994). In this study, some of the adoptees otherwise classified as securely attached showed inappropriate social behavior toward the stranger. These behaviors were consistent with earlier anecdotal reports of indiscriminately friendly behavior toward strangers on the part of institutionalized children. This is one example in which the classification system developed with a normative group may not capture salient aspects of attachment-related behavior in atypical groups. Home–institution comparisons may be confounded by the classification of "false secures" (see also Rutter, Chapter 2, this volume).

However, in this sample, children who were secure had lower CBCL scores than those who were insecure, and disorganized/controlling attachment accounted for much of this effect; children who were in the controlling group were 2.2 times more likely than those who were secure to score above the clinical cutoff. Furthermore, 7 out of 10 children who scored above the clinical cutoff on the CBCL were in this attachment group.

Study 3: Children of Mothers with Anxiety Disorders

So far, we have considered two risks for disrupting attachment and increasing risk for behavior problems: poor health and deprivation of early attachment experiences. The third risk we consider is that of having a parent with a psychiatric disorder. Manassis, Bradley, Goldberg, Hood, and Swinson (1994) studied a small group of $1\frac{1}{2}$- to 5-year-olds ($N = 20$) being raised by mothers diagnosed with an anxiety disorder ($N = 18$).

In this sample, AAIs with the mothers showed them to be uniformly insecurely attached, with unresolved (the adult analogue of disorganized) the predominant classification ($N = 14$). However, for seven of these mothers, the alternative classification was secure. The distribution of attachment for the children also was unusual (Figure 6.5). As predicted from maternal attachment, the children were classified predominantly as disorganized or controlling. Four, however, were judged as securely attached. Mothers of securely attached children reported fewer recent stressful life events, fewer depressive symptoms, and a greater sense of competence than did mothers of insecurely attached children. Three of the children met DSM-III-R (American Psychiatric Association, 1987) criteria for anxiety disorders: all were insecurely attached (one avoidant and two disorganized). All had mothers with "unresolved" attachment classifications.

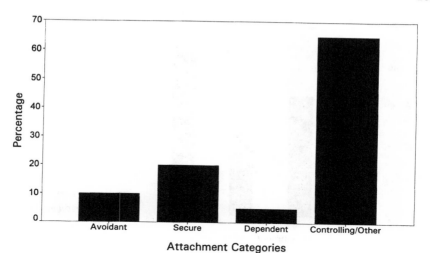

FIGURE 6.5. Distribution of attachment patterns for children of anxiety-disordered mothers (N = 20).

Study 4: Infants Referred to Clinic Services

It is rare that children under 3 years old are diagnosed with a psychiatric disorder. In fact, various editions of the *Diagnostic and Statistical Manual of Mental Disorders* provide very few diagnoses applicable to children this young. However, mental health interventions focus increasingly on the early years. Targeted populations include those at high risk as well as those whom parents, physicians, or daycare providers judge to require attention. The C. M. Hincks Treatment Centre in Toronto runs an intervention program for infants and parents called Watch, Wait and Wonder (Cohen, Lojkasek, & Muir, 1996). The intervention encourages the parent to observe the infant and to be responsive rather than initiating. The parent's experience in these sessions is discussed with a therapist/observer. Because the intervention focuses on the parent–child relationship, it seems reasonable that one aspect of evaluating its efficacy would be to see whether it results in changed attachments. An ongoing study of this type is being conducted; thus far, only the preintervention data have been examined. A comparison group of 41 infants was recruited through newspaper advertisements for this particular project (Lojkasek, 1995). Figure 6.6 shows the preintervention attachment distributions for the clinic and comparison groups. They are remarkably similar and unlike the normative distributions in much of the infancy literature. Once again, there is a paucity of avoidant attachments and a plethora of disorganized ones.

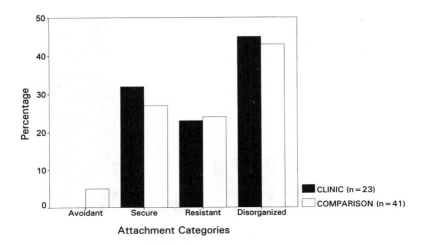

FIGURE 6.6. Distribution of attachment patterns, Watch, Wait and Wonder clinic and comparison group.

Although subjects in the comparison group were not judged to have obvious behavioral problems on assessment, they are more like the clinic sample in distribution of attachment patterns than like other normative infant samples. These data raise an interesting question as to what is a "normal" sample and how to find it. It may be that because it was based in a treatment center this study attracted mothers with concerns about their infants to participate, in search of help or reassurance. The "dismissing" mothers likely to have avoidant infants may be unlikely to express needs for help in such circumstances.

Study 5: Boys with Gender Identity Disorder

The last study (Birkenfeld-Adams, 1996) includes two groups of clearly diagnosed boys: one with gender identity disorder (gender identity group; N = 22) and a clinic comparison group that includes a mixture of diagnoses (other clinic group; N = 12). In addition, the investigators recruited a volunteer group of "normal" controls (N = 20). On screening with the CBCL, 7 children in the normal group were found to score above the clinical cutoff on the CBCL. Therefore, the controls appear in two configurations: Normal 1 is the full group; Normal 2 is the group with the high-CBCL-scoring cases deleted.

Figure 6.7 shows that the clinic groups (gender identity and other clinic) are less likely to be securely attached than are the normals. There also are differences between the gender identity group and the other clinic group; subjects in the gender identity group are more likely to be classified as having dependent attachments than are the other clinic subjects, a group which is notable for its absence of dependent attachments. The gender identity group is equally distributed across avoidant, secure, and dependent categories, whereas the other clinic group is predominantly avoidant and controlling. Comparison of the two normal groups shows that removal of children with high CBCL scores creates a shift in the direction predicted by attachment theory: Normal 2 has more secure and fewer avoidant attachment subjects than does Normal 1.

Comparisons across Samples

Four tables (Tables 6.1–6.4) summarize data from all samples discussed thus far. These are, admittedly, crude comparisons. Some of these groups are small and reporting data in percentages to make these comparisons is questionable. However, data on attachment in clinically diagnosed children as well as these risk groups are rare, so this is primarily a hypothesis-generating exercise. As a way of quantifying the observed patterns, I assumed that the expected ordering for any type of insecure attachment is that it will be lowest in the normative groups and highest in the diagnosed groups (with risk groups in the middle); I computed rank order correlations

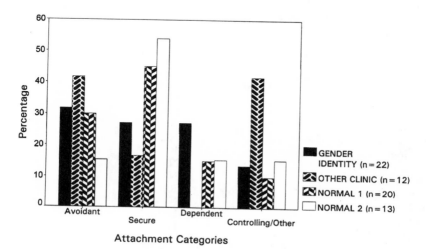

FIGURE 6.7. Distribution of attachment patterns for gender identity disorder study.

between the predicted and observed ordering of groups. For these analyses, only the Normal 1 group in the gender identity study was included.

When groups are ordered by the percent of insecurity in the sample (Table 6.1), they generally show the assumed ordering, Spearman $\rho = .69$, $p < .05$. A notable exception in the ordering is that children of anxious mothers rank close to the top, higher than expected.

When groups are ordered by percent of avoidance (Table 6.2), the relationship between risk status and avoidance is not significant, $\rho = .22$. Some diagnosed and risk groups are particularly low on avoidance, ranking below the normative samples. Others, particularly the two clearly diagnosed groups (the gender identity group and their psychiatric [other clinic] controls), rank very highly, as expected.

TABLE 6.1. Percent Insecure across Samples

Group[a]	Status[b]	% insecure
Healthy infants	N	33
GID normal controls 2	N	46
Chronically ill infants	R	48
GID normal controls 1	N	55
Adoptees	R	61
WWW comparison infants	N	67
WWW clinic infants	D	68
GID	D	73
Children of anxious mothers	R	80
GID psychiatric controls	D	83

[a]GID, gender identity disorder; WWW, Watch, Wait and Wonder.

[b]N, normative; R, risk; D, diagnosed.

TABLE 6.2. Percent Avoidant across Samples

Group[a]	Status[b]	% avoidant
Adoptees	R	0
WWW clinic infants	D	0
WWW comparison infants	N	5
Children of anxious mothers	R	10
Healthy infants	N	12
GID normal controls 2	N	15
Chronically ill infants	R	21
GID normal controls 1	N	30
GID	D	32
GID psychiatric controls	D	41

[a]GID, gender identity disorder; WWW, Watch, Wait and Wonder.

[b]N, normative; R, risk; D, diagnosed.

When groups are ordered by percent of resistance/dependence (Table 6.3), there is no relation between risk status and resistance/dependence, $\rho = .03$. The normative groups cluster in the middle, at the level consistent with published norms. The two clearly diagnosed groups are at opposite ends of the continuum, the gender identity group being highest and the psychiatric controls lowest. Risk groups are relatively dispersed.

Finally, we examine the percent of disorganized/controlling or insecure–other attachment across groups. In Table 6.4, risk status and attachment are again related, $\rho = .62$, $p < .05$. Most of the normative groups fall within the 10% to 15% range that Main and Solomon (1986) suggested as the expected range for normative data when they first described disorganized attachment in infancy. Most of the risk and clinic groups

TABLE 6.3. Percent Dependent/Resistant across Samples

Group[a]	Status[b]	% dependent/resistant
GID psychiatric controls	D	0
Children of anxious mothers	R	5
Chronically ill infants	R	8
Healthy infants	N	10
GID normal controls 2	N	15
GID normal controls 1	N	15
WWW clinic infants	D	23
WWW comparison infants	N	24
Adoptees	R	24
GID	D	27

[a]GID, gender identity disorder; WWW, Watch, Wait and Wonder.
[b]N, normative; R, risk; D, diagnosed.

TABLE 6.4. Percent Disorganized/Controlling/Insecure–Other across Samples

Group[a]	Status[b]	% disorganized
GID normal controls 1	N	10
Healthy infants	N	12
GID	D	13
GID normal controls 2	N	15
Chronically ill infants	R	29
Adoptees	R	40
WWW comparison infants	N	41
GID psychiatric controls	D	41
WWW clinic infants	D	45
Children of anxious mothers	R	65

[a]GID, gender identity disorder; WWW, Watch, Wait and Wonder.
[b]N, normative; R, risk; D, diagnosed.

exceed this. The gender identity group is a notable exception here, ranking lower than expected, whereas children of anxious mothers rank higher than expected.

IMPLICATIONS AND FUTURE DIRECTIONS

What can we conclude from these comparisons? First, they reinforce the notion that as we move along a continuum of risk to clear diagnosis, the likelihood of secure attachment decreases and the likelihood of disorganized, controlling, and insecure–other attachment increases. Because these are normally rare patterns and, in the case of the disorganized and insecure–other categories, not clearly defined strategies, this is consistent with the notion that clinic samples include attachment patterns that fall outside of the established schemes. Further differentiation within these categories based on clinic samples may prove to be more useful than are the normatively derived classification schemes in linking attachment and psychopathology.

The fact that avoidance and resistance were not related to risk or clinical status is consistent with this suggestion. However, this does not preclude the possibility that avoidant or resistant/dependent attachment styles may be linked to the etiology of specific disorders. Among the groups available, distinctions between internalizing and externalizing problems are difficult to make. For example, the psychiatric controls in the gender identity study included a mixture of diagnoses; the Watch, Wait and Wonder group often had feeding or sleeping problems which belong to neither category. Examination of well-defined clinic groups may allow clear tests of predictions linking avoidant and resistant attachment with specific disorders. Meanwhile, the observation that a particular form of insecurity is extremely low or absent in a diagnosed group may indicate that a particular attachment strategy, even an insecure one, serves as a protection against particular behavior disorders. For example, Adam, Sheldon-Keller, and West (1995) concluded that avoidant attachment served a protective function for suicide in adolescents. Thus, while we generally think of secure attachment as protective, forms of insecure attachment also are protective. This is consistent with the underlying assumption of attachment theory that patterns of attachment *are* adaptations to the child's caregiving environment.

Do these findings tell us about early attachment as a possible influence in the emergence of behavior problems? In all of the diagnosed groups, attachment was assessed concurrently. In our own longitudinal sample, we found that concurrent attachment and behavior problems at 4 years of age were not related, while infant attachment predicted some aspects of behavior problem reports at age 4. In addition, attachment from infancy to age 4 was less stable than expected. This should make us wary about making inferences about the contribution of early attachment to later behavior disorders from concurrent data. We also must consider that when we look at concurrent attachment in psychiatric samples we may be examining the effects of disorder on attachment rather than the other way round.

What information could help us disentangle cause and effect in these kinds of data sets? Data on stability of attachment from infancy through childhood is clearly relevant. Do children who receive high scores on behavior problem checklists have more or less stable attachments than those who receive low scores? Or are they no different from other children in stability of attachment? On the assumption that behavior problems may influence attachment as well as distort its measurement, I would guess that these children are less stable, but if in fact they were shown to be relatively stable in attachment history, this would enhance our confidence in extrapolating infant attachment from concurrent measures in clinic samples.

Could parental attachment status be an alternative marker of early childhood attachment in clinical samples? The AAI was designed primarily to identify parents who form specific types of relationships with infants. Adult attachment has shown good short-term stability but we do not know whether this stability extends from offspring's infancy into the preschool years. However, suppose we found that concurrent attachment of children with behavior disorders was significantly less concordant with that of the parent than is true in normative samples. This would lend credibility to the notion that children's concurrent attachment in clinic samples is not a good marker of earlier attachment and is more likely a feature or consequence of disorder. At the same time, it encourages us to consider the parent's attachment status as a plausible marker of the earlier experience, particularly if accompanied by evidence of stability of AAI classifications over an extended period of the offspring's childhood.

Pre- and posttreatment assessment of attachment in clinic samples, particularly those in which treatment targets parent–child relationships, also could provide evidence for the direction of effects in linking attachment and behavior disorders. One reason for the lack of attachment data in clinic samples is that our current assessment procedures are not cost effective in clinical settings. They remain expensive and time consuming, though powerful laboratory procedures. Berger (1994) is currently developing methods by which observations at a well-baby examination could be used to classify early attachment. Perhaps at some time in the future we will be able to go back to infant health records for our clinic samples to find a record of early attachment!

It would be remiss to leave the impression that all the work in this

enterprise needs to be done in expanding and improving our understanding and database regarding attachment. Although childhood
behavior disorders have received increasing attention in each revision
of the *Diagnostic and Statistical Manual of Mental Disorders,* the fact
remains that childhood behavior disorders have not been well defined
in diagnostic manuals. As a nonclinician, I have relied heavily on
standardized parent and teacher reports and the traditional distinction
between internalizing and externalizing disorders. High correlations
between the Internalizing and Externalizing scales of the CBCL and
research on comorbidity (as discussed earlier) suggest that this may not
be the most useful way of conceptualizing childhood disorders for the
questions we are asking. Attempts to link attachment and childhood
behavior disorders will benefit as much from advances in diagnosing
and conceptualizing behavior disorders as they will from advances in
attachment research per se.

REFERENCES

Achenbach, T. M. (1991). *Manual for the Child Behavior Checklist/4–18 and
    1991 profile.* Burlington: University of Vermont.
Achenbach, T. M. (1992). *Manual for the Child Behavior Checklist/2–3.*
    Burlington: University of Vermont.
Adam, K., Sheldon-Keller, A., & West, M. (1995). Attachment organization and
    vulnerability to loss, separation, and abuse in disturbed adolescents. In S.
    Goldberg, R. Muir, & J. Kerr (Eds.), *Attachment theory: Social, developmen-
    tal and clinical perspectives* (pp. 309–342). Hillsdale, NJ: Analytic Press.
Ainsworth, M. D. S., Blehar, M., Waters, E., & Wall, S. (1978). *Patterns of
    attachment.* Hillsdale, NJ: Erlbaum.
American Psychiatric Association. (1987). *Diagnostic and statistical manual of
    mental disorders* (3rd ed., rev.). Washington, DC: Author.
Bates, J. E., & Bayles, K. (1988). Attachment and the development of behavior
    problems. In J. Belsky & T. Nezworski (Eds.), *Clinical implications of
    attachment* (pp. 253–300). Hillsdale, NJ: Erlbaum.
Bates, J. E., Maslin, C. A., & Frankel, K. A. (1985). Attachment security and
    mother–child interaction and temperament as predictors of behavior problem
    ratings at age three years. In I. Bretherton & E. Waters (Eds.), Growing points
    of attachment theory and research. *Monographs of the Society for Research
    in Child Development, 50*(1–2, Serial No. 209), 167–193.
Beckwith, L., & Rodning, C. (1991, April). *Stability in attachment classification
    from 13 to 36 months.* Paper presented at the meeting of the Society for
    Research in Child Development, Seattle, WA.
Berger, S. (1994, September). *Applying an attachment framework to psychosocial
    screening of infants in primary care pediatrics.* Paper presented at the meeting
    of the Society for Behavioral Pediatrics, Minneapolis, MN.

Berlin, L. (1993, March). *Attachment and emotions in preschool children.* Paper presented at the meeting of the Society for Research in Child Development, New Orleans, LA.

Birkenfeld-Adams, A. (1996). *Quality of attachment in young boys with gender identity disorder.* Doctoral dissertation in progress, York University, Downsview, Ontario, Canada.

Blokland, K. (1993). *Infant attachment and emotional expression in 3-year-olds.* Unpublished master's thesis, University of Toronto.

Bowlby, J. (1969). *Attachment and loss: Vol. 1. Attachment.* New York: Basic Books.

Cadman, D., Boyle, M., Szatmari, P., & Offord, D. R. (1987). Chronic illness, disability, and mental and social well-being: Findings of the Ontario Child Health Study. *Pediatrics, 79,* 805–813.

Carlson, V., Cicchetti, D., Barnett, D., & Braunwald, K. (1989). Disorganized/disoriented attachment relationships in maltreated infants. *Developmental Psychology, 25,* 525–531.

Cassidy, J. (1994). Emotion regulation: Influences of attachment relationships. In N. Fox (Ed.), The development of emotion regulation: Biological and behavioral considerations. *Monographs of the Society for Research in Child Development, 59*(1–2, Serial No. 240), 228–249.

Cassidy, J., & Berlin, L. (1994). The insecure/ambivalent pattern of attachment: Theory and research. *Child Development, 65,* 971–991.

Cassidy, J., & Kobak, R. R. (1988). Avoidance and its relevance to other defensive processes. In J. Belsky & T. Nezworski (Eds.), *Clinical implications of attachment* (pp. 300–326). Hillsdale, NJ: Erlbaum.

Cassidy, J., & Marvin, R. S., with the Attachment Working Group of the MacArthur Network on the Transition from Infancy to Early Childhood. (1992). *Attachment organization in three- and four-year-olds: Coding guidelines.* Unpublished manual, University of Virginia at Charlottesville.

Cohen, J. (1992). A power primer. *Psychological Bulletin, 112,* 155–159.

Cohen, N. J., Lojkasek, M., & Muir, E. (1996, April). *Outcome of two interventions for troubled infant–mother relationships.* Paper presented at the International Conference of Infant Studies, Providence, RI.

Crittenden, P. M. (1985). Social networks, quality of parenting, and child development. *Child Development, 56,* 85–96.

Crittenden, P. M. (1995). Attachment and psychopathology. In S. Goldberg, R. Muir, & J. Kerr (Eds.), *Attachment theory: Social, developmental and clinical perspectives* (pp. 363–406). Hillsdale, NJ: Analytic Press.

Donovan, W., & Leavitt, L. (1985). Physiologic assessment of mother–infant attachment. *Journal of the American Academy of Child Psychiatry, 24,* 65–70.

Erickson, M. F., Sroufe, L. A., & Egeland, B. (1985). The relationship between quality of attachment and behavior problems in a preschool high-risk sample. In I. Bretherton & E. Waters (Eds.), Growing points of attachment theory and research. *Monographs of the Society for Research in Child Development, 50*(1–2, Serial No. 209), 147–166.

George, C., Kaplan, N., & Main, M. (1984). *Attachment interview for adults.* Unpublished manuscript, University of California at Berkeley.

Goldberg, S., Gotowiec, A., & Simmons, R. J. (1995). Infant–mother attachment and behavior problems in healthy and chronically ill preschoolers. *Development and Psychopathology, 7,* 267–282.

Goldberg, S., Lojkasek, M., Minde, K., & Corter, C. (1990). Predictions of behavior problems in 4-year-olds born prematurely. *Development and Psychopathology, 2,* 15–30.

Goldberg, S., Washington, J., Birenbaum, A., & Simmons, R. J. (1994, July). *Attachment in health and illness: Infancy to preschool.* Paper presented at the Symposium on Attachment in the preschool years, International Society for the Study of Behavioral Development, Amsterdam.

Greenberg, M. T., Speltz, M. L., DeKlyen, M. C., & Endriga, M. C. (1991). Attachment security in preschoolers with and without externalizing problems: A replication. *Development and Psychopathology, 3,* 413–430.

Lavigne, J., & Faier-Routman, J. (1992). Psychological adjustment to pediatric physical disorders. *Journal of Pediatric Psychology, 17,* 133–158.

Lewis, M., Feiring, C., McGuffog, C., & Jaskir, J. (1984). Predicting psychopathology in six-year-olds from early social relations. *Child Development, 55,* 123–136.

Lojkasek, M. (1995). *Characteristics of the primary attachment relationship of clinic infants and their mothers.* Unpublished doctoral dissertation, York University, Downsview, Ontario, Canada.

Lyons-Ruth, K., Alpern, L., & Repacholi, B. (1993). Disorganized infant attachment classification and maternal psychological problems as predictors of hostile–aggressive behavior in the preschool classroom. *Child Development, 64,* 572–585.

Lyons-Ruth, K., Connell, D., Grunebaum, H., & Botein, S. (1990). Infants at social risk: Maternal depression and family support services as mediators of infants' development and security of attachment. *Child Development, 61,* 85–98.

Main, M., Kaplan, N., & Cassidy, J. (1985). Security in infancy, childhood and adulthood: A move to the level of representation. In I. Bretherton & E. Waters (Eds.), Growing points of attachment theory and research. *Monographs of the Society for Research in Child Development, 50*(1–2, Serial No. 209), 66–106.

Main, M., & Solomon, J. (1986). Discovery of an insecure-disorganized/disoriented attachment pattern. In T. B. Brazelton & M. W. Yogman (Eds.), *Affective development in infancy* (pp. 95–124). Norwood, NJ: Ablex.

Main, M., & Solomon, J. (1990). Procedures for identifying infants as disorganized/disoriented during the Ainsworth Strange Situation. In M. T. Greenberg, D. Cicchetti, & E. M. Cummings (Eds.), *Attachment in the preschool years* (pp. 121–160). Chicago: University of Chicago Press.

Manassis, K., Bradley, S., Goldberg, S., Hood, J., & Swinson, R. P. (1994). Attachment in mothers with anxiety disorder and their children. *Journal of the American Academy of Child and Adolescent Psychiatry, 33,* 1106–1113.

Offord, D. R., Boyle, M. H., Fleming, J. E., Monroe-Blum, H., & Rae-Grant, N.

(1989). Ontario Child Health Study: Summary of selected results. *Canadian Journal of Psychiatry, 34,* 483–491.

Radke-Yarrow, M., Cummings, E. M., Kuczynski, L., & Chapman, M. (1985). Patterns of attachment in 2- and 3-year-olds in normal families and families with parental depression. *Child Development, 56,* 884–893.

Renken, B., Egeland, B., Marvinney, D., Mangelsdorf, S., & Sroufe, L. A. (1989). Early childhood antecedents of aggression and passive-withdrawal in early elementary school. *Journal of Personality, 57,* 257–281.

Rosenthal, R. (1991). *Meta-analytic procedures for social research.* London: Sage.

Sabbagh, R. (1994). *Attachment and behavior to strangers in Romanian orphans adopted in Canada.* Unpublished master's thesis, University of Toronto, Canada.

Spangler, G., & Grossmann, K. E. (1994). Biobehavioral organization in securely and insecurely attached infants. *Child Development, 64,* 1439–1450.

Speltz, M. L., Greenberg, M. T., & DeKlyen, M. C. (1990). Attachment in preschoolers with disruptive behavior: A comparison of clinic-referred and non-problem children. *Development and Psychopathology, 2,* 31–46.

Sroufe, L., & Waters, E. (1977). Heart rate as a convergent measure in clinical and developmental research. *Merrill–Palmer Quarterly, 23,* 3–27.

van IJzendoorn, M. H., Goldberg, S., Kroonenberg, P. M., & Frenkel, O. (1992). The relative effects of maternal and child problems on the quality of attachment: A meta-analysis of attachment in clinical samples. *Child Development, 63,* 840–858.

van IJzendoorn, M. H., & Kroonenberg, P. M. (1988). Cross-cultural patterns of attachment: A meta-analysis of the Strange Situation. *Child Development, 57,* 147–156.

Wartner, U., Grossmann, K., Femmer-Bombik, E., & Suess, G. (1994). Attachment patterns at age 6 in south Germany: Predictions from infancy and implications for preschool behavior. *Child Development, 65,* 1014–1027.

Waters, E. (1978). The reliability and stability of individual differences in infant–mother attachment. *Child Development, 49,* 483–494.

7

The Role of Attachment Processes in Externalizing Psychopathology in Young Children

MARK T. GREENBERG
MICHELLE DεKLYEN
MATTHEW L. SPELTZ
MARYA C. ENDRIGA

The idea that social relationships both affect and are affected by developing psychopathology in childhood is fundamental to most modern theories of development. Furthermore, theorists from object relations (Mahler, Pine, & Bergman, 1975; Winnicott, 1965) and ego psychology (Freud, 1965, 1981) have hypothesized that the child's earliest and closest relationships would most impact the development of mental health and illness. However, it was not until John Bowlby (1969/1982, 1973) focused the fields of child development and child psychiatry on the study of infant and child attachment that researchers began to study the connections between the child's closest relationships and the development of various forms of behavioral disorder. In this chapter, we review what is known about the relations between attachment and externalizing problems in the preschool years and provide new findings from our ongoing research. In doing so, we pose the following questions. First, what can attachment theory contribute to the understanding of externalizing problems in preschoolers? Second, how can attachment theory and research contribute to more effective models for diagnosis and treatment of these disorders?

We organize these thoughts around a series of studies that we (Mark

Greenberg, Matthew Speltz, and Michelle DeKlyen) began in 1986, and in which we were later joined by Marya Endriga. We present these ideas and results as a personal journey of understanding, rather than as a finished product. To do so, we first provide a brief review of early externalizing problems.

EARLY EXTERNALIZING PROBLEMS

The term "externalizing" has been used generally to summarize a core set of negativistic, defiant, and hostile behaviors including noncompliance, aggression, tantrums, and other intense or immature emotional responses to limit setting; early and later forms of delinquency also are included in this category. There are three DSM-IV (American Psychiatric Association, 1994) diagnostic categories of particular relevance to externalizing problems: oppositional defiant disorder (ODD), attention-deficit/hyperactivity disorder (ADHD), and conduct disorder (CD), which are referred to collectively as the "attention deficit and disruptive behavior disorders." As CD rarely is seen before age 6 or so, most preschoolers with externalizing symptoms fit criteria for ODD, ADHD, or a combination of the two disorders.

The social and economic costs of these types of disorders are staggering (Kazdin, 1985). By early childhood, referrals for externalizing problems represent the largest group of children served at mental health centers (Offord, Boyle, & Racine, 1991). These early problems also show considerable stability in childhood. Campbell (1991) reported that about half of the externalizing children in a longitudinal preschool clinic sample also met criteria for a disruptive disorder at school age and that about two-thirds of this half were again diagnosable at age 9. Furthermore, epidemiological research suggests that preschool externalizing behaviors may be a common pathway by which a wide range of adolescent and adult disorders of both an externalizing and internalizing nature develop (Fisher, Rolf, Hasazi, & Cummings, 1984; Lerner, Inui, Trupin, & Douglas, 1985). Thus, the study of such children when first brought to a clinical treatment setting may provide clues to the early nature and progression of a variety of forms of subsequent psychiatric dysfunction.

Although it is believed that both organic (biological) and environmental/ecological conditions might potentiate or exacerbate these early externalizing disorders, the exact nature of their roles is poorly understood, and it is assumed that there are multiple pathways by which varying risk factors play a role (Greenberg, Speltz, & DeKlyen, 1993). Nevertheless, both the quality of parenting and the nature of the home environment are implicated strongly in most cases (McMahon & Forehand, 1988; Rutter,

1985a). In addition, research has indicated that children with externalizing psychopathology often show deficiencies in the development of impulse control, emotion regulation, and executive function (i.e., planning, strategy formation, and working memory; Cook, Greenberg, & Kusche, 1994; Dodge, 1986; Moffitt, 1993). In many cases, these difficulties in thought and behavioral regulation are hypothesized to arise from a combination of deprived or disturbed environmental conditions and early and current relations with significant others.

INITIAL CLINICAL OBSERVATIONS

When I (M.T.G.) completed graduate school in the mid-1970s I was interested in two topics. The first was how attachment processes changed during the preschool years and the second was how infant and preschool parent–child attachment relationships influenced the development of behavior disorders. These interests were energized in my graduate clinical training when I worked with both normal and developmentally challenged children who were referred to clinics because of early disruptive behavior problems. Observation of these cases led me to the following working assumptions:

1. In many cases these children *were* very difficult to deal with and parents were at a total loss as to what to do to either decrease noncompliance and disruption or to increase prosocial behavior. In some cases the parents were already "afraid" of their children and attributed to them characteristics that implied vengeance or vindictiveness on the child's part (see Lieberman, Chapter 9, this volume, on parental attributions).

2. In many cases there were numerous family factors, both historical and current (e.g., intergenerational violence, marital distress, high life stress), that contributed to the present situation. In some cases the parents also were angry and potentially explosive.

3. Even if successful in the short term, behavioral parent training programs such as reinforcement systems, time out, and other parenting strategies were unlikely to be sustained very long, especially in cases marked by intergenerational difficulties or by parental psychiatric disorder.

4. Although these children were portrayed as if they were primarily disobedient, disruptive, and aggressive, they appeared on observation with their parents also to be extremely needy, dependent, and anxious. This often was not noticed by the parents.

5. Given my attachment training with Robert Marvin and Mary Ainsworth, the more I focused on the behavior of the child in relation to the mother, the more it became apparent that, for some preschoolers, many

of the symptoms of "opposition" appeared to be attempts, albeit strange and alarming, to get their parents to interact with them, that is, to get the parents to maintain attention, proximity, and contact.

My clinical supervisor allowed me to run informal Strange Situations as part of my diagnostic assessment, which provided clinically useful information. However interesting, they were a small part of a bigger story of both the etiology and treatment of these cases.

INFANT ATTACHMENT AND LATER BEHAVIOR PROBLEMS

Nearly all previous research linking attachment and externalizing psychopathology has focused on *infancy* attachment and its relation to subsequent behavioral adjustment in normative or high-risk samples. For example, findings from the Minnesota High Risk Project (e.g., Egeland, Kalkoska, Gottesman, & Erickson, 1990; Erickson, Sroufe, & Egeland, 1985; Sroufe, Egeland, & Kreutzer, 1990) indicate that insecure attachments across infancy are associated with later behavior problems of an externalizing nature, especially for boys who also experience chaotic life event changes and hostile or neglectful parenting in the postinfancy years. These findings support a transactional model in which insecurity is not viewed as synonymous with disorder, but rather as a risk factor interacting with other vulnerabilities in the child and the family ecology. We believe that attachment process may be an important risk factor, but neither a necessary nor a sufficient cause for later externalizing problems (Greenberg et al., 1993). As Rutter (1985b) has noted:

> Early events may operate by altering sensitivities to stress or in modifying styles of coping, which then protect from, or predispose towards, disorder in later life only in the presence of later stress events. The suggestion, then, is not that any direct persistence of good or ill-effects but rather that patterns of response are established that influence the way the individual reacts to some later stress or adversity. (p. 363)

The notion that attachment is unlikely to have direct effects, but rather it acts as a risk factor, fits well with the data Goldberg has reviewed (Chapter 6, this volume); other researchers, studying *low-risk* samples, have *not* found direct associations between infant attachment and later childhood behavior problems.

Attachment theory posits that sensitive and responsive parenting during infancy leads the child to develop a cognitive–affective working model (expectancy) that he or she will be cared for and responded to when necessary. Although most of these early interactions are nonverbal and physical in nature, major changes occur between the ages of 2 and 5 years in the child's capabilities, needs, and goals in relation to attachment functions (Cicchetti, Cummings, Greenberg, & Marvin, 1990; Greenberg & Speltz, 1988). Further, these changes influence transactionally the caregiver's behaviors and goals, and thus alter both the process and structure of the parent–child attachment relationship during the postinfancy years. This structural change has been characterized as the Phase IV goal-corrected partnership (Bowlby, 1982; Marvin, 1977).

During Phase IV, the relationship is aided by the process of joint verbal planning, which supports the child's rudimentary coping/defensive repertoire and thereby reduces the child's anxiety regarding separation. Through verbal discussion of internal states and plans, the child is provided with a short-term, situationally based working model of his or her relationship. In this manner, planning increases the child's autonomy by providing a reality-based, intersubjective plan of action. It should be obvious that the affective nature of joint planning both affects and is affected by the child's current feelings of security. Moreover, the preschooler–parent attachment relationship clearly is influenced by both earlier experiences and affects associated with the parent. There has been little study of the developmental processes occurring in the attachment relationship during the transition to Phase IV.

As during infancy, it is important that the parent be responsive to the preschooler's needs during situations of high emotional arousal (i.e., fear, anger, sadness) that occur during separations and reunions. All children, regardless of their degree of attachment security, experience these emotions. When the parent is able to respond to the child's emotional expression with empathy and labeling, they teach the young child that emotional expressions will not overwhelm the parent and that these affects are sharable and tolerable experiences (Malatesta-Magai, 1991). Thus, the "good-enough" parent is one who does not become agitated or disorganized by their child's display of strong affect, but rather is able to accept their preschooler's expression of affect while also modeling for the child new ways to express emotions. In Winnicott's (1965) terms, the parent provides a "holding environment" that affords boundaries and support for more mature forms of emotional expression and control.

In relationships characterized by behavioral and emotional problems, children often express negative affect (Campbell, 1990; Patterson, 1982); however, these expressions usually are interpreted by the parent as intolerable and/or frightening and they often are stimuli for the elicitation of coercive cycles. A pattern is then established in which the parent indicates to the child that these negative or conflicting affects are intolerable or "bad" and the parent does not assist the child in developing internalized control or more mature forms of emotional expression. Although parents of children with behavior problems may show deficiencies in strategies for child control/discipline (Patterson, 1986), a more fundamental problem for some parents may be their inability to be sensitive and responsive to their child's needs for security and attention. Further, we have hypothesized that some of the behaviors labeled as "problems" may themselves be necessary strategies to engage the attachment/caretaking behaviors of some parents—strategies that may have some functional value for the child in such relationships, although probably maladaptive in the social world at large.

During the early 1980s at the University of Washington, Matthew Speltz and I began to discuss such children. His specialty was the treatment of preschool conduct problems and he took a primarily social learning approach using parent training. He was well versed in the Hanf (1969) model of parent training and Patterson's (1982) model of the coercive trap, in which the child comes to control the parent through persistent nuisance behaviors (nagging and acting out) that parents give in to, and thus unwittingly reinforce. The child learns that if he persists in his negative, defiant behaviors he will usually get his way.

Emerging out of radically different training traditions (in the literature, attachment theorists and social learning theorists engaged in heated polarized discussions throughout the 1970s [Ainsworth, 1972]), we began to try to integrate these two perspectives. As we watched children together, I began to see how the "operants" between parent and child developed into coercive patterns, and Matt thought more about the developmental implications of oppositional behavior. We began to theorize that in some of these children, nuisance behaviors (hitting siblings, stubbornness, provocations) were their primary strategy for eliciting the parent's attention and proximity. That is, some of the very symptoms of opposition were in fact functioning for the child to help them maintain their attachments with otherwise unresponsive parents. Thus, we began to see that there were two levels of analysis—the operants that influenced the details of sequential interactions, and the broader effects of these behaviors on the attachment relationship.

Like many interesting questions in developmental psychopathology, this issue seemed extremely difficult to study. There were no methodologies at that time for assessing attachment quality in preschoolers; there was no methodology for studying attachment processes in parents. There had been little clinical discussion on this topic that was not utilizing an operant or social learning model. Even more startling was the fact that Bowlby's model, although derived from his own clinical work and intended as a model for clinical use, had engendered no investigation of how attachment processes might contribute to the development of psychopathology.

STUDY I

During the mid-1980s, under the aegis of the MacArthur Foundation, a conceptual coding system for assessing attachment processes in the preschool years was developed (Greenberg, Cicchetti, & Cummings, 1990). In coordination with the developing model of preschool attachment that was evolving in the MacArthur group, we began to collect data on preschoolers with and without externalizing problems. Between 1987 and 1991 we collected data on two samples of children. Each sample had 50 children. Half of these children were recruited through Children's Hospital Child Psychiatry Outpatient Clinic; they were consecutive referrals of 4 to 6-year-old children who met DSM-III-R (American Psychiatric Association, 1987) criteria for ODD (some also meeting other diagnostic criteria in addition, such as for ADHD). The other 25 were comparison children, matched on a variety of demographic criteria, who did not show any significant behavior problems. In both studies, children were from predominant middle-class, European-American, two-parent families. In Study 1, 28% were females and clinic and comparison groups were group-matched. Study 2 was composed only of boys and each clinic and comparison participant was case-matched on age, family structure, and family socioeconomic status. In the first study our main goal was to study the children's reactions to a short, 3-minute separation and reunion and to see if the behavior problem sample could be distinguished from the controls (see Speltz, Greenberg, & DeKlyen, 1990, for details).

Assessment of Attachment

The quality of parent–child attachment was coded from videotapes of interactions between mother and child during the 3-minute separation and 3-minute reunion periods. Because of the wide age range of the children, it was necessary to use two different coding systems. For those children 5 years or older, the tapes were coded according to a system developed for rating 5- to 7-year-olds (Cassidy, 1988; Main & Cassidy, 1988). For children under age 5, the newly developed MacArthur system for preschoolers (Cassidy & Marvin, 1989) was utilized. In both systems, physical proximity and contact, as well as the nature of verbal exchanges, were used in classifications and ratings. Although the criteria for coding and the designation of subgroups are somewhat different for the two systems, both their rating scales and the major attachment classifications are constructed in a similar manner. Both coding systems include five main classifications: secure, insecure–avoidant, insecure–controlling, insecure–ambivalent, and insecure–other.

A brief description of the classifications follows. Complete versions of these systems are available elsewhere (Cassidy & Marvin, 1989; Main & Cassidy, 1988).

Secure

The child initiates positive interaction (nonverbal or verbal), proximity, or contact with the parent or responds positively to initiations by the parent. The child appears to have a special relationship with the parent, is pleased to see the parent, and is relaxed throughout the reunion. One distinction between the two coding systems in this classification is that older children are more likely to discuss personal information or spontaneously share what they did during the separation; this is not necessarily characteristic of younger children. During reunion, the very secure child initiates interaction or contact with the parent that is affectionate and warm. There is little or no avoidance or ambivalence. There are a number of subcategories that can be characterized as moderately secure.

Insecure–Avoidant

There is a great similarity across age groups in this pattern. In both systems, the child displays a strategy of maintaining *neutrality* with the parent. This may be accomplished in a variety of ways, including maintaining or increasing physical distance, ignoring parental behavior and initiations, the absence of spontaneous and/or personal conversation, or continuing engagement with the toys. The child may occasionally orient to the mother or reply, but the child's responses are short, minimal, and neutral in affective content.

Insecure–Ambivalent/Dependent

The child appears excessively dependent upon the parent. This may include displays of immature behavior (e.g., whining); wanting to be picked up or held, but then displaying resistant behavior (wriggling away or other signs of discomfort); and passivity. Immature behavior may be accompanied by direct and open hostility, petulance, willfulness, or temper tantrums. The child often is upset by the separation and appears preoccupied with the parent at the expense of exploration. This pattern differs from the "C" pattern of infants not only in terms of new behaviors (e.g., talking like a baby, acting coy, emphasizing immaturity), but also because mild-to-moderate avoidance also may occur (especially in the eldest children).

Insecure–Controlling

The dominant characteristic is that the child takes direct control of the interaction upon reunion. This role reversal, in which the child assumes a role more appropriate for the parent, is shown in two quite different subpatterns. In the *controlling–punitive* subcategory, the child acts in a punitive or hostile manner that is humiliating or rejecting of the parent. This could include telling the parent to leave or ordering the parent around during the reunion. This hostile, angry behavior is differentiated from that of the *insecure–ambivalent* child in that it does not highlight the child's dependency. The second subcategory, *controlling–caregiving,* is marked by overly solicitous behavior in which the child attempts to take care of the parent. This pattern may be accompanied by overly bright greetings, extreme cheerfulness, and nervousness on the part of the child. This is to be distinguished from the secure child, who may also be helpful and cooperative. In the 3- to 4-year classification system, one additional subcategory, *controlling–general,* is scored when the child takes control of the interaction in a way that is not clearly either punitive or caregiving, or that is a combination of both.

Insecure–Other (Unclassified)

This category is utilized to describe the behavior of children who are clearly insecure but do not fit the avoidant, ambivalent, or controlling classification descriptions. This may be either because the child shows unusual behaviors (e.g., extreme fearfulness, depression, or sexualized behavior) or a combination of insecure patterns.
     Three of the categories (secure, avoidant, and ambivalent) are developmentally more mature versions of Ainsworth's original three-category system (Ainsworth, Blehar, Waters, & Wall, 1978). It has been hypothesized that the insecure–controlling classification is a developmental transformation of the insecure–disorganized/disoriented "D" classification (Main, Cassidy, & Kaplan, 1985). There is no known correspondence between the current insecure–other and infancy classifications.

Rating of Attachment Security

In addition to the classificatory system, both the 3 to 4-year and 5 to 6-year systems utilize a 9-point scale to rate security of attachment, ranging from 1, "very insecure," to 9, "very secure."
     Figure 7.1 shows the attachment classifications for clinic and comparison groups. We found that 72% of the comparison children were

classified as secure, versus only 16% of the clinic group, χ^2 (1, N = 50) = 15.9, p < .001. The clinic children also received significantly lower scores on the attachment security rating scale, $F(1,49)$ = 19.5, p < .001. There were four very interesting findings. First, 16% of clinic children were scored as having a secure attachment. Thus, similar to Campbell's study (1991) on preschoolers with attention-deficit disorder (ADD), there was a definite portion of the sample in which, despite severe symptomatology, the underlying relationship with the parent appeared to be responsive and trusting. Second, a large proportion of insecure clinic boys were controlling and punitive, a category that is seen with little regularity in comparison samples. Further, Main et al. (1985) had hypothesized that this controlling pattern was the developmentally advanced version of infant disorganization. Interestingly, although the description of the controlling classification appears quite similar to the symptoms of ODD, there were no differences in parent ratings of levels of problems between differing attachment classifications in the clinic group. That is, insecure-controlling children were not showing higher levels of externalizing symptoms than were other

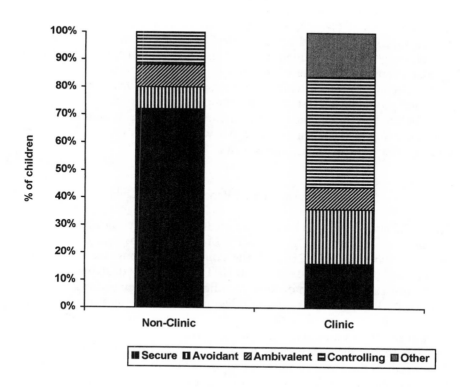

FIGURE 7.1. Study 1 child attachment classification by group.

insecure or secure clinic children. A third interesting finding was that there appeared to be a gender effect. Although only one-third of our subjects were girls, girls who were clinic subjects were less likely to be insecure than were clinic-referred boys, χ^2 (1, N = 24) = 13.5, p < .01. Finally, when a separate set of coders looked at the behavior of the child when their mothers were gone, the clinic children showed higher levels of separation distress; they appeared more anxious and were more likely to search or call for their mothers.

STUDY 2

Given these promising findings, we began immediately to gather a second cohort of 50 children, collecting more extensive data on attachment processes. First, we moved from a one-separation observation to one in which there were two short separations and reunions between the child and mother. Second, with the advent of new measures to assess the internal working models or representations of attachment, we broadened our assessment of attachment. Michelle DeKlyen conducted Adult Attachment Interviews (AAIs; George, Kaplan, & Main, 1984) with our mothers. Marya Endriga assessed the preschooler's working models using a modified version of the Attachment Story Completion Task (ASCT) developed by Inge Bretherton and her colleagues (Bretherton, Ridgeway, & Cassidy, 1990). Because of the difficulty in gaining a sufficient number of girls with behavior problems we restricted this sample to boys only.

Each of these independent assessments of attachment relations will be presented first. Then, their concordance will be examined to gain a more clinical view of attachment assessment.

Observed Attachment Behavior of the Child

Figure 7.2 shows the attachment classifications for the clinic and comparison groups. In the clinic group, 80% of the children were classified as insecure, whereas only 28% of the comparison group were classified insecure, χ^2 (1, N = 50) = 14.3, p < .001. The frequency distribution of the five major categories also differed significantly between groups, χ^2 (4, N = 50) = 15.4, p < .001. As shown in Figure 7.2, there was a much greater frequency of insecure–controlling (32% vs. 4%) and insecure–other classifications (16% vs. 8%) in the clinic group.

Separation distress was assessed using a 25-item checklist that we developed on the basis of our informal observations of specific separation behaviors shown by subjects in the earlier study. It assessed continuous versus interrupted play, crying, active search for mother, room departure, and

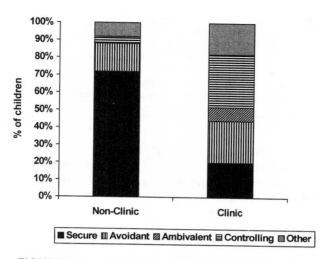

FIGURE 7.2. Study 2 child attachment classification by group.

language content and affect. There was a significant interaction between clinic status and attachment classification, $F(1,46) = 4.0$, $p < .05$. In the comparison group, secure ($M = 4.1$, $SD = 3.6$) and insecure ($M = 4.9$, $SD = 3.9$) boys had nearly equivalent low levels of separation distress. However, in the clinic group, insecure boys had distress scores ($M = 11.0$, $SD = 8.2$) that were more than twice as high as those of the secure boys ($M = 4.8$, $SD = 4.2$). This finding suggests that children in a clinic population show extreme heterogeneity in separation distress, with a large percentage showing significant distress on separation. Validating the earlier clinical observations, many of the clinic children appeared anxious, yet parental attributions were likely to focus on child aggression. In addition, among the small percentage of clinic children who were secure, separations appeared to be handled with ease (see Goldberg, Chapter 6, this volume, for similar observations).

Maternal Representations of Attachment

During the same visit, mothers were interviewed using the AAI. The tapes were transcribed and all information regarding clinic status was removed from the transcripts. The transcripts were coded independently by Michelle DeKlyen, who met reliability criteria after training with Mary Main. Table 7.1 shows the major categories of adult attachment and their hypothesized correspondence to child classifications (see Main, Cassidy, & Kaplan, 1985). Figure 7.3 displays the maternal attachment classifications of clinic and comparison mothers. Mothers of clinic children were more likely to have a form of insecure representation ($p < .005$).

TABLE 7.1. Adult Attachment and Hypothesized Correspondence to Child Attachment Classifications

Childhood	Adulthood
Secure	Autonomous–free
Avoidant	Dismissing
Ambivalent–resistant	Preoccupied/enmeshed
Disorganized	Unresolved

We then examined concordance between the mother's classification and the child's classification (see Figure 7.4). First, we assessed overall concordance between secure versus insecure classifications and found that 82% of cases were concordant between mother and child. We then examined point-by-point correspondence to test the hypothesis of specific linkages of the four-category system indicated in Table 7.1. The findings indicated concordance in 70% of the cases, with a kappa of .50. Insecure–dismissing adults were more likely to have children showing avoidance. Mothers who showed unresolved attachments were more likely to have children showing insecure–controlling or insecure–other patterns (see DeKlyen, 1992, 1996, for further information). The finding of high concordance between the AAI and the observation of attachment behavior upon reunion in the preschool years lends construct validity to the use of

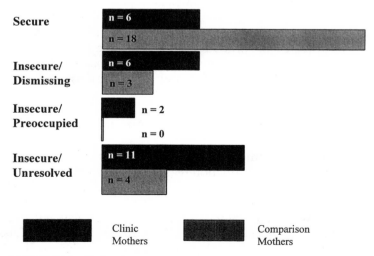

FIGURE 7.3. Mothers' attachment classifications: clinic versus comparison.

reunion as an assessment of attachment in 4- to 5-year-old children. This is because the AAI has been shown to both predict (over a 1-year period) and concurrently relate to infant attachment behavior as assessed in the Strange Situation (van IJzendoorn, 1995).

Child Attachment Representation

Finally, we attempted to examine the attachment representations of the child. To do so, we utilized the ASCT (Bretherton et al., 1990). The task consists of a series of stories that are told to the children using a family of small dolls and various props. Each story is begun by the experimenter, who sets up the story and takes it to a certain point; then the experimenter says to the child, "Show me what happens now." The child is able to move the figures and verbally tell how the story will end. We made a number of changes from the original procedure. First, because we wanted to differentiate attachment-related story reactions from more general reactions, we created a few neutral stories without attachment content. We did this because we were concerned that children who are aggressive with toys might be aggressive across both neutral and attachment-related stories. If so, we might get a handle on which responses were attachment related versus more general. Table 7.2 provides the story stems for the attachment-related and neutral stories. We completed two different types of ratings from the story responses. The first was an overall 9-point assessment of emotional openness. This rating was adapted from Kaplan (1988), who used a similar rating on a different measure of representation, the Separa-

		ADULT ATTACHMENT CLASSIFICATION			
		Secure	Insecure/ Dismissing	Insecure/ Preoccupied	Insecure/ Unresolved
Child–Mother Attachment	Secure	19 (38%)			4 (8%)
	Insecure/ Avoidant	3 (6%)	6 (12%)		1 (2%)
	Insecure/ Dependent			1 (2%)	1 (2%)
	Insecure/ Controlling/ Other	2 (4%)	3 (6%)	1 (2%)	9 (18%)

FIGURE 7.4. Concordance between mother and child attachment classification.

tion Anxiety Test (Slough & Greenberg, 1990). A high score on this rating (6 or above) meant the child was able to share openly his or her feelings and provide adequate coping in the story contexts. A low score (4 or below) indicated either an inability to deal with stories through physical or verbal avoidance, or a very aggressive, silly, or bizarre response to the story stems. The second type of ratings were 5-point scales that rated each attachment story on the child's (1) quality of coping (constructiveness of response to attachment issue), (2) avoidance of story content (both verbal and nonverbal behavior), (3) aggression (shown between play figures), and (4) silly/bizarre responses that were incongruent with story content (see Endriga, 1991, for further information regarding coding). A final 9-point rating assessed the child's level of engagement with the interviewer. A new set of coders who were blind to clinic status and all other information was utilized.

The findings on the ASCT "doll stories" are complex and at first sight confusing. First, the clear information: insecure children, both clinic and control, showed higher levels of aggression in the attachment stories ($M = 2.3$, $SD = .85$) than did the secure children ($M = 1.46$, $SD = .65$), $F(1,46) = 4.2$, $p < .05$. Similarly, insecure children in both subsamples showed lower levels of engagement with the interviewer ($M = 6.0$, $SD = 1.3$) than did the secure children ($M = 7.4$, $SD = 1.1$), $F(1,46) = 5.2$, $p < .05$. Also as expected, there were no differences in story responses between attachment groups for the neutral stories. These findings make sense and follow from our hypothesis that insecure children would show poorer coping with the story content.

TABLE 7.2. The Attachment Story Completion Task[a]

Attachment issue stories	
Hurt knee	Child climbs a rock, falls off, hurts knee, and cries.
Monster in bedroom	Child is sent to bed and cries out that there is a monster in the bedroom.
Departure	Parents leave for overnight trip. Grandmother stays with children.
Exclusion	Parent comes home from work and wants time alone with other parent.
"Neutral" issue stories	
Park & slide	Children play on a slide while parents watch nearby.
McDonald's	Family drives to eat at McDonald's.
Toy train	Family plays together outside with a toy train.

[a]Revised version of the ASCT created by Bretherton, Ridgeway, and Cassidy (1990).

Surprisingly, clinic children did not show lower emotional openness, more aggression, or more avoidance than did nonclinic children. Furthermore, when we examined separately the clinic and comparison groups, we found a surprising difference in the relationship between ratings on the ASCT and ratings of attachment security from the observed reunions, as shown in Table 7.3. As the theory would suggest, children in the comparison sample with higher security ratings during reunion showed better coping and less avoidance, less aggression, and fewer silly/bizarre responses on the ASCT. Thus, the ASCT ratings were related significantly in the expected direction to the rating of attachment security during the observed reunions. However, in the clinic group there was no relationship at all between security ratings on reunion and responses to the doll stories; clinic children who showed more secure behavior on reunion did not respond differently to the stories than did less secure clinic children. Our first reaction to this data was to conclude that there was no relationship here. However, a problem with a nonsignificant correlation is that what it signifies is not clear without further examination. It could mean that there is no association between these two measures of attachment or that there is a positive association for some subjects and a negative association for other individual cases.

This led us to forgo correlational analysis and instead take a more clinical, person-oriented view of the data, where the unit of analysis was the individual case (Rutter, 1988). We wanted to know how often the different attachment measures were discrepant and the clinical meaning of these discrepancies. This issue of concordance and discrepancy is a complicated topic, as it is likely that some discrepancies are real; that is, different assessments actually lead to different findings. On the other hand, some discrepancies may be due to differing types of error variance. One example is errors in coding; remember that coder agreement is only in the .80s for each of these measures. Some discrepancies may be due to "person

TABLE 7.3. Relation between ASCT Ratings and the Rating of Attachment Security at Reunion

ASCT rating	Security rating	
	Clinic (*n* = 25)	Nonclinic (*n* = 25)
Coping	.05	.35[*]
Avoidance	−.10	−.38[*]
Aggression	.02	−.44[**]
Silly/bizarre	.27	−.53[**]

Note. ASCT, Attachment Story Completion Test.
[*]$p < .05$; [**]$p < .01$.

factors"; that is, something may have happened to the person recently that makes the assessment invalid (e.g., a child might be sick, extraordinarily tired, just had a fight with the parent before coming to the lab, etc.). This error variance is part of what a clinician factors into an evaluation and diagnosis and why clinical assessment is seen as an ongoing process, rather than as a one-time event. In contrast, "blind" coders are denied this contextual information in research studies so that they are not "biased." Finally, because the coding of both the AAI and reunion behavior are categorical codes, there are always cases that are "borderline," in which it is a judgment call as to whether a person should be coded as insecure or as secure; this is where most unreliability arises.

Given these provisos and shortcomings of controlled research, we asked the following questions:

1. How concordant are these three attachment assessments?
2. What does this tell us about their convergent and construct validity?
3. What can they tell us about clinic children who are secure on reunion?

We defined a case as concordant if both the reunion and the AAI were coded as secure (categorical classifications) and the ASCT emotional openness rating was 6 or above, *or* if both the AAI and reunion were coded insecure and the ASCT rating was 4 or below. If an ASCT was given a rating of 5 (this is the midpoint and considered a borderline), we then looked at the ratio of coping to avoidant responses to place it in either the secure or insecure grouping (a positive coping to avoidant ratio was considered secure).

Figure 7.5 provides a summary of the findings for the comparison sample. There was agreement in 56% of the cases (14 of 25) among all three assessments. Of discordant cases, most (7 of 11) showed agreement between the reunion and AAI but not the ASCT. In six of seven cases in which the ASCT did not agree with the other assessments, the ASCT classification was "insecure" whereas the other two classifications were as "secure." Thus, it appeared that the ASCT (at least given our scoring of emotional openness) was likely to overscore children as insecure. In four of the six cases in which the ASCT was discrepant and insecure, the children showed a positive ratio of coping to avoidant responses despite being rated low on emotional openness (an unusual state for low emotional openness ratings). Further, in two cases it appeared that the child was extremely tired or very tentative throughout all our testing, including IQ and other nonsocial tests that occurred before the ASCT. Thus, the ASCT, at least for normal preschool boys, appeared to overrate insecurity in some cases. In three cases reunion and ASCT agreed but the AAI did not. In two of these cases, the mother looked secure, whereas both child assessments looked insecure. The first case involved a cross-racial adoption which might partly explain the discrepancy; the second case was one in which both the AAI and reunion coders noted low confidence in their classification; that is, this was a borderline case that was difficult to classify. Finally, there was one case in which the reunion was coded as insecure and both AAI and ASCT were coded as secure: the reunion classification was clearly a borderline case. In such cases, the clinical information on the ASCT and AAI, had it been known, might have altered the interpretation of the reunion behavior.

Figure 7.6 presents similar data for the clinic sample. There was a very similar three-way concordance of 53% (12 of 23 cases). Of discordant cases, once again the great majority were those in which the reunion and AAI agreed and the ASCT did not. In six of these seven cases, the ASCT was rated secure whereas the others were not. This was just the opposite of the comparison sample: in the clinic sample the ASCT responses looked "better" than did the reunion behavior. In two cases the reunion and ASCT agreed and were both insecure, but the AAI did not; in both cases it

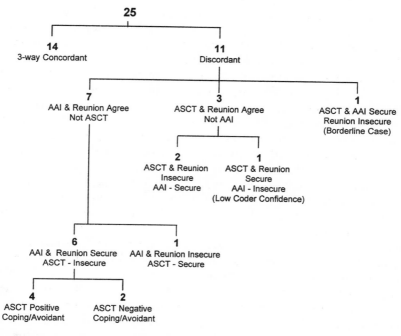

FIGURE 7.5. Concordance between three attachment measurements: comparison sample.

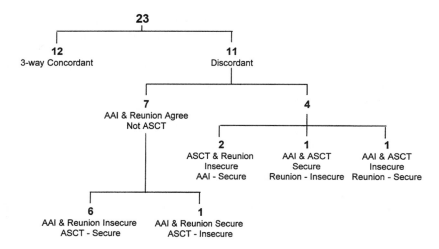

FIGURE 7.6. Concordance between three attachment measurements: clinic sample.

appeared that the child's behavioral problems and insecurity might be unrelated to the mother's AAI status.

What did the more clinical, case-by-case analysis yield? First, in about 55% of the cases, all three assessments point toward either security or insecurity. That is, all assessments regarding attachment provided veridical information. This is clearly greater than chance, and high considering the reliability of each measure is less than 90%. However, we still do not know if they are measuring the same construct or somewhat differing constructs that are highly related. Determination of construct validity requires either strong convergent validity or a definite "gold standard." As we did not have longitudinal data from infancy, it is necessary to rely on convergent validity. Given both the high agreement among the present measures as well as the documented construct validity of the AAI (van IJzendoorn, 1995), it appears that the reunion data is in fact a valid assessment of childhood attachment. Second, many of the instances in which there was not concordance concerned the ASCT. In both the clinic and comparison samples, in about 30% of the cases the ASCT did not agree, but disagreements were in the opposite directions in the two subgroups. For the children without behavior problems, the "doll stories" looked worse or produced more insecure categorizations than did the other assessments. For children with behavior problems, the "doll stories" often looked better or produced more secure classifications than did the other assessments. There are a number of hypotheses that we have about these discrepancies. First, for nonproblem boys, playing with these dolls may naturally bring out a good number of aggressive fantasies—especially given that the dolls that most preschool boys in our culture play with are aggressors (Ninja Turtles, Transformers, Power Rangers). Thus, for some normal boys, the doll stories may elicit aggressive fantasies or themes that are unrelated to attachment issues, but are nevertheless scored as insecure. When reviewing the tapes of the ASCT it appeared that this might have been true, but only in a few cases. Second, as stated above, the fact that the ASCT was conducted late in a long session in which some children became quite tired may have led these "fatigued" children to give curt responses that were scored as avoidant.

But what about the clinic boys? Why did they not show (i.e., act out) more aggression and avoidance? Perhaps some of the boys were consciously controlling their play in this "test" situation—using "scripted" information instead of revealing their attachment-related representations. This may have been due to the fact that they knew they had been taken to the doctor because of their misbehavior. Unfortunately, we did not systematically assess what the "clinic" parents told their children about this visit or about expectations for behavior. It is possible that normal boys may be more likely to "sublimate" the aggressive impulses through play with toys, whereas problem boys may be more likely to act them out in "real life."

Although there was less concordance between the reunions and the child's internal working model as assessed by ASCT, there was agreement in 66% of the cases. Further, there was no difference in the number of agreements between clinic and comparison samples. The fact that there was no difference is surprising given the correlation matrix previously discussed (Table 7.3). Although the correlation matrix shows a much better fit between the reunions and ASCT in the comparison as compared with the clinic samples, this is *not* so if we look at the number of matches into the broad classes of secure and insecure. Further examination of data reveals that the difference is that when there *was* a mismatch between reunion and ASCT in the clinical sample, it was widely discrepant. This was not so in the comparisons; when they were discordant, they were numerically closer in rank. This provides an example of how misleading correlations can be and the value of a person-oriented analyses; in the clinical sample there was no correlation, yet 60% of the cases matched into secure versus insecure. In attachment research there has been an overreliance on statistical analysis to confirm or disconfirm ideas, rather than a focus on how different sources of data might fit meaningfully together to understand individuals.

Secure Attachment in a Clinic Population

Approximately 20% of the clinic children were scored as secure. In 1990, we hypothesized that maybe these clinic secures had externalizing problems that might be due to temporary exacerbations of family stresses, and this would explain their security. As a result, we predicted that they might have both a different etiology and course of disorder. In the present study we have looked more carefully at these cases. As results have indicated, these children may be a more complex group than we had anticipated. Greenberg, Speltz, DeKlyen, and Endriga (1991) presented brief case summaries of these five children and their families. Three of the five cases did fit our original hypothesis that externalizing symptoms might result from recent psychosocial stressors that were not complicated by either a history of poor parent–child interaction or by significant family psychopathology. Interestingly, in all three cases the mothers were independently assessed as secure on the AAI. In contrast, two other subjects presented more complicated histories of both early medical and/or behavior problems and family histories of disorder and trauma. Thus, in some cases with secure attachments, biological vulnerabilities may combine with psychosocial stressors to present with more difficult and long-term disorders. It is clear that studies of much larger samples of clinic children will be necessary to better characterize the profiles of secure children with clinic status. We are now conducting a new study in which 90 clinic and 90 comparison subjects are being followed for a 3-year period.

The findings of our Study 2 cohort provide a strong replication of the original study, demonstrating a high rate of insecure attachments among clinic-referred boys and their mothers. The percentage of clinic boys who showed controlling and insecure–other attachment patterns was remarkably similar to the percentage of the first cohort. Further, there was strong correspondence between the independent assessment of attachments in the parents and the reunion patterns of the children. There was moderate to high concordance between theoretically related attachment categories in both clinic and comparison dyads. Of further interest is the subgroup of clinic boys showing insecure–controlling reunions; in five of these eight cases, their mothers were unresolved and reported either childhood trauma or the loss of attachment figures in a way that suggested strongly unresolved or disorganized metacognition in relation to such loss. These findings are quite consistent with the theoretical formulations of Main and Hesse (1990). The assessment of the child's working model was less concordant with both reunion and the AAI. There is clearly a need for further work in the assessment of representational models in preschoolers.

CLINICAL IMPLICATIONS

The understanding of differences between clinic children showing different patterns of attachment has practical implications for both case formulation and treatment (Speltz, 1990). As our clinic boys all presented with relatively similar levels of problem behavior, standard "diagnosis" from DSM-III-R or DSM-IV provides little in the way of conceptualization or treatment planning. Attachment assessments within the family may provide another level of analysis by which to formulate subgroups, that is, relationship-based patterns that may have differing prognoses and varying levels of treatability. Some treatment decisions might be better based upon the additional information provided by child and parent attachment classification than by child diagnosis alone. For example, the dyads in our clinic group containing children and/or mothers with secure attachments might be good candidates for social learning-oriented parent training programs (e.g., Forehand & McMahon, 1981). These mothers, unencumbered by preoccupation, disorientation, or denial of the importance of past relationships, may be better able to learn and use the "here and now" skills important in current relationships. In contrast, parents with unresolved loss or trauma, or dismissing or preoccupied attachment, or children with more complex diagnostic features, may require the extended and highly individualized approach described by Speltz (1990) and others (Fraiberg, Adelson, & Shapiro, 1975; Greenspan, 1981). Given the correspondence between AAI and reunion behavior, our findings would suggest that the parent's failure to provide the necessary structure for healthy parenting may be influenced by his or her experiences of trauma or loss of past attachment figures and a failure to reorganize these internal models in relation to this loss or trauma (Main & Hesse, 1990).

The present findings lend further support to the validity of the attachment construct at this age and to the association between familial attachment processes and preschool externalizing problems. At this point the causal direction of effects between attachment processes and preschool externalizing problems is unclear and it may be idiosyncratic to each case (see Goldberg, Chapter 6, this volume, for further discussion). In some cases the earlier, insecure attachment during infancy may be a risk factor that is part of a multicausal process leading to later behavior problems (Sroufe, 1983). In other cases, insecure attachment may be either secondary or unrelated to the presenting problems (as suggested by the clinic-referred children whom we found with secure attachments) and thus not part of the risk etiology, but rather operating as a protective factor that might mitigate against further disorder or assist in the treatment process. Finally, it might be the case that in some clinic-referred children, the *quality* of earlier or later attachment is less important than some problem in the *transition* from early physical/proximal attachment to the symbolic/distal strategies more typical of older children. For example, even the secure infant or toddler may experience difficulty in partnership functions or joint planning activities as the result of limitations in symbolic representation, language, or communication skills. Such developmental problems might engender an immature dependence upon the physical regulation of attachment functions (Speltz, 1990).

We believe that the study of attachment processes in clinical populations may lead to an enlightened understanding of both attachment processes and developmental trajectories of some forms of psychopathology. By bringing a developmental perspective to bear on clinical issues one can begin to chart the trajectories of children with similar surface symptoms, but different etiologies and family circumstances. To answer such questions we have initiated a longitudinal study of a larger sample in which the developmental trajectories of clinic-referred and comparison children with varying attachments will be followed across the early school years.

REFERENCES

Ainsworth, M. D. S. (1972). Attachment and dependency: A comparison. In J. C. Gewirtz (Ed.), *Attachment and dependency* (pp. 97–137). Washington, DC: Winston.

Ainsworth, M. D. S., Blehar, M. C., Waters, E., & Wall, S. (1978). *Patterns of attachment.* Hillsdale, NJ: Erlbaum.

American Psychiatric Association. (1987). *Diagnostic and statistical manual of mental disorders* (3rd ed., rev.). Washington, DC: Author.

American Psychiatric Association. (1994). *Diagnostic and statistical manual of mental disorders* (4th ed.). Washington, DC: Author.

Bowlby, J. (1973). *Attachment and loss: Vol. 2. Separation.* New York: Basic Books.

Bowlby, J. (1982). *Attachment and loss: Vol. 1. Attachment* (2nd ed.). New York: Basic Books. (Original work published 1969)

Bretherton, I., Ridgeway, D., & Cassidy, J. (1990). Assessing internal working models of the attachment relationship. In M.T. Greenberg, D. Cicchetti, & M. Cummings (Eds.), *Attachment in the preschool years: Theory, research and intervention* (pp. 273–308). Chicago: University of Chicago Press.

Campbell, S. B. (1990). The socialization and social development of hyperactive children. In M. Lewis & S. Miller (Eds.), *The handbook of developmental psychopathology* (pp. 125–156). New York: Plenum.

Campbell, S. B. (1991). Longitudinal studies of active and aggressive preschoolers: Individual differences in early behavior and outcome. In D. Cicchetti & S. L. Toth (Eds.), *Rochester Symposium on Developmental Psychopathology: Vol. 2. Internalizing and externalizing expressions of dysfunction* (pp. 57–90). Hillsdale, NJ: Erlbaum.

Cassidy, J. (1988). Child–mother attachment and the self in 6 year olds. *Child Development, 59,* 121–134.

Cassidy, J., Marvin, R. S., & the MacArthur Working Group on Attachment. (1989). *Attachment organization in three and four year olds: Coding guidelines.* Unpublished scoring manual.

Cicchetti, D., Cummings, E. M., Greenberg, M. T., & Marvin, R. S. (1990). In M. T. Greenberg, D. Cicchetti, & M. Cummings (Eds.), *Attachment in the preschool years: Theory, research and intervention* (pp. 3–49). Chicago: University of Chicago Press.

Cook, E. T., Greenberg, M. T., & Kusche, C. A. (1994). The relations between emotional understanding, intellectual functioning, and disruptive behavior problems in elementary school-aged children. *Journal of Abnormal Child Psychology, 22,* 205–219.

DeKlyen, M. (1992). *Childhood psychopathology and intergenerational relations in the representation of attachment: A comparison of normal and clinic-referred disruptive preschoolers and their mothers.* Unpublished doctoral dissertation, University of Washington at Seattle.

DeKlyen, M. (1996). Disruptive behavior disorders and intergenerational attachment patterns: A comparison of normal and clinic-referred preschoolers and their mothers. *Journal of Consulting and Clinical Psychology, 64,* 357–365.

Dodge, K. A. (1986). A social information processing model of social competence in children. In M. Perlmutter (Ed.), Cognitive perspectives on children's social behavior and behavioral development. *Minnesota Symposia on Child Psychology* (Vol. 18, pp. 77–125). Hillsdale, NJ: Erlbaum.

Egeland, B., Kalkoska, M., Gottesman, N., & Erickson, M. (1990). Preschool behavior problems: Stability and factors accounting for change. *Journal of Child Psychology and Psychiatry, 31,* 891–909.

Endriga, M. C. (1991). *Attachment Story Completion Task (modified version) coding manual.* Unpublished manual, University of Washington.

Erickson, M. F., Sroufe, L. A., & Egeland, B. (1985). The relationship between quality of attachment and behavior problems in preschool in a high-risk sample. In I. Bretherton & E. Waters (Eds.), Growing points in attachment theory and research. *Monographs of the Society for Research in Child Development, 50*(1–2, Serial No. 209), 147–186

Fisher, M., Rolf, J. E., Hasazi, J. E., & Cummings, L. (1984). Follow-up of a preschool epidemiological sample: Cross-age continuities and predictions of later adjustment with internalizing and externalizing dimensions of behavior. *Child Development, 55,* 137–150.

Forehand, R. L., & McMahon, R. J. (1981). *Helping the noncompliant child: A clinician's guide to parent training.* New York: Guilford Press.

Fraiberg, S., Adelson, E., & Shapiro, V. (1975). Ghosts in the nursery: A psychoanalytic approach to the problems of impaired infant–mother relationships. *Journal of the American Academy of Child Psychiatry, 14,* 387–422.

Freud, A. (1965). *The writings of Anna Freud: Vol. 6. Normality and pathology in childhood: Assessments of development.* New York: International Universities Press.

Freud, A. (1981). *The writings of Anna Freud: Vol. 8. Psychoanalytic psychology of normal development.* New York: International Universities Press.

George, C., Kaplan, N., & Main, M. (1984). *Attachment interview for adults.* Unpublished manuscript, University of California at Berkeley.

Greenberg, M. T., Cicchetti, D., & Cummings, M. (Eds.). (1990). *Attachment in the preschool years: Theory, research and intervention.* Chicago: University of Chicago Press.

Greenberg, M. T., & Speltz, M. L. (1988). Contributions of attachment theory to the understanding of conduct problems during the preschool years. In J. Belsky & T. Nezworski (Eds.), *Clinical implications of attachment* (pp. 177–218). Hillsdale, NJ: Erlbaum.

Greenberg, M. T., Speltz, M. L., DeKlyen, M., & Endriga, M. C. (1991). Attachment security in preschoolers with and without externalizing problems: A replication. *Development and Psychopathology, 3,* 413–430.

Greenberg, M. T., Speltz, M. L., & DeKlyen, M. (1993). The role of attachment in the early development of disruptive behavior problems. *Development and Psychopathology, 5,* 191–213.

Greenspan, S. I. (1981). *Psychopathology and adaptation in infancy and early childhood: Principles of clinical diagnosis and preventive intervention.* New York: International Universities Press.

Hanf, C. (1969, March). *A two-stage program for modifying maternal controlling during mother–child interaction.* Paper presented at the annual meeting of the Wester Psychological Association, Vancouver, Canada.

Kazdin, A. E. (1985). *Treatment of antisocial behavior in children and adolescents.* Homewood, IL: Dorsey.

Kaplan, N. R. (1988). *Individual differences in six-year-olds' thoughts about separation: Predicted from attachment to mother at one year.* Unpublished doctoral dissertation, University of California at Berkeley.

Lerner, J. A., Inui, T. S., Trupin, E. W., & Douglas, E. (1985). Preschool behavior can predict future psychiatric disorders. *Journal of the American Academy of Child Psychiatry, 24,* 42–48.

Mahler, M. S., Pine, F., & Bergman, A. (1975). *The psychological birth of the child.* New York: Basic Books.

Main, M., & Cassidy, J. (1988). Categories of response to reunion with the parent at age six: Predictable from infant attachment classifications and stable over a one-month period. *Developmental Psychology, 24,* 415–426.

Main, M., Cassidy, J., & Kaplan, N. (1985). Security in infancy, childhood and adulthood: A move to the level of representation. In I. Bretherton & E. Waters (Eds.), Growing points in attachment theory and research. *Monographs of the Society for Research in Child Development, 50*(1–2, Serial No. 209), 66–104.

Main, M., & Hesse, E. (1990). Adult lack of resolution of attachment-related trauma related to infant disorganized/disoriented behavior in the Ainsworth Strange Situation: Linking parental states of mind to infant behavior in a stressful situation. In M. T. Greenberg, D. Cicchetti, & M. Cummings (Eds.), *Attachment in the preschool years: Theory, research and intervention* (pp. 339–426). Chicago: University of Chicago Press.

Malatesta-Magai, C. (1991). Emotional socialization: Its role in personality and developmental psychopathology. In D. Cicchetti & S. L. Toth (Eds.), *Rochester Symposium on Developmental Psychopathology: Vol. 2. Internalizing and externalizing expressions of dysfunction* (pp. 203–224). Hillsdale, NJ: Erlbaum.

Marvin, R. S. (1977). An ethological–cognitive model for the attenuation of mother–child attachment behavior. In T. Alloway, L. Krames, & P. Pliner (Eds.), *Advances in the study of communication and affect: Attachment behavior* (Vol. 3, pp. 25–60). New York: Plenum.

McMahon, R. J., & Forehand, R. (1988). Conduct disorders. In E. J. Mash & L. G. Terdal (Eds.), *Behavioral assessment of childhood disorders* (2nd ed., pp. 105–153). New York: Guilford Press.

Moffitt, T. E. (1993). The neuropsychology of conduct disorder. *Development and Psychopathology, 5,* 135–151.

Offord, D. R., Boyle, M. C., & Racine, Y. A. (1991). The epidemiology of antisocial behavior in childhood and adolescence. In D. J. Pepler & K. H. Rubin (Eds.), *The development and treatment of childhood aggression* (pp. 31–54). Hillsdale, NJ: Erlbaum.

Patterson, G. R. (1982). *A social learning approach to family intervention: III. Coercive family process.* Eugene, OR: Castalia.

Patterson, G. R. (1986). Performance models for antisocial boys. *American Psychologist, 41,* 432–444.

Rutter, M. (1985a). Family and school influences on behavioral development. *Journal of Child Psychology and Psychiatry, 26,* 349–368.

Rutter, M. (1985b). Resilience in the face of adversity: Protective factors and resistance to psychiatric disorder. *British Journal of Psychiatry, 147,* 598–611.

Rutter, M. (Ed.). (1988). *Studies of psychosocial risk.* New York: Cambridge University Press.

Slough, N. M., & Greenberg, M. T. (1990). Five-year-olds' representations of separation from parents: responses from the perspective of self and other. *New Directions for Child Development, 48,* 67–84.

Speltz, M. L. (1990). The treatment of preschool conduct problems: An integration of behavioral and attachment concepts. In M. T. Greenberg, D. Cicchetti, & M. Cummings (Eds.), *Attachment in the preschool years: Theory, research and intervention* (pp. 399–426). Chicago: University of Chicago Press.

Speltz, M. L., Greenberg, M. T., & DeKlyen, M. (1990). Attachment in preschoolers with disruptive behavior: A comparison of clinic-referred and nonproblem children. *Development and Psychopathology, 2,* 31–46.

Sroufe, L. A. (1983). Infant–caregiver attachment and patterns of adaptation in preschool: The roots of maladaptation and competence. In M. Perlmutter (Ed.), *Minnesota Symposia on Child Psychology* (Vol. 16, pp. 41–83). Hillsdale, NJ: Erlbaum.

Sroufe, L. A., Egeland, B., & Kreutzer, T. (1990). The fate of early experience following developmental change: Longitudinal approaches to individual adaptation in childhood. *Child Development, 61,* 1363–1373.

van IJzendoorn, M. H. (1995). Adults' attachment representations, parental responsiveness, and infant attachment: A meta-analysis on the predictive validity of the Adult Attachment Interview. *Psychological Bulletin, 117,* 387–403.

Winnicott, D. W. (1965). *The maturational process and the facilitating environment.* New York: International Universities Press.

8

Morality, Disruptive Behavior, Borderline Personality Disorder, Crime, and Their Relationships to Security of Attachment

PETER FONAGY
MARY TARGET
MIRIAM STEELE
HOWARD STEELE
TOM LEIGH
ALICE LEVINSON
ROGER KENNEDY

This chapter aims to bring together progress within two fields of inquiry with a common root, but which have grown apart over recent years: attachment research and criminology. The chapter commences with a brief overview of essential observations from the study of crime, highlighting the well-established role of the family in crime. We also attempt to establish a "prima facie" case for a link between the two fields while highlighting some of the challenges in bringing the fields to bear upon one another. We examine in detail four areas: first, we attempt to show that one of the crucial components of the acquisition of morality, the understanding of the other's point of view, crucially depends on a background of secure attachment. Second, we illustrate the complex relationship between early disruptive behavior and attachment on the one hand and its longitudinal sequelae, delinquent behavior, on the other. We suggest that the developmental challenge of creating a coherent internal working model of relationships may be compromised by suboptimal parenting and the difficulty thus created for the child may result in disruptive behavior, particularly aggression. Third, we marshal evidence suggestive of an attachment disorder in delinquent groups from both individual and population studies. The transition of attachment in adolescence highlights its abnormalities and causes a developmental surge in criminality. The fourth section draws on work from a related psychiatric group, borderline personality disorder, which manifests a combination of disordered attachments, sexual or physical maltreatment, and a reduced capacity to envision the mental states of the other. A similar pattern of results is reported from a study of a prison population. In the final section of the chapter we draw the threads together and propose an attachment theory model of delinquent behavior which assumes that adverse psychosocial environments undermine the creation of coherent internal working models of attachment relationships and the development of an adequate capacity to understand others in terms of their psychological states. Both of these factors can be seen as depriving these individuals of the normally available psychological mechanisms that protect adolescents from criminal activities.

SOME PERTINENT FACTS ABOUT CRIME

The Prevalence of Crime

According to all respected authorities, crime has been on the increase in the Western world since World War II (e.g., Smith, 1995a). Historical trends indicate that this relatively recent increase followed falling rates of crime in the late 19th and early 20th centuries, which in its turn was predated by a veritable epidemic of criminal behavior in the early 19th century (Archer & Gartner, 1981; Gurr, 1977a, 1977b, 1981; Monkkonen, 1981; Wilson & Herrnstein, 1985).

There are, however, indications that crime is on the decrease in the United States. The number of murders in New York City fell by 25% in 1995, according to FBI and New York Police Department sources. Overall in the United States, most serious crimes declined over the last year (by 12% for murders, 10% for robbery, and 5% for all violent crime). The cities benefiting most are those big centers that faced the greatest problems in the last few years: New York, Houston, and Washington, DC. Smaller cities, by contrast, are still showing rising levels of criminality. It is generally accepted that the current drop in serious crime in big cities is due to demographic trends, with fewer young men to commit crimes (Easterlin,

1968; Field, 1990). The population of the United States is aging and many offenders are behind bars; the prison population of the United States has tripled since the 1980s. This does not mean that the problem can be set aside. As there are 40 million children under 10 years of age in the United States, there will be 500,000 additional teenagers by early in the 21st century. As approximately 6% of midteenage males become persistent offenders, the next century may be expected to see about 30,000 more young villains regularly committing crimes.

The prevalence of crime is greatest in the midteenage years, although the number of offenses per offender appears not to vary with age (Farrington, 1986). Criminality is thus a developmental phase and crime itself is largely a developmental issue. Although the proportion of women involved in crime is increasing (Heidensohn, 1996), it remains principally a male preserve. Looking at historical trends in crime is helpful because a number of commonly cited explanations of criminal behavior are contradicted by detailed exploration of historical trends. For example, "modernization" (Mayhew, 1992) in and of itself is unlikely to have led to the rise in crime, as the most advanced industrial nation in the northern hemisphere, Japan, also has by far the lowest crime rates (Bayley, 1991). Social and economic conditions, including income differentials, are often inversely related to crime rates (Smith, 1995b). Trends in housing conditions, poverty, and unemployment, while linked to crime at the individual level, run counter to trends in crime (Field, 1990; Orsagh & Witte, 1981, Smith, 1995a, 1995b).

Social Change and the Family

The exception to this trend is changes in the social institution of the family, which has gone through major transitions in the 1960s and 1970s brought about by increasing differentiation and individualization. There have been a number of relevant changes: (1) the delay in making life relationship commitments (Boh, 1989; Hoffmann-Nowotny, 1987); (2) the increasing fragility of such commitments, which tend to last for shorter periods (Schmid, 1984); (3) the diversification of family forms and cohabitation before marriage and after the breakup of marriages (Chesnais, 1985; Keilman, 1987; Kiernan & Estaugh, 1993; Sardon, 1990); (4) the decrease in household size (Behnam, 1990; Chesnais, 1985; Keilman, 1987); (5) an increase in extramarital births (Kiernan & Estaugh, 1993) and single-parent and stepfamily households (Cseh-Szombathy, 1990; Popenoe, 1987; Roll, 1992); (6) the decrease in family size (Chesnais, 1985); and (7) the increase in divorce rates (Burns, 1992; Haskey, 1983; Kiernan, 1988), making it increasingly likely that children will experience multiple transitions in the structure and functioning of families (Festy, 1985; Kiernan, 1988; White & Booth, 1985).

The strain of change shows on the family. There are few epidemiological facts which are as accurately represented in the media, and therefore in popular culture, as the sad fate of the family in late 20th-century Western society. It is generally known that almost 50% of children born in the United States between 1980 and 1989 will experience the divorce of their parents. The figure in the United Kingdom is likely to be close to this in the 1990s; the number of children involved in divorce and custodial parents' remarriage increased from 145,000 in 1981 to over 160,000 in 1991. The proportion of children in Britain in single-parent care was less then 10% 20 years ago but is over 20% now. Over 90% of these children are living with single mothers who are likely to be at work or to be deprived economically.

The social structure of work commitment and family life are poorly aligned in most Western cultures. A number of again, relatively well-publicized observations speak eloquently to this. For example, 30% of men and 40% of women claim to feel "used up" at the end of a working day. "Downsizing," common across many industries in the 1980s and 1990s, has increased work loads further. Unemployment, or at least the threat of it, is likely to increase pressure even more. Mothers are still the primary providers of child care, yet their role in the workplace has become increasingly central since the 1960s. The average mother's "second shift" is at least 15 hours of housework and childcare. According to one report, working men spend on average 5 hours in "primary child care" per week, whereas nonworking men spend 5.5 hours, nonworking women spend 12 hours, and working mothers spend on average only a little over 6 hours. Employment halves the time mothers make available solely for their child, but unemployment of fathers increases the time they might give to their child only marginally. Because of the increased proportion of women in the workforce, the time that parents have for primary child care has decreased substantially in recent years.

The impact of this set of social changes depends entirely on the quality of alternative child care available to working families. The provision is far from ideal. Two major studies in the United States provide substantial grounds for concern. Observation of nursery-type daycare facilities reveals that infants and toddlers spend 50% of their time wandering aimlessly and even older toddlers are occupied for only 33% of their time. It is not surprising that only 30% are regularly engaged in, and are perhaps capable of, cooperative pretend play. The child placed with relatives or childminders is little better off. Only 40% of care providers plan activities for the child. Only 20% of relatives looking after a child (usually grandmothers) appear to give consideration to the child's daytime activity. Independent ratings suggest that only 9% provide "good care" and over one-third are rated as providing inadequate care. For children looked after in their relative's home, the latter figure goes up to 69%.

This generally unfavorable picture is shown at its bleakest in the problem of unplanned adolescent pregnancies. The risks of such pregnancies are well known: (1) low quality prenatal care, (2) lower likelihood of reducing nicotine intake, (3) less compliance with immunization schedules, (4) increased risk of child abuse and neglect, (5) lower birth weight, (6) higher infant mortality. Teenage pregnancy has a high cost to society. Teenage mothers face financial deprivation and long-term dependence on social security, which undoubtedly contribute to adverse sequelae such as increased risk of poor health and emotional and behavioral problems in the child, and a repetition of the pattern of early pregnancy in the next generation.

This could all be taken as moral panicmongering. Alternatively, it may be seen as a nostalgic harping back to times long gone when "men were men, women were women, parents were parents," and political correctness referred to not belonging and never having belonged to the Communist party. There is little evidence to substantiate the assumption of any recent worsening of parenting. One of the most interesting findings of the Carnegie Task Force on Meeting the Needs of Young Children (1994) is precisely how little the situation has changed. For example, in 1950, 45% of parents regularly read to their children; in 1990 the figure is more or less unchanged at 47%.

Nevertheless, figures produced by UNICEF on the social health of children from 1970 to 1989 do indicate some worrying trends. When figures for the best-ever level of infant mortality, spending on education, teenage suicide, and income distribution are combined and contrasted with 1970, 1980, and 1989 levels to provide a single index of change in the social health of children across all industrialized countries, most countries are able to show improvements or at least no deterioration over this period. Unfortunately, the notable exceptions are the United Kingdom and the United States, both of whose current levels of social health are at about 33% of best-ever levels and seem to have deteriorated significantly since 1980. Thus, while parents probably continue to behave as they have always done, society around them has changed to make the task of childrearing more challenging.

Family Structure and Crime

Could the changing trends in family structure (smaller families, disappearance of larger family units, weaker ties with traditional families, consensual unions as opposed to marriages, children born outside of marriages, frequent family dissolutions, remarriages, frequent family relocations, etc.) be an important part of an explanation for the increased rates of crime? As large, rather than small, family size appears to be a risk factor with regard to educational achievement and attainment (Alwin & Thornton, 1984; Blake, 1981; Glenn & Hoppe, 1982; Hernandez, 1986; Mott & Haurin, 1982), the current trend for decreased family size may be regarded as a favorable underlying influence. The impact of divorce on children's psychosocial development has been extensively investigated over recent years (see Amato & Keith, 1991; Barber & Eccles, 1992; Cherlin et al., 1991; Emery, 1982; Hetherington, 1988; Wallerstein, 1991). It appears that divorce has important negative financial implications for families (Duncan & Hoffman, 1985; Weiss, 1984; Weitzman, 1985), with consequent elevation of emotional difficulties in both parents and children (Elder, Conger, Foster, & Ardelt, 1992) and increased probability of entrance into deviant subcultures during adolescence (Voydanoff & Majka, 1988). Amato and Keith (1991), in their meta-analysis of 92 studies of the impact of divorce on children, found small but significant effects on psychological adjustment, self-concept, and social adjustment, as well as on academic achievement. The effects were smaller in the United States than in European studies, probably because of the greater social acceptability of divorce. It is nevertheless unlikely that increased divorce rates are themselves to blame for increased conduct problems in children. In a number of longitudinal investigations conduct problems were shown to be linked to parental conflict before the divorce (Block, Block, & Gjerde, 1986; Buchanan, Maccoby, & Dornbusch, 1991; Cherlin et al., 1991; Kline, Johnston, & Tschann, 1991). Thus it is high levels of parental conflict, rather than divorce or family structural changes per se, that place children at risk of conduct problems.

In summary, although crime is increasing (if demographic variables are controlled for), it is difficult to identify social-structural variables which might directly account for this increase. Family process, particularly interparental conflict, may be associated with short-term problems. Although a case could be made that economic and social changes have imposed constraints upon family interactions which might determine developmental outcomes (see, e.g., Bronfenbrenner, 1979; Bronfenbrenner & Crouter, 1983), it is unclear if the quality of parenting in families which might have stayed together a few decades ago would have been better for the child than is the current family environment. It is unlikely that we will be able to substantially advance our understanding of these social trends without studying the interpersonal and emotional factors associated with family functioning.

THE THEORY OF ATTACHMENT

Attachment theory concerns the nature of early experiences of children and the impact of these experiences on aspects of later functioning of particular relevance to crime. Variables often regarded as critical in explanations of variations in crime, such as self-esteem, mastery and control, the interconnectedness of individuals and groups, and the different attitudes societies have toward children, may all be approached from the viewpoint of attachment theory in terms of patterns of childrearing. Patterns of child rearing may be more or less conducive to the development of secure attachments. Secure attachment patterns may lead to the development of capacities conducive to "healthy" beliefs and social bonding and thus preclude the development of delinquence.

The question we attempt to address here is how deprivation, in particular early deprivation, comes to affect the individual's propensity toward crime. As part of this question we are naturally also concerned to understand how such adverse consequences may be avoided. The key assumption made by attachment theory is that individual social behavior may be understood in terms of generic mental models of social relationships constructed by the individual. These models, although constantly evolving and subject to modification, are strongly influenced by the child's experiences with the primary caregivers. Let us now turn to the details of the theory.

Attachment and Other Theories of Crime

In 1969, Bowlby (1969/1982) identified three psychological states associated with the disruption of early attachment in the first 3 years of life. Following on from the acute distress of the protest state, the despair state is characterized by preoccupation, withdrawal, and hopelessness. Most pertinent, from our viewpoint, is Bowlby's third state, detachment, which is thought to follow prolonged separation. Detachment represents an apparent recovery from protest and despair, but there is no resumption of normal attachment behavior following the refinding of the object. The infant is apathetic and may totally inhibit bonding. There is an intensification of interest in physical objects and a self-absorption which is only thinly disguised by superficial sociability.

In 1946, Bowlby linked affectionless psychopathy to the absence of a maternal object and a biological predisposition. The term "affectionless" is perhaps unfortunate in the light of the common clinical experience that emotional detachment from others in the past and present does not stop psychopathic characters from repeatedly and aggressively engaging with objects (Meloy, 1992). In primary psychopathy (Hare & Cox, 1987; Meloy, 1988a) the violence is predatory; it is planned, purposeful, and only apparently emotionless. By contrast, affective violence is not predatory; rather, it is a reaction to a perceived threat and is accompanied by heightened emotional (autonomic) arousal (Meloy, 1988b). The attachment system may be involved in both predatory and affective acts of violence; whereas in the former case the individual seeks the object, and the purpose of such proximity seeking is primarily destructive, in the latter case proximity triggers an intense defensive reaction of a violent kind. Violence and crime are, for Bowlby, disorders of the attachment system. They are permitted by lack of concern for others (consequent on the inhibition of bonding) and are motivated by distorted desires to engage the other in emotionally significant interchange. In this section we shall attempt to place attachment theory of crime in the context of other theories of violent and criminal behavior.

Risk Factors for Crime and Attachment: The "Prima Facie" Case

Many of the factors which appear to place young people at risk of criminality are known. Here we shall identify some factors shown to be associated with behavioral problems to illustrate the pertinence of attachment theory to the problem of crime. There are a number of reviews of factors that exist within communities, families, schools, and peer groups which are suggestive of a strong association between attachment and crime (Reiss & Roth, 1993; Tolan & Guerra, 1994; Yoshikawa, 1994).

Community Risk Factors

Even normal school transitions predict increases in problem behaviors. The moves between middle and high school and between elementary and middle school are accompanied by increases in antisocial behavior (Gottfredson, 1986). Such transitions may be seen as disruptions of attachment to other children, provoking an experience of loss and consequent detachment. On the whole, communities with high rates of mobility tend to have more severe crime problems. It is individuals whose attachment history is compromised who are also most likely to find making connections in new communities difficult and are less likely to have the resources to deal with the impact of frequent moves. There is also good evidence to suggest that neighborhoods where people have little attachment to the community, where, for example, rates of vandalism are high, manifest the highest crime rates (Murray, 1983; Wilson & Hernstein, 1985). Not only are unstable attachment histories more common in these neighborhoods, thus reducing the overall likelihood of strong attachments to the community, but also insecure attachment may manifest itself in later childhood as a lowered sense of control over the personal and physical environment (Bates, Maslin, & Frankel, 1985). The disorganization of neighborhoods may thus be the cumulative consequence of individuals incapable or unwilling to make emotional investments in others, including social institutions such as churches, schools, and families, which in turn are critical in the transmission of prosocial values and norms (Herting & Guest, 1985; Sampson, 1987).

Family Risk Factors

Families manifesting serious behavioral problems tend to "breed" children who display similar difficulties (e.g., Bohman, 1978). The very same problems are likely to undermine sensitive caregiving. More centrally, poor family management practices, particularly the failure to supervise and monitor children and exposure to severe, harsh, or inconsistent punishment, is known to increase the risk of delinquent behavior (Farrington, 1991; Kandel & Andrews, 1987; Peterson, Hawkins, Abbott, & Catalano, 1994; Thornberry, 1994). Such parenting, of course, also leads to disorganized patterns of attachment (Cicchetti & Beeghly, 1987; Main & Hesse, 1990).

School Risk Factors

Academic failure beginning in late elementary school is associated with delinquency, probably mediated by the experience of failure rather than as a direct consequence of cognitive capacity (Farrington, 1991; Moffitt, 1993). Securely attached children perform better at school and have superior relationships with their teachers than do insecurely attached children (Grossmann & Grossmann, 1991; Sroufe, Carlson, & Shulman, 1993). It would not be surprising if children with insecure attachment histories who are ineffective with peers and socially rather incompetent (Sroufe et al., 1993) would also find it more difficult to feel committed to school and to see the role of student as a viable part of their lives. Such lack of commitment to school places children at higher risk for problem behaviors (Johnston, 1991). There is good evidence from studies using schools as their unit of analysis to suggest that schools are an important determinant of crime rates, even after student mix and geographical area have been controlled for (Mortimore, Sammons, Stoll, Lewis, & Ecob, 1988; Rutter, Maughan, Mortimore, Ouston, & Smith, 1979; Smith & Tomlinson, 1989). Schools, as all social institutions, may vary in their capacities to activate representational systems associated with secure attachment. After all, children's relationships with teachers may be readily and reliably characterized in attachment theory terms (Sagi et al., 1985).

Individual and Peer Group Factors

There is by now overwhelming evidence for the association between the use of alcohol and aggression, including violent crime, as well as the use of illicit drugs and a broad range of criminal activities (Chaiken & Chaiken, 1990; Evans, 1990; Fagan, 1990; Gordon, 1990). The association is subject to a number of theoretical interpretations (Fagan, 1990): (1) aggression as a direct consequence of the action of pharmacological agents, such as ethanol, at the brain level; (2) aggression as a consequence of the effect of intoxicants on personality structure; (3) aggression as a socially conditioned manifestation of intoxication; (4) aggression as a consequence of the same underlying psychological (developmental) pathology as substance abuse. Time series data showing covariation of alcohol consumption and crime appear to support a direct relationship between the two (Smith, 1990; Wiklund & Lidberg, 1990). Data from the U.S. studies (reviewed by Chaiken & Chaiken, 1990) also identifies a special group of predatory criminals whose antisocial acts are drug related. However, the bulk of adolescent crime is not preceded by alcohol and drug use, and both crime and alcohol and drug use could be linked to underlying psychological or family-based dysfunction. Sampson and Laub (1993) see weak attachment (e.g., a poor marital relationship) as the cause of both alcohol abuse and crime and their case studies illustrate how the breakdown of the attachment (marital) relationship can be closely connected with excessive drinking in children. There has been a substantial rise over the past decades in most countries in the use of alcohol and drugs among young people (see Silbereisen, Robins, & Rutter, 1995, for a review). This increase has paralleled the social-structural changes which challenge parenting and the development of secure attachments in our children. Alchohol abuse may well be an attachment-related problem, and thus a mediator of increased rates of crime.

Attachment theory assumes that internal representations of relationships develop from early schemas which are modifiable, yet likely to be reinforced by later experience. Children whose expectations of others are distorted by early experience may be expected to gradually drift to join the company of other youngsters who share these maladaptive expectations.

Delinquent groups are known to represent an independent risk factor for crime (Barnes & Welte, 1986; Cairns, Cairns, Neckerman, Gest, & Gariepy, 1988; Farrington, 1991). This association is one of the most consistent predictors of delinquent behavior, and the notion of gangs or delinquent peer groups as ways young people find to manage social inadequacies is being explored (Elliott, 1994; Elliott, Huizinga, & Menard, 1989).

Loeber and Hay (1994) have proposed a compelling model for the integration of genetic (constitutional) and environmental factors, proposing that peer group relationships serve to consolidate the relationship between aggression and criminality. Children manifesting early conduct problems are rejected by their nondeviant peer groups who attribute aggressive motives to them even when they are behaving normally; in turn, these children see others' behavior as aggressive in intent even when the motivation was neutral (Dodge, 1991). Peer groups are not the causes of delinquent behavior (as Sutherland & Cressey, 1978, suggested); rather, they help to reinforce the individual's existing predispositions (Rowe, Woulbroun, & Gulley, 1994; Sampson & Laub, 1993). Gangs are attachment figures; they fulfill many of the functions of the caregiver. Attachment theory is relevant to gang membership because it provides, however maladaptively for society, the only expression of the youngster's biological need for bonding which is available to him or her. Attachment may be either a mediator or a further factor which influences an individual's peer group behavior and acceptance (Grossmann & Grossmann, 1991) and in addition to or in combination with attribution biases may influence the final developmental outcome.

Some Problems in Linking Literatures

Whereas the association between attachment theory and risk factors for crime is, as we have seen, highly suggestive, it would be unwise to consider the prima facie case without also considering some of the difficulties which face a conceptual analysis of this sort. As was clear from the previous overview, data are not yet available to answer many important questions considering the potential role of attachment. For example, although there is evidence of a specific link between cognitive capacity and delinquency (Moffitt, 1993) and there are some data linking attachment security and cognitive development (Carlson & Sroufe, 1995), in most studies of crime the causes of intellectual impairment are not considered. In most areas of risk studies, the absence of a comprehensive causal framework hampers integration.

Even where a broader theoretical framework is available, attachment-related formulations have yet to find an appropriate place within them. There are too many rival formulations (even within the same theoretical tradition) of explaining crime to permit the easy integration of attachment constructs. For example, some of the most promising ideas in this field have come from investigators interested in the biological determinants of personality. A number of workers have argued that one dimension (impulsivity) provides a good account of antisocial behavior (Gottfredson & Hirschi, 1990; Quay, 1988; Rowe & Osgood, 1990). Others argue that criminality is determined by two personality dimensions: (1) impulsivity and anxiety related to oversensitivity of the behavioral activation system, and (2) dysfunction of the behavioral inhibition system (Gray, 1982, 1990; Lahey, McBurnett, Loeber, & Hart, 1994). Yet others argue for three dimensions: low harm avoidance (anxiety), high novelty seeking (impulsivity), and low reward dependence (psychoticism; Cloninger, 1987; Eysenck & Gudjonsson, 1989). Whereas there may be a link between patterns of attachment and temperament (Fox, Kimmerly, & Schafer, 1991; Goldsmith & Alansky, 1987; Kagan, 1984, 1989; Lamb 1987), temperamental theories of crime are too equivocal to permit ready integration.

Linking attachment work with some theories confronts us with complex "levels of analysis" problems. For example, we indicated before that ecological approaches to crime which have demonstrated large differences in crime rates between different geographical areas classified in terms of quality of housing (Hope & Hough, 1988), the perceived characteristics of particular areas (Gottfredson & Taylor, 1988; Wilson & Kelling, 1982), or the demographic characteristics of its inhabitants (Sampson & Wooldredge, 1987; Schuerman & Kobrin, 1987) may also be understood in terms of the aggregated attachment capacity of those living in particular high-risk communities. Data collection at the "area" level of analysis is incompatible with information gathering at the individual level; thus, linking attachment concepts with such results may entail insurmountable difficulties. Similar problems emerge in trying to link attachment theory to data on delinquency from educational institutions. There are no data which link statistics at the school level with individual-based data concerning the strength of the bond between student and teacher, or with differences in representations of the relationship with the teacher in schools differing in rates of delinquency.

Links with some theories may appear viable on the surface but even here we can anticipate difficulties of terminology. For example, Hirschi's (1969) social bonding theory links crime to the failure to form attachments, but these refer to social institutions rather than to individuals, thus the research generated in this tradition is barely relevant to modern attachment theory. Social learning theories of deviance also lean heavily on dysfunctions of the parent–child relationship as the root of antisocial behavior (Patterson, DeBarsyshe, & Ramsey, 1989; Reid & Patterson, 1989). However, although these theories trace disruptive behavior to the earliest years in many cases, the data gathering inspired by these theories is normally restricted to school-aged children already showing disruptive behavior.

In sum, whereas superficial links between attachment theory and crime may be readily made, it will require substantial research and conceptual effort to validate the theoretical link which John Bowlby established over half a century ago. In this chapter we shall take a step toward this goal in advancing the view that attachment may protect the individual from criminal behavior by reducing vulnerability to high-risk environments. We shall attempt to demonstrate that secure attachment facilitates the development of mental capacities which both reduce the motivation for criminal behavior and inhibit the individual's potential to commit acts of aggression. We will cover in detail four related areas: (1) moral development, (2) disruptive behavior, (3) delinquent behavior, and (4) borderline personality disorder (BPD). Each of these areas of development is of direct relevance to crime, and in each there is evidence linking patterns of attachment to the developmental processes which underpin them.

ATTACHMENT AND MORALITY

The Development of Morality

Morality is acquired early. Kagan (1981), in his studies of the development of morality in North American and Fijian children, found that between 18 months and 26 months of age children acquire a new set of functions related to cleanliness, integrity of property, harm to others, and toileting, centered on their sensitivity to adult standards and their ability to meet these. Turiel (1983) demonstrated that children can distinguish *social conventions* from *morality* as early as their fourth year. They recognize the difference between rules which are based on consensus (e.g., whether the teacher should be addressed by her first or second name) and where prescriptive judgments of justice, rights, and welfare are involved (e.g., causing distress to another child by bullying). Hoffmann (1984) suggested that empathy forms the basis for morality, and that morality consists of feelings of obligation to foster the welfare of others. Children's awareness that others may feel differently develops during the third and fourth years of life together with an increased willingness to offer appropriate help. Can the quality of awareness of others be influenced by attachment-related factors?

Prosocial Behavior and Styles of Parenting

Pro- as well as antisocial behavior is likely to be a function of the nature of the parent–child relationship. Qualities of parenting linked by research to secure attachment (warmth, sensitive and responsive mothering) appear also to feature in the facilitation of prosocial behavior in children. Miller, Eisenberg, Fabes, Shell, and Gular (1989) report an interesting study of 4- to 5-year-old children and their mothers. Children who showed more sympathy in social situations had mothers who independently indicated that, should their child hurt a peer, they would use reasoning techniques with their children to nurture the development of sympathy in their child; by contrast, mothers whose children tended to show less sympathy felt equally strongly about such incidents, but indicated that they would respond with negative control practices. Thus, the mother's intent to understand the child's motivation at such times of intense affect appears to generate a capacity for sympathy in the child, whereas an unempathic attempt to induce concern appears to be counterproductive. Barnreim (1988), cited in Eisenberg and Mussen (1989), also reported that parents who provided authoritative parenting (i.e., were disciplining but warm, providing their child with many positive experiences) were more likely to rear children who showed sympathetic and cooperative behaviors. An interesting longitudinal study reported by Franz, McClelland, Weinberg, and Peterson (1994) showed the transgenerational nature of this aspect of childrearing. Mothers of these individuals (now in their 30s) had been interviewed when their child was 5 years old. Those whose mothers modeled sympathetic care to a dependent other but were intolerant of aggression were, in adulthood, more likely to report high levels of empathic concern. Another aspect of the child's behavior pattern may contribute to this: avoidant infants are known to be less likely to engage cooperatively in joint tasks (Main, Kaplan, & Cassidy, 1985).

However, the link is by no means a simple one. Some types of parent–child relationships known to be linked to insecure attachments also play a role in the development of prosocial behaviors. For example, concern for the other is not invariably associated with the experience of an empathic object. Toddlers whose mothers suffer from bipolar illness are especially likely to react with empathic concern when they witness distress (Zahn-Waxler, Cummings, McKnew, & Radke-Yarrow, 1984) and are more likely to narrate stories that emphasize responsibility and involvement in other people's problems (Zahn-Waxler, Kochanska, Krupnick, & McKnew, 1990). Such children appear to show elevated rates of prosocial behavior in response to the needs of their depressed mothers. Within Zahn-Waxler's model, this increased empathy may lead to pathological outcomes, possibly contributing to patterns of depression in childhood

(Zahn-Waxler, Cole, & Barrett, 1991). As we shall see, attachment theory may be helpful in explaining this pattern of findings.

Attachment and the Point of View of the Other

There is accumulating evidence that secure attachment implies greater awareness of the mental states of others. The abandonment of egocentrism and development of understanding of another's mental state is not an all-or-nothing phenomenon; rather it is a process of gradual development. It may indeed start in early infancy in a biological preparedness to attend to people as entities (e.g., Nelson, 1987) and to see personal, human causation as distinct from physical, mechanical causation (see Bertenthal, Proffit, Spetner, & Thomas, 1985; Poulin-Dubois & Shultz, 1988). An understanding of others as having intentional subjective experiences is evident early in the second year from studies of joint perception (e.g., Butterworth, 1991), attention to emotional reactions (Adamson & Bakeman, 1985), and social referencing (Sorce, Emde, Campos, & Klinnert, 1985). Three-year-olds appear to understand how desires are involved in emotions such as happiness (Wellman & Banerjee, 1991) and consider desires imputed to characters as potential explanations of their behavior (Bartsch & Wellman, 1989; Moses & Flavell, 1990). Only 4-year-olds evidence consistently the capacity to consider the beliefs of the other (Perner, Leekam, & Wimmer, 1987; Wellman & Bartsch, 1988). We may imagine that the development of the psychological processes underpinning a child's "theory of mind" do not simply follow a biologically predetermined course, but instead are deeply nested in the relationship which the child develops with his caregivers.

There are a number of tasks that cognitive psychologists use to assess when the child achieves "theory of mind competence." There are several reasons to expect that securely attached children would do better on theory of mind (metacognitive) tasks. In a pioneering study, Main (1991) found that the metacognitive capacities of secure infants were superior to those of children with insecure histories. In our own cross-sectional study (Fonagy, Redfern, & Charman, in press) we found that children who were rated secure on the Separation Anxiety Test (a projective test of insecurity) were more likely to pass the "Ellie-the-elephant" theory of mind task (Harris, Johnson, Hutton, Andrews, & Cooke, 1989). This association remained statistically significant when verbal intelligence and social maturity were controlled for. The limitation of both these studies, however, is that measures of infant security and theory of mind were obtained concurrently. To demonstrate that the awareness of the mental state of the other is a developmental achievement which is more likely to be acquired in the context of a secure attachment relationship (i.e., when the child feels at liberty to explore the mind of the other), a longitudinal design is preferable.

We used our longitudinal sample of 100 parent–child pairs to test this hypothesis. Both parents had been assessed before the birth of their first child on the Adult Attachment Interview (AAI; George, Kaplan, & Main, 1996) and were tested with their infant in the Strange Situation at 12 months of age (with mother) and 18 months (with father) (see Fonagy, Steele, & Steele, 1991; Steele, Steele, & Fonagy, 1996). We examined the association between the outcome of the theory of mind task described above and parent attachment classification, as well as child attachment at 12 to 18 months and 5 to 6 years of age. Our findings imply that secure attachment in the first year of life (particularly to mother) facilitates the acquisition of a theory of mind.

Understanding the point of view of the other by no means implies a willingness to act on this understanding under most circumstances. Research on childhood social interaction tends to highlight the pragmatic self-interest of children, in terms of both their friendship behavior (Shantz, 1983) and their morality (Rest, 1983). Nevertheless, the superior awareness of securely attached children of the mental world of others may not only signal a more rapid evolution of morality, but also may protect them in a number of ways from acting violently. Firstly, awareness of the merely representational nature of mental states may be a protective factor in situations in which stress is created by the actions of others. They may be better able to interpret and predict such actions in terms of the mental state of the perpetrator, and thus restrict the potentially catastrophic nature of such actions. Second, being aware of the mental experience of the other may inhibit them from being perpetrators of malevolent acts themselves (see below). Third, the capacity to reflect on mental states may facilitate the development of social relationships with peers and adults (e.g., teachers) which in its turn may protect the child through facilitating bonds to social institutions and avoiding unhelpful peer relationships. Thus, secure attachment is likely to contribute to social situations which are inconsistent with the backgrounds of young people likely to turn to violence and crime.

EARLY DISRUPTIVE BEHAVIOR PROBLEMS AND ATTACHMENT

Early Experience and Crime

Early childhood characteristics are rarely considered by criminologists (Caspi, Darryl, & Glen, 1989; Farrington, 1989; Gottfredson & Hirschi, 1990; Sampson & Laub, 1990). Criminal behavior peaks in the teenage years but high-rate offenders begin deviant behavior early in their lives, well before traditional sociological variables (e.g., labor markets, community, peer groups, marriage) "could play much of a role" (Wilson & Herrnstein, 1985, p. 311). Olweus (1979) reported substantial stability between early aggression and later criminality ($r = .68$). Childhood aggressiveness predicts later antisocial behavior consistently across a number of situations: criminality, spouse abuse, traffic violations, self-reported physical aggression (Huesmann, Eron, Lefkowitz, & Walder, 1984). In Sampson and Laub's (1990) report of the Gluecks' data (500 delinquent boys and 500 individually matched controls), childhood temper tantrums at 10 to 17 years ($M = 14$ years) predicted adult criminality for up to 18 years. The systematic study of the relationship between preschool behavior and the early onset of delinquent behavior is just beginning (Farrington et al., 1990; Tonry et al., 1991). In the Dunedin Multidisciplinary Health Developmental Study, motor problems and parent-rated behavioral problems at ages 3 and 5 years predicted delinquency at age 11 in boys (White, Moffitt, Earls, Robins, & Silva, 1990). Robins (1991), in overviewing the study, points out that antisocial disorder at age 13 was predicted by "externalizing behavior" at age 3 and behavior problems at age 5. The best predictors of delinquency across studies tend to be early conduct problems such as aggression, stealing, truancy, and lying (Loeber & Stouthamer-Loeber, 1987), the majority showing continuity from early teens. Childhood conduct problems and delinquency are the consequence of the same underlying processes (Gottfredson & Hirschi, 1990; Reiss & Roth, 1993; Rowe, 1990).

Alongside the continuity there is, of course, substantial discontinuity. Many adult criminals have no history of juvenile delinquency (McCord, 1980), and most delinquent children do not grow up to be antisocial (Gove, 1985). In the Epidemiologic Catchment Area Study (Robins & Regier, 1991) only 26% of individuals who met the childhood criteria for antisocial personality also met the adult criteria. The Dunedin study reveals that although there is a correlation between behavioral problems at age 5 and persistent antisocial behavior at age 11, and between antisocial behaviors at age 11 and criminal offenses at age 15 (White et al., 1990), the correlations between early childhood behavioral problems and criminality at the age of 15 were weak. Thus, while there is a considerable degree of continuity from one stage to the next, the predictive power of behavioral problems in early childhood can become diluted, hinting at a variety of possible environmental (protective or vulnerability) influences along the way.

The issue of continuity raises the issue of the genetic determination of delinquency. Findings of Reiss et al. (1995) may go some way toward clarifying this ambiguity concerning genetics and the role of early environment. In a major study of 708 families with mono- and dizygotic twins and similarly aged full siblings, half siblings, and stepsiblings, they demonstrated that the environment predictive of conduct problems was not that shared between siblings (based on the behavior of parents with both children). Rather, the specific behavior of the parent with the specific child constituted the critical environmental contribution. Of three dimensions of parenting (conflict–negativity, warmth–support, and monitoring–control) the first two in particular marked differential parenting of siblings. The specific level of conflict–negativity or warmth–support directed toward one child substantially correlates with that child's antisocial behavior. Furthermore and interestingly, a high level of conflict directed toward one sibling can lead to lower-than-expected levels of antisocial behavior in the other. These findings confirm that families are important in the causation of antisocial behavior, but the importance lies in *specific* parent–child relationships. Furthermore, even such relationships cannot be evaluated in isolation without reference to the behavior of the same parent with other children in the same family. The relative contribution of genetic and environmental factors cannot be evaluated unless the specific child–parent relationship is considered in addition to family characteristics. This finding is clearly of relevance to the study of attachment and resonates with some of our longitudinal data reported below.

Pathways from Early to Late Childhood

Recent studies have attempted to identify more specific pathways from early childhood to antisocial behavior in adulthood. It appears that, for boys in particular, early manifestation of behavioral problems is strongly linked to later problems (Loeber & Hay, 1994). The Pittsburgh Youth Study (Loeber, Keenan, Green, Lahey, & Thomas, 1993) has demonstrated at least three pathways from early problems to conduct disorder: (1) *authority conflict* starts with stubborn, oppositional behavior which leads to defiance and later total avoidance of authority (e.g., running away); (2) *covert acts* similarly can escalate with development taking on increasingly serious implications and ending in confrontation with the law; and (3) *aggression* can also increase in severity with development, with quite serious ultimate implications. Any one person may simultaneously follow more than one of these pathways to offending. Some combinations of these pathways may entail greater risks of later serious offending than do others; early aggression, for example, is a common precursor to violence in adolescence and young adulthood (Farrington, 1978; Magnusson, 1987; Magnusson, Stattin, & Duner, 1983).

Can attachment theory account for this continuity as well as for the steep increase in antisocial behavior in adolescence? An attachment theory perspective assumes that the nature of bonds changes at the time of adolescence. The parent–child bonds which predominate in early childhood are reconfigured as bonds to social institutions and adult figures which represent them (teachers, employers, etc.). The underlying structures remain the same. The need to reconfigure internal representations of relationships in this way may makes all adolescents prone to antisocial behavior for brief periods. The period of change represents a developmental moment of detachment when neither old nor new patterns are fully active.

This is a normal process of transition to be found in all our lives. The situation is, however, far more serious for those whose early attachments and consequent working models of social relationships are compromised or distorted by adverse early experience. Whereas the absence of appropriate parent–child bonding may express itself as oppositional, avoidant, secretive, and aggressive behaviors in childhood, we assume that the failure to transfer these attachments to social institutions in adolescence and young adulthood would bring with it quite different consequences (see Sampson & Laub, 1993). The absence of a strong attachment to the parent in the early years may be masked by the adults' physical capacity to control the child. The absence of parental control through emotional ties may not become fully manifest until the individual's behavior requires internal controls through morality, empathy, caring, and commitment. These are the very processes which, as we have seen in the previous section, can be compromised by insecure attachment. The weakening of parental influence thus creates a control vacuum in adolescence. They stay unattached to the structures provided by society to assist in controlling oneself, and they remain so for substantial periods because the psychological structures that normally underpin such bonds are inadequately developed.

A related question, but one which is perhaps much harder to answer, is why individuals in their mid-twenties normally start to desist from criminal behavior. Attachment theory suggests that those individuals who are ultimately able to make appropriate bonds, notwithstanding their early failure to do so, would be likely also to return to the path of normal development. There is a certain amount of data to support such a proposition. Sampson and Laub (1993) reported that individuals who found a marital partner and were able to commit themselves to social or educational roles reduced their chances of reconviction. Zoccolillo, Pickles, Quinton, and Rutter (1992) reported that individuals whose early attachments had been disrupted by a prolonged period in a children's home were less likely to show deviant behavior if they were able to attach themselves to a nondeviant spouse. Quinton, Pickles, Maughan, and Rutter (1993), analyzing the same data set, found that the positive effect of a supportive cohabiting relationship was more likely to be available to individuals without early behavioral problems. Thus, whereas attachment does appear to be a protective factor for antisocial behavior, it is one which is more likely to be accessible to individuals whose propensity to form such relationships is greater to start with.

The Role of Parenting

Environmental influences which undermine the development of secure attachment are also antecedents to disruptive behavior problems. Among the most important are life stress and family adversity (Spieker & Booth, 1988), parental psychopathology (Lyons-Ruth, Zoll, Connell, & Grunebaum, 1989), and social support satisfaction (Crnic, Greenberg, & Slough, 1986). Qualities of parenting which are associated with secure attachment (warmth, sensitive and responsive mothering) appear to be the inverse of the behavior of parents of disruptive children (Isabella & Belsky, 1991). Forehand, Lautenschlager, Faust, and Graziano (1986) reported a direct link between parental depression, ineffective management techniques, and the development of childhood noncompliance. The interactions of uninvolved, unresponsive mothers with aversively demanding 10-month-old infants foreshadowed noncompliance and coercive cycles of power-assertive interactions in the third and fourth years of life (Martin, 1981). Lack of maternal responsiveness and infant demandingness were predictive of disruptive child behavior in interaction.

The well-established association between inconsistent power-assertive and somewhat neglectful parental monitoring and antisocial behaviors in children (Dishion, 1990; Loeber & Dishion, 1984; Olweus, 1984; Patterson & Stouthamer-Loeber, 1984) may be mediated by dysfunctional representations of interpersonal relationships. Not only do negative expectations of the caregiver dominate the internal working model, but the self-soothing capacities acquired in normal infant–caregiver interactions are lacking, leaving the child vulnerable to stress arousal. In the literature it emerges that in addition to inconsistency of parenting and severity of punishment (Loeber & Dishion, 1983; McMahon & Forehand, 1988; Sampson & Laub, 1993) and the coerciveness of parent–child interaction (Patterson, 1982, 1986), the absence of a positive, warm, and affectionate bond between parent and child may play an important role in the etiology of disruptive behaviors (Loeber & Stouthamer-Loeber, 1986; Pettit & Bates, 1989; Robinson, 1985; Rutter, 1985a; see also Greenberg, DeKlyen, Speltz, & Endriga, Chapter 7, this volume). Encouraging positive parent–child relations has a beneficial effect in the treatment of early noncompliance (Speltz, Greenberg, & DeKlyen, 1990; Strayhorn & Weidman, 1991) and in resilience to childhood adversity (Crockenberg & Litman, 1990; Werner & Smith, 1982). Attachment theory suggests that such environmental influences enhance the individual's general capacity for affect regulation. Attachment theory also shifts the focus from the observation of parent–child interaction to the representation of the parent–child relationship in the child's mind (Main et al., 1985). There is good evidence that secure attachment with a caregiver is related not only to greater compliance and reciprocity (Richters & Walters, 1991), but also to better peer relations, self-control, and sociability in the preschool years (Greenberg & Speltz, 1988).

Longitudinal Studies of Attachment and Disruptive Behavior

A number of longitudinal studies have attempted to identify a simple relationship between attachment status in the second year of life and disruptive behavior problems in 4- to 6-year-olds (Bates, Bayles, Bennett, Ridge, & Brown, 1991; Fagot & Kavanagh, 1990; Lewis, Feiring, McGuffog, & Jaskir, 1984). None of these studies reported a simple relationship between attachment and externalizing problems, although in one study (Lewis et al., 1984) insecure boys appeared to have more externalizing problems. One shortcoming of these studies (Greenberg, Speltz, & DeKlyen, 1993) is that they concentrated on the influence of attachment as a possible independent cause of early disruptive behavior problems, whereas prevailing models of disruptive behavior identify a combination of risk factors which may be necessary for such problems to develop.

The Minnesota Mother–Child Project followed a high-risk sample whose subjects' attachment classifications were made in the second year of life. Renken, Egeland, Marvinney, Mangelsdorf, and Sroufe (1989) used a combination of variables including quality of parental care, life stress, and Strange Situation classification at 12 and 18 months of age to predict teacher ratings of aggressiveness at 8 years of age. Aggressive boys were more likely than others to have been avoidant, although it should be noted that the modal classification of aggressive boys was secure at both 12 and 18 months. Harsh parental treatment and stressful life events were related to later aggression for boys and girls, but avoidant attachment was a significant predictor only for boys. Assessments of attachment were predictive, but even securely attached infants developed behavioral problems if the transactional patterns between mother and child were unsupportive, inconsistent, uninvolved, or confused. Insecure children were protected if their mother was warm, supportive, and appropriate at limit setting at age 3½ years. Thus, the subsequent variation in parent–child relationship and family circumstances appears to be critical in determining whether or not the developmental pathway set by early mother–infant relationship is continued or abandoned.

The development of a method for assessing attachment between 3 and 6 years of age (Cassidy & Marvin, 1989; Main & Cassidy, 1985) has given an additional boost to the study of the relationship of attachment and disruptive disorders. Two studies have shown insecurely attached boys to be more aggressive, disruptive, and attention seeking than are securely attached boys (Cohn, 1990; Turner, 1991). Two substantial clinic-based investigations show that boys meeting the criteria for oppositional defiant disorder manifested insecure attachment in over 80% of cases, compared with an age-, social class-, and family composition-matched group where the prevalence of insecurity was less that 30% (Greenberg, Kusche, & Speltz, 1991; Speltz et al., 1990).

There is both a conceptual and a methodological problem associated with these investigations in that the assessment of attachment security in the modified Strange Situation may be strongly influenced by disruptive behavior; thus, the attachment assessment cannot be considered to be independent of the diagnosis. Studies are not yet available which demonstrate a link between infant attachment in the second year and child attachment at age 5.

How Does Insecure Attachment Lead to Disruptive Behavior?

This question may be answered in a number of ways. Aggression may become a response to inadequate parental sensitivity. Greenberg and his colleagues (1993) propose that insecurely attached children might develop internal working models of relationships (IWMs) "in which relationships are generally viewed as characterized by anger, mistrust, chaos and insecurity" (p. 201). The avoidant child may have learned to expect hostility from early experience, and the persistence of the IWM leads to preemptive aggression in later situations. This would account for the attributional biases which have been noted in aggressive children (Dodge, 1991). In fact, Suess (1987), cited in Renken et al. (1989), found evidence that anxious, avoidant infant attachment is a predictor of a later tendency to attribute hostile intent in an ambiguous social situation.

Shaw and Bell (1993) propose that temperamentally difficult infants of nonresponsive mothers may be at particular risk in that nonresponsive parenting exacerbates the irritability or demandingness of the infant, which exacerbates the mother's difficulty in parenting (Martin, 1981). Avoidance of the mother develops as a strategy to avoid being blocked from access to her, and approaches decline in frequency toward the middle of the second year (Main et al., 1985). Increased mobility together with more frequent episodes of undirected anger and negative reactions may provoke the mother of an avoidant infant to view their child's behavior as demanding and difficult. There is empirical support for such a bias in the perception of infant difficulty (Bates et al., 1985; Sanson, Oberklaid, Pedlow, & Prior, 1991). In this way an insecure–avoidant infant not only may become more noncompliant and negative, but also, in the face of mother's continued rebuff of his or her contact approaches, may strive to engage the mother through negative behavior, to which she responds with "unpleasant efforts to control" (p. 611).

Disruptive behaviors may thus be viewed as strategies initially adopted by children who receive nonoptimal care to maximize parental attention (see Greenberg et al., Chapter 7, this volume; Greenberg & Speltz, 1988). These are amplified through transactional processes, ending up in the coercive interaction pattern noted in such families. Insecure attachment may also reduce the child's predisposition toward socialization (Richters & Walters, 1991), thus reducing the child's prosocial orientation. The insecurity of parental representations of attachment may have an independent impact upon the child apart from its influence on the child's own attachment system. For example, parents with unresolved experiences of loss or abuse may at times act in ways which are frightening for the child (Main & Hesse, 1990), as such lack of resolution is assumed to be linked to states of dissociation (Main & Hesse, 1992).

By the age of 24 months, the avoidant dyad may be predisposed to a coercive style of interaction. It must be harder to control a child whose bond to the caregiver is insecure, as a major means of control (threat of loss of love) has a significantly reduced potency. In the fourth year, the characteristics of the dyadic process will be generalized. For example, the child may extend his expectations of interaction to the school situation. Coercive intervention strategies become more extreme and therefore almost by necessity less consistent; harsh or threatening punishments cannot be employed to address every instance of rule violation. The avoidant child's motivational system is extrinsic, aiming to maximize rewards and minimize punishment. Enhanced feelings of self-control associated with intrinsic motivation fail to emerge.

Limitations of Attachment Models of Early Disruptive Disorder

There are several limitations to the attachment theory models of disruptive disorders considered above.

1. Insecure attachment is unlikely to be a direct cause, as the vast majority of children with this pattern of relationships do not manifest any

kind of psychological disorder. Also, insecure attachment patterns have been shown to be prevalent in childhood disorders different in etiology, presentation, course, and outcome from disorders of conduct (e.g., depression, generalized anxiety state, borderline personality disorder).

2. There are many children with secure attachments in pathological groups.

3. There are few studies of infancy linking attachment status to ecological variables in a developmental context (Robins, 1991). Relatively few studies bridge the two traditions of attachment theory: the one rooted in psychoanalytic observation at the micro level (Bowlby, 1969/1982) and the ecological approach to attachment focused on social factors (Bronfenbrenner, 1979).

4. There is a striking absence of studies in the literature which address the impact of the child's attachment to the father and the role of paternal representations of attachment.

It may be more consistent with the literature to suggest that insecure attachment is a risk factor, whereas secure attachment may be a protective factor against the kind of biological and experiential factors which may be operative in early conduct problems (see Rutter, 1985b, 1987, 1988). The large number of secure children with psychopathology remains a difficulty even for a resilience model.

An Alternative Approach to the Study of Psychopathology and Attachment

Our approach to the study of psychopathology and infant attachment aims to move away from the more traditional examinations of the association of patterns of attachment and pathological outcomes. Rooted in the work of Anna Freud (1965), we are inclined to see attachment patterns as mechanisms of defense mustered by the child to cope with the idiosyncratic styles of interaction of his caregivers (Fonagy, Steele, & Steele, 1993). In this framework there can be no simple relationship between attachment classification and psychological disturbance, the latter becoming a manifest problem only once the mechanisms of defense have proved inadequate to the task of protecting the child from anxiety. Pathology is the malfunctioning of attachment strategies, rooted in conflict between mutually exclusive strategies, their maladaptive evolution, and their incoherent internal organization. They are neither cause nor consequence, yet they are important as pieces within the complex puzzle of early disruptive behavior. The link between attachment strategies encoded in IWMs and psychopathology can be found in the interrelationship of IWMs. Such an approach would also be more consistent with recent genetic evidence which highlights the significance of the nonshared environment (Reiss et al., 1995).

Our own longitudinal study of attachment in the second year of life has followed 100 infants whose parents were assessed with the AAI before the birth of the child, and who were tested in the Strange Situation at 1 year and 18 months and the modified Strange Situation at 5 to 6 years of age. In the second year we found that attachment to father was relatively independent of infant–mother attachment and that both were well predicted by the respective parent's attachment classification (Steele et al., 1996). The development of a singular IWM of attachment relationships is the developmental task of the preschool years.

The analysis of the relationship between symptomatology at 5 to 6 years on the Child Behavior Checklist (CBCL; Achenbach, 1991, 1992), and the interrelationship of child and parent attachment classifications across our three sets of attachment measures yielded a number of findings relevant to a link between antisocial behavior and attachment. One striking finding was that whereas asymmetry in the patterns of attachment to the parents *in infancy* (secure with mother and insecure with father or vice-versa) did not seem to foreshadow later problems, if the attachment pattern was still asymmetrical in relation to mother and father at the 5- to 6-year-old assessment, the child was more likely to tend toward delinquent, oppositional behavior. Secure or insecure attachment to either parent did not strongly predict pathology, whereas the asymmetry between attachment patterns did. The suboptimal patterns of parenting discussed above may lead to delinquent behavior which compromises the possibility of a single integrated model of attachment with both parents. Alternatively, the child's difficulty in resolving different representations of relationships may in itself be the cause of behavioral problems. Surprisingly, early matching of father's IWM was more significant for problem-free development than was the matching of mother's IWM.

ATTACHMENT IN DELINQUENT GROUPS

Attachment-Related Assessments

Projective tests discriminate reasonably well between the representational system of violent/criminal and nonviolent, noncriminal individuals and confirm an overriding pattern of detachment from human relationships in the former group. Gacono and Meloy (1992) investigated 60 DSM-III-R (American Psychiatric Association, 1987) antisocial personality disorder (APD) prisoners of both psychopathic and nonpsychopathic types using projective techniques. In Rorschach protocols APD was associated with a lack of affectional relatedness, a relatively high frequency of "hard," nonhuman or part-human objects, and a failure to represent whole people. Idealization was rare and predominantly directed toward nonhuman objects. These tendencies were stronger in psychopathic than in nonpsychopathic individuals.

In a further study, Weber, Meloy, and Gacono (1992) studied adolescents with conduct disorders, using dysthymic inpatients as a comparison group. Conduct-disordered adolescents manifested the emotional detachment and devaluation observed in the prison population of psychopaths, but to a lesser degree. Conduct-disordered adolescents showed very weak desire for relationships compared with depressed adolescents, and were indifferent to people as whole, real, and meaningful individuals.

Bruhn and Davidow (1983) demonstrated that the earliest childhood memories reported by delinquents could be distinguished from a matched, nondelinquent sample of youngsters. One of the strongest distinguishing features was the way other people were represented in early memory. Delinquents recalled them in terms of whether they helped or hindered their activities, but not as three-dimensional characters. The nondelinquents were much more likely to embellish their portraits of others by recalling personality traits and other distinguishing characteristics. Davidow and Bruhn (1990) replicated this study with 71 delinquents matched with 71 nondelinquents with controls for age, socioeconomic status, and family constellation. Particularly striking was the amount of description of "the other." The majority of delinquents gave minimal or moderate descriptions, whereas nondelinquents tended to give extensive portraits of the other. In a similar vein, parents were recalled as not available to help, offering minimal assistance, or as causing injury. Davidow and Bruhn (1990) note a qualitative difference in the description of the other person: in a delinquent individual the description tends to be self-referred as well as negative (e.g., "He was mean to me"). In the control group, the other person is described as a separate human being (e.g., "My father was jumpy and nervous").

Population Studies

Epidemiological studies of clinical populations inspired by social control theory have provided a rich source of data relevant to attachment theory. Social control theory (Durkheim, 1951; Hirschi, 1969; Kornhauser, 1978) proposes that crime and deviance will result when an individual's *bond to society* is weak or broken. As discussed earlier, individuals strongly attached to social institutions are less likely to engage in antisocial and criminal behavior than are weakly attached individuals (Sampson & Laub,

1990). Hirschi's (1969b) formulation suggests that there are four components to the social bond: attachment, commitment, involvement, and
belief. Studies based on social control theory tend to measure attachment
in superficial ways. Nevertheless, the results are consistent with the
contention of this chapter that criminality involves disturbance of attachment processes.

Mutual attachment appears also to be protective in a closely related
problem area, drug abuse. A series of studies carried out by Brook and
colleagues offered convincing evidence that aspects of mutual attachment
may insulate young people from drug use (Brook, Whiteman, Brook, &
Gordon, 1981, 1984; Brook, Whiteman, & Gordon, 1983; Brook, Whiteman, Gordon, & Brook, 1984, 1985; Norem-Hebeisen, Johnson, Anderson, & Johnson, 1984). Brook, Whiteman, and Finch (1993) studied drug
use over a 10-year period in 400 children and showed that earlier child
aggression appeared to predict drug use. It led to adolescent unconventionality and difficulty in later attachment relationships, which in turn led
the young person to drug abuse. Aggression, assessed on the basis of
maternal reports, included anger, noncompliance, temper tantrums, and
aggression with siblings; this was a powerful predictor of low attachment
and, to a lesser extent, of unconventionality and drug use. We have already
explored the relationship between aggression and early attachment. In
agreement with the claim that such aggression is closely linked to dysfunctional IWM of relationships, the Brook et al. (1993) study found that weak
parent–child attachment (measured by questionnaire) at 13 to 18 years of
age led to unconventionality (rebelliousness, lack of responsibility, and
tolerance of deviance), which in turn led to drug use. This suggests that
parent–child attachment has an important reciprocal role. Aggression, as
we have seen, may be the outcome of inadequate early attachment relationships, but may also cause a weakening of the parent–child bond in this
way contributing importantly to the development of deviance.

Cross-sectional and longitudinal studies on the relationship between
family factors and delinquency highlight the dynamic nature of family
influences, broadly in agreement with attachment theory. Loeber and
Stouthamer-Loeber's (1986) meta-analytic review identified four "para-
digms" for the transmission of adverse family influences:

1. The *neglect* paradigm entails both lack of appropriate supervision
   and lack of involvement resulting from insufficient interaction.
2. The *conflict* paradigm manifests in escalating child–parent conflict
   consequent to inconsistent disciplinary rejection of the child by the
   parent, and the parents by the child.
3. The *deviance* paradigm denotes a parental tendency to hold attitudes or manifest behaviors which are delinquent and deviant.

4. The *disruption* paradigm entails discord between the parents, separation, and/or loss with consequent neglect and conflict.

Neglect was the most powerful predictor of delinquent outcomes, followed by conflict and deviance (both intermediate), and disruption was the weakest predictor. Broadly speaking, the review identified socialization variables (such as parental involvement, rejection, and supervision) as more important than background family variables (such as parental absence). The fact that socialization variables were stronger predictors in longitudinal investigations than in cross-sectional ones suggests that the impact of these variables emerges only with time, an assumption which is fully consistent with attachment theory.

Only a handful of studies have succeeded in linking traditional work on attachment with these large-scale epidemiological findings concerning the ecology of crime. For example, Shaw and Vondra (1993) demonstrated that risk factors normally considered to be related to delinquency and criminality (e.g., parental criminality, overcrowding, quality of relationship with a significant other) were more commonly observed together in families of insecure infants. These challenging findings suggest that infant security and risk factors considered relevant to the child's adoption of a deviant developmental trajectory may be inter-related. At the present state of knowledge it is not possible to determine which may be of primary significance.

As mentioned above, the integration of the large-scale, epidemiological investigation and the single-case orientation of clinical work is problematic from an epistemological viewpoint. Very often the bare facts of epidemiological associations are precisely that: bare. For example, the influence of marital relationships on criminality is hard to understand in the absence of information regarding the meaning of the relationship to the individual. From a clinical viewpoint, we know that an individual may have an extremely strong attachment to a fraught, sadomasochistic relationship. Measures such as the AAI, which assesses the subject's current state of mind with regard to the relationship, will need to be developed for epidemiological use if the impact of adult attachment relationships on criminality are to be appropriately assessed.

CRIMINAL BEHAVIOR AND BORDERLINE PERSONALITY DISORDER

The Link between Borderline Personality Disorder and Criminality

Although a significant proportion of individuals with criminal records meet diagnostic criteria for borderline personality disorder (BPD; Gunn,

Maden, & Swinton, 1991; Taylor, 1986), it would be foolhardy to claim that they are the same thing. From an attachment theory perspective, we may, however, identify commonalities at the level of psychic mechanism between individuals in the two groups. Recently, Meloy (1992) made a systematic attempt to link the object relations theory approach to BPD with a wide variety of violent criminal behavior. For example, he explored cases of ego-dystonic, sudden violent acts which appear to be impulsive rage reactions without a prodromal period. These acts would be exemplified by intermittent explosive disorder, whose typical victim is a spouse, lover, boyfriend, or girlfriend, or more chronic obsessive preoccupations with the future victim where depression, helplessness, and a conscious sense of tension build up over a period of months and years to be "released" by a violent act. A small-scale, controlled study showed sudden murderers to be apparently ambivalently attached to dominant mothers and to experience their fathers as rejecting, negative, and hostile (Weiss, Lamberti, & Blackman, 1960). The fragmentation of the self structure through splitting and projective identification makes such individuals vulnerable to injuries to the perception of the self (criticisms, insults, belittling rejection), which are common precipitants of the violent act (Blackman, Weiss, & Lamberti, 1963). Ruotolo (1968) came to the same conclusion in a clinical investigation of five sudden murderers. Some authors stress the symbolic meaning of either the violent act or the victim (Revitch & Schlesinger, 1978, 1981; Wertham, 1966). The violent act is directed against a split-off part of the self with which the individual projectively identifies. Rather than pursuing Meloy's excellent analysis, we would like to explore the applicability of our own attachment theory formulations of BPD to certain types of criminal behavior.

Borderline Personality Disorder and Attachment

The most frequently noted shared characteristic of individuals considered to be borderline is an impairment of attachment relationships (intrapsychic as well as external) identified within and outside the therapeutic relationship. The attachment relationships they describe appear to be fundamentally disordered, short-lived, and chaotic, yet extremely intense. They make attachment bonds, including a strong relationship with their therapist, yet the attachment is never without problems, discord, complaint, disarray, destruction, and damage. They manifest an interpersonal hypersensitivity which leads to dramatic alterations in their relationships, a fragmentation of their sense of identity, an overwhelming affective response, and mental disorganization. These features are particularly evident in the transference. Their submissiveness can suddenly turn to disparagement and rage of remarkable intensity. The trigger may be the mildest criticism or the slightest rebuff in the face of what appear to be unreasonable demands for understanding or gratification.

In an ongoing study we administered AAIs to a sample of 85 consecutively admitted nonpsychotic inpatients at the Cassel Hospital in London, which is run along the principles of a psychoanalytic therapeutic community (Fonagy et al., 1996). About 40% of the patients met diagnostic criteria for BPD on the basis of the the Structured Clinical Interview for DSM-III-R, Axis II (SCID-II; Spitzer, Williams, Gibbon, & First, 1990). The distribution of AAI classifications, arrived at totally independently of the diagnostic process, did not distinguish BPD from other personality disorder diagnoses, although the number of entangled (particularly E3) classifications was greater than was expected.

In addition to rating the AAIs on the dimensions described by Mary Main, we also scored these transcripts on our own reflective function scale, which aims to assess an individual's capacity and readiness to understand mental states and to contemplate these in a coherent manner. The scale is based partly on Main's (1991) seminal chapter on metacognitive monitoring and single versus multiple models of attachment. The reflectiveness scale operationalizes the notion of individual differences in adults' metacognitive capacities. The term "reflective" (rather than "self-reflective") is used to underscore that the scale extends to the assessment of the clarity of an individual's representation of the mental states of others, as well as of their own mental states. The operationalization is based on the literature on the evolution of metacognitive knowledge (Flavell, Green, & Flavell, 1986), as well as on more recent contributions under the heading of "a theory of mind" (see Baron-Cohen, Tager-Flusberg, & Cohen, 1993). We asked raters to note the frequency of statements in AAI narratives in a number of categories: (1) those involving a special mention of mental states; (2) sensitivity to the characteristics of mental states; (3) sensitivity to the complexity and diversity of mental states; (4) special efforts at linking mental states to observed behaviors; (5) appreciation of possibility of change in mental states. The rater's manual is available from the authors by request.

Borderline patients' interviews were differentiated by a combination of three characteristics: (1) higher prevalence of physical or sexual abuse reported in the AAI narratives than that for non-BPD subjects, (2) significantly lower ratings on the reflective function scale, (3) a significantly higher rating on the lack of resolution of abuse, but not on the loss scale of the AAI. These findings are consistent with our assumption that *individuals with experience of severe maltreatment in childhood who respond to this experience by an inhibition of reflective self function are less likely to resolve this abuse, and are more likely to manifest borderline psychopathology.*

Childhood maltreatment may or may not have long-term sequelae, and the determinants of the outcome are only partially understood. Here we propose that if children are maltreated but they have access to a meaningful attachment relationship which provides the intersubjective basis for the development of mentalizing capacity, then they will be able to resolve (work through) their experience and the outcome of the abuse will not be severe personality disorder. We do not expect that their reflective processes will protect them from episodic psychiatric disorder, such as depression, and epidemiological data suggests that victims of childhood maltreatment are at an elevated risk for many forms of Axis I disorder. However, if the maltreated child has no social support of sufficient strength and intensity for an attachment bond to develop which could provide the context for developing the capacity to envisage the psychological state of the other (even in intense relationships), then the experience of abuse will not be reflected on or resolved. Naturally, the unresolved experience of abuse diminishes the likelihood of meaningful relationships which, in a self-perpetuating way, further reduces the likelihood of a satisfactory resolution of the disturbing experience through the use of reflective processes. In fact, a pattern may be established whereby suspicion and distrust generalizes and leads to a turning away from the mental state of most important objects and an apparent "decoupling" of the "mentalizing module," leaving the person bereft of human contact. This may account for the "neediness" of borderline personality disordered individuals; yet no sooner do they become involved with another than the malfunctioning of their inhibited mentalizing capacity leads them into terrifying interpersonal confusion and chaos. Within intense relationships their inadequate mentalizing function rapidly fails them, they regress to the intersubjective state of the development of mental representation, and they are no longer able to differentiate their own mental representations from those of others and both of these from external reality. These processes combine and sufferers become terrorized by their own thoughts about the other experienced (via projection) *in the other,* particularly their aggressive impulses and fantasies ; these become crippling and most commonly they reject or arrange to be rejected by their object. A similar model may help in understanding aspects of criminality, particularly violence.

Reflective Function in Criminals

An inhibition of the capacity to envision the state of mind of the other may be assumed to disable the normal aversive emotional reaction which we experience when we observe distress in others, particularly when the distress was caused by ourselves. The development of moral behavior may crucially depend on this negative emotional state, without which the distinction between conventional and moral behavior (Turiel, 1983) may never be established.

Blair (1992) examined the attributions made by criminals diagnosed as showing antisocial personality disorder (APD) and other criminals without a diagnosis. He compared their responses to a number of stories which could normally be expected to evoke guilt, happiness, sadness, or embarrassment in the protagonists. The happiness story concerned an individual winning the lottery and the sadness story a person placed last in a competition; the embarrassment stories involved three forms of audience condition (no audience, passive audience, or negative audience) with the embarrassing acts being, for instance, dropping a tray of food. The guilt stories were also divided into three groups: person harm (a man punches another man), object harm (a man smashes up public property), and unintentional harm (to either property or person). Differences emerged in both the intentional and unintentional person harm stories: in both cases APD individuals made fewer guilt attributions and more indifferent attributions than did nondiagnosed criminals. Both groups made fewer guilt and more indifferent attributions than did normal control subjects. Attributions of happiness and sadness emotions were not different between the groups.

Despite its small sample, this study offers preliminary support for the contention that certain criminals lack the capacity to envision the state of mind of victims in distress. On the basis of the investigations of BPD we are inclined to assume that these difficulties arise because of failures of the primary attachment relationships. We have some preliminary evidence that is consistent with this point of view. As with borderline patients, a history of maltreatment is present in 80% to 90% of juvenile offenders, and approximately a quarter of those with histories of severe maltreatment are likely to have criminal convictions. We have suggested that attachment to individuals and social institutions may be critical in reducing the risk of delinquency, and adjustment processes are severely disrupted by childhood maltreatment (Main & Hesse, 1992). More specifically, if attachment to the primary caregiver is intimately linked to the acquisition of reflective capacity (see previous section on moral development), the latter may be a key mediator in predisposing an individual to criminality, particularly to violent offenses. We may suppose that those individuals who were never exposed to interpersonal relationships wherein the acquisition of a reflective capacity would have been facilitated, or who were exposed to caregiving environments wherein their only route to adaptation was the inhibition of mentalizing, are most likely to develop insecure attachments and to manifest low reflective capacities, thus removing essential inhibitions on criminal activities. The capacity to envision the mental state of the potential victim may be essential in preventing us from deliberately harming other beings.

To put these ideas to test, Levinson and Fonagy (submitted) collected AAIs from 22 prisoners (convicted or on remand with a diagnosable psychiatric disorder) and matched them with two control groups on age, gender, social class, and IQ: a noncriminal, psychiatric inpatient control group matched for DSM-III-R diagnoses (Axis I/II), and a normal control group recruited from a medical outpatient department. The findings are as follows:

1. There were significantly more secure attachments in the normal control group, and the two clinical groups did not differ from each other in terms of overall level of security.

2. Thirty-six percent of the prison group versus 14% of the psychiatric group were classified as "dismissing," with normal control subjects in between (23%).

3. Forty-five percent of prisoners versus 64% of psychiatric controls were classified as "preoccupied," with only 14% of noncriminal controls receiving this classification.

4. Eighty-two percent of psychiatric patients, but only 36% of prisoners and 0% of nonclinical controls, received "unresolved" classifications.

5. Eighty-two percent of prisoners and only 36% of psychiatric patients and 4% of normal control subjects had been abused (two-thirds of abuse was physical, one-third was sexual in both clinical groups).

6. Neglect was more prevalent in the prison group but rejection was more frequently reported by psychiatric patients.

7. Current anger with attachment figures was dominant in psychiatric patients but was relatively more intense among prisoners.

8. Prisoners had significantly lower ratings on the reflective function scale (RF) than did either psychiatric patients or those from the nonclinical group, but RF ratings of normal subjects were still significantly higher than those of psychiatric patients.

9. When the prison group was split into those with violent index offenses (murder, malicious wounding, grievous bodily harm, armed robbery, indecent assault to child) versus those with nonviolent ones (possession, importation, obtaining property by deception, theft, handling stolen goods), the rating on reflectiveness of the former group was significantly lower than it was for the latter.

The pattern of results is consistent with our assumption that criminality arises in the context of weak bonding with individuals and social institutions and the relatively ready dismissal of attachment objects.

Criminal behavior may be seen as a socially maladaptive form of resolving trauma and abuse (which were almost ubiquitous in our small sample). Violent acts are committed *in place of* experienced anger concerning neglect, rejection, and maltreatment. Committing antisocial acts is facilitated by a nonreflective stance regarding the victim, which may be of particular significance in cases in which the victim is clearly identifiable, as in violent acts against another person.

This is only a pilot investigation, but the results are promising to the extent that they link attachment-related narratives to the nature of the offense committed. Naturally, an important alternative account to the one proposed here may be that it was these crimes which caused the disorganization of the attachment system and it was the psychological impact of crime which permeated the interviews of the violent group. The less serious offenses may have made less impact on the representation of relationships.

THE ROLE OF REFLECTIVENESS AND ATTACHMENT IN CRIMINAL BEHAVIOR

We propose that crimes, at least in adolescence, are often committed by individuals with inadequate mentalizing capacities as part of their pathological attempt at adaptation to a social environment in which mentalization is essential. We assume that these individuals did not have access to meaningful attachment relationships which would have provided them with the intersubjective basis for developing a metacognitive capacity capable of organizing and coordinating their IWMs. The disavowal of the capacity to represent mental states (momentary or permanent) may be a key component of crime against the person. Thus, violence against another may not be possible unless the mental state of the other is insufficiently clearly represented for this to block the violent act. Violence is a solution to psychological conflict because metacognitive capacity is limited, and ideas and feelings are experienced in physical, often bodily, terms.

Thus, the current implementation of an attachment theory of crime is in essence a social control theory (Sampson & Laub, 1993). It starts from the need to explain why most people do not normally commit crime, rather than why some people commit crimes and violent acts. We assume that crimes against people are normally inhibited by the painful psychic consequences of identifying with the victim's mental state and the equally uncomfortable awareness of the beliefs and feelings of important others. Without this level of social awareness, it is hard to see how informal sanctions by family, peers, neighbors, school, or employer could be exercised. Mentalizing capacity is also essential for some of these social agencies (particularly school and family) to exercise their socializing function. Tomassello, Kruger, and Ratner (1993) demonstrated that mentalizing capacity was essential to culture-based learning, wherein knowledge transmitted was available only through active understanding of the mental state of those transmitting it. Thus, mentalizing ability is seen here as a prerequisite to socialization, the internalization of rules and values and their integration into a coherent system of self-evaluation (Bandura, 1991).

There are at least four ways in which a failure of mentalization can lead to a moral disengagement:

1. If we accept that mentalizing capacity lies at the core of self-awareness, those with reduced ability to envision the mental states of others will also have a less well-established sense of their own identity. While this may be a source of substantial discomfort, it may also serve to reduce an individual's sense of responsibility for their own actions. Such individuals may more readily feel that they are not responsible for their actions because they genuinely lack a sense of agency (of intentionality) within which an experience of personal responsibility may be located. By the same token, thinking about others may impinge on individuals with fragile self representations in a far more threatening way than most of us normally experience.

2. We have already noted the importance of mentalizing capacity to anticipating the consequences of an action in the minds of both victim and observer. Limitations upon mentalizing might permit the individual to disregard or at least to misrepresent the psychological consequences of an act on others.

3. A further, related process may entail the devaluing or dehumanizing of the victim, which permits treating other people like physical objects.

4. The limitations of metacognitive capacity may result in a fluidity of the entire mental representational system within which ideas may be readily reconstructed and actions reinterpreted. Thus, unacceptable conduct may be reconstrued as acceptable in a selective and self-serving manner.

There is a second aspect which concerns the changed significance and meaning of behaviors and mental states for the individual with limited mentalizing capacity which may, speculatively, be linked to acts of criminality and violence. This highlights the adaptive value of violent acts within the internal world of such individuals. For example, the concrete nature of mental representations may create a situation where unpalatable ideas may be felt to be removed by destroying the physical object which embodies that idea (Fonagy & Target, 1995). Aggression may serve as a defense to safeguard the self from thoughts and fantasies which it cannot protect itself against through mental manipulation (Fonagy, Moran, & Target, 1993). Similarly, aggression in disruptive children may be an adaptation to the activation of discordant IWMs by a caregiver, through disruption of the relationship. In more severe disorders, this defense might come to be integrated within the working model of relationships of self with others; thus, aggression may become a part of self-assertion. The violent act can then be seen to be aimed at destroying symbolic representation. The assault on the perpetrator's fragile sense of self has to be removed. As one murderer put it: "Either he or I must die, something has to give" (Meloy, 1992, p. 58).

To summarize our model: we assume that certain psychosocial environments, particularly those characterized by high conflict and negativity and low warmth and support, threaten (perhaps constitutionally) vulnerable children. Their IWMs of their caregivers will be limited because of the lack of the critical component, the capacity to see the other's behavior as motivated by mental states, particularly in the context of intense, affectively charged interactions. In the context of such emotionally charged situations, these individuals might revert to mental models of self–other interaction wherein both are depicted as essentially physical rather than as psychological, mentalizing entities. This state of affairs is most likely to arise for individuals whose core self structure includes a relatively fragile mentalizing component. We assume that in early childhood (and subsequently) these individuals did not have access to relationships where they could see themselves as intentional beings motivated by mental states in the eyes of their caregiver. Thus, they were deprived of a relationship in which they could have felt sufficiently safe to explore the mind of the other, to find within it an image of themselves as thinking and feeling beings. Their limited and hostile IWMs are therefore overwhelmingly powerful, unchecked by the attenuating influence of a metacognitive capacity. Physical experience has a motivational immediacy because there is no insight into the merely representational basis of human interaction. The failure of mentalizing, however, offers them concrete solutions to intrapsychic and social problems. They are limited in their ability to form bonds with the social world and its institutions, as these are based in a multitude of ways upon the assumption of human intentionality. But in its place, they can control, distance, or indeed bring into proximity subjective states through physical, principally bodily, experiences. As self-cohesion is limited by the deficit in the core psychological self, by the inhibition of their capacity to reflect on and integrate mental experiences these individuals avail themselves of the opportunity to use bodily experiences (alcohol, drugs, physical violence, and crime) to provide them with a sense of consolidation and a coherent identity.

In many instances, after the turmoil of adolescence, when working models of self–other relationships are transferred from the primary caregivers to the social world, some of these individuals encounter situations and persons which enable them to rebuild their limited reflective capacity. These are the lucky ones, perhaps the ones without a genetic predisposition which undermines close interpersonal ties. In the context of these attachment relationships, many may be able to undo the damage created by their early deprivation and form reflective models of themselves and others, which both reduce the motivation for violent acts and arguably create a powerful block against these. However, for those who, through social happenstance or genetic predisposition, are deprived of such critical interpersonal relations in their young adulthood, the life of violence and crime may be perpetuated beyond the adolescent years. To these individuals, society has surprisingly little to offer.

Let us consider finally the implication of this model for the likely effect of formal sanctions for criminal behavior. Smith (1995a) argues that formal systems of social controls are likely to be effective only in the context of strong informal social control systems where individuals might fear separation from their social networks (attachment bonds) through efficient systems of detection and consequent incarceration. By contrast, when informal social control is low and awareness of mental states in self and other is limited by early disruptions to attachment relationships, imprisonment is unlikely to be an effective deterrent because the loss of relationships is felt as a meaningless threat; "others" views of the self are poorly constructed and weakly invested, and increased contact with similarly handicapped others may be an attraction rather than a disincentive. In fact, the inhumane and mechanical world of most prisons may be an attractive alternative to the discomfort of many social situations to such individuals. The dehumanizing atmosphere of prisons may further weaken the individual's mentalizing capacity and would therefore be expected to increase the probability of further offenses. As is well known, this has been the observed pattern of outcomes across many studies (e.g., Sampson & Laub, 1993).[1]

NOTE

1. The lack of effectiveness of incarceration as a deterrent should not be exaggerated. Farrington and Langan (1992) reinterpreted the divergent trends in the prevalence of property and violent crimes in the United States and the United Kingdom in terms of differences in custodial sentences handed out in these two countries. The increased risk of custodial sentences appears to have worked, at least to some degree, to reduce the rate of both types of crime in the United States, whereas the reduced risk of custodial sentences for property offenses was associ-

ated with increase in this category of crime in the United Kingdom over the same period.

REFERENCES

Achenbach, T. (1991). *Manual for the Child Behavior Checklist/4–18 and 1991 profile.* Burlington: University of Vermont.

Achenbach, T. (1992). *Manual for the Child Behavior Checklist/2–3.* Burlington: University of Vermont.

Adamson, L. B., & Bakeman, R. (1985). Affect and attention: Infants observed with mothers and peers. *Child Development, 56 , 582–593.*

Alwin, D. F., & Thornton, A. (1984). Family origins and the schooling process: Early versus late influence of parental characteristics. *American Sociological Review, 49,* 784–802.

Amato, P. R., & Keith, B. (1991). Parental divorce and the well-being of children: A meta-analysis. *Psychological Bulletin, 110,* 26–46.

American Psychiatric Association. (1987). *Diagnostic and statistical manual of mental disorders* (3rd ed., rev.). Washington, DC: Author.

Archer, D., & Gartner, R. (1984). *Violence and crime in cross-national perspective.* New Haven, CT: Yale University Press.

Bandura, A. (1991). Social cognitive theory of moral thought and action. In W. M. Kurtines & J. L. Gewirtz (Eds.), *Handbook of moral behavior and development: Vol. 1. Theory* (pp. 45–103). Hillsdale, NJ: Erlbaum.

Barber, B. L., & Eccles, J. S. (1992). Long-term influence of divorce and single parenting on adolescent family- and work-related values, behaviors and aspirations. *Psychological Bulletin, 111,* 108–126.

Barnes, G. M., & Welte, J. W. (1986). Patterns and predictors of alcohol use among 7–12th grade students in New York State. *Journal of Studies on Alcohol, 47,* 53–62.

Baron-Cohen, S., Tager-Flusberg, H., & Cohen, D. J. (1993). *Understanding other minds: Perspectives from autism.* Oxford: Oxford University Press.

Bartsch, K., & Wellman, H. M. (1989). Young children's attribution of action to beliefs and desires. *Child Development, 60,* 946–964.

Bates, J. E., Bayles, K., Bennett, D. S., Ridge, B., & Brown, M. M. (1991). Origins of externalizing behavior problems at eight years of age. In D. J. Pepler & K. H. Rubin (Eds.), *The development and treatment of childhood aggression* (pp. 93–120). Hillsdale, NJ: Erlbaum.

Bates, J. E., Maslin, C. A., & Frankel, K. A. (1985). Attachment security, mother–child interaction, and temperament as predictors of behavior problem ratings at age three years. In I. Bretherton & E. Waters (Eds.), Growing points of attachment theory and research. *Monographs of the Society for Research in Child Development, 50*(1–2, Serial No. 209), 167–193.

Bayley, D. H. (1991). *Forces of order: Policing modern Japan* (2nd ed.). Berkeley: University of California Press.

Behnam, D. (1990). An international inquiry into the future of the family: A UNESCO project. *International Social Science Journal, 126,* 547–552.

Bertenthal, B. I., Proffit, D. R., Spetner, N. B., & Thomas, M. A. (1985). The development of infant sensitivity to biomechanical motions. *Child Development, 56,* 531–543.

Blackman, M., Weiss, J., & Lamberti, J. (1963). The sudden murderer III: Clues to preventive interaction. *Archives of General Psychiatry, 8,* 289–294.

Blair, R. J. B. (1992). *The development of morality.* Unpublished PhD dissertation, University of London.

Blake, J. (1981). Family size and the quality of children. *Demography, 18,* 421–442.

Block, J. H., Block, J., & Gjerde, P. F. (1986). The personality of children prior to divorce: A prospective study. *Child Development, 57,* 827–840.

Boh, K. (1989). European family life patterns—a reappraisal. In K. Boh, M. Bak, C. Clason, M. Pankratova, J. Qvortrup, G. B. Sgritta, & K. Waerness (Eds.), *Changing patterns of European family life: A comparative analysis of 14 European countries* (pp. 265–298). London: Routledge.

Bohman, M. (1978). Some genetic aspects of alcoholism and criminality. *Archives of General Psychiatry, 35,* 269–276.

Bowlby, J. (1982). *Attachment and loss: Vol. 1. Attachment.* New York: Basic Books. (Original work published 1969)

Bowlby, J. (1946). *Forty-four juvenile thieves: Their character and homelife.* London: Balliere, Tyndall & Cox.

Bronfenbrenner, U. (1979). *The ecology of human development.* Cambridge, MA: Harvard University Press.

Bronfenbrenner, U., & Crouter, A. C. (1983). The evolution of environmental models in developmental research. In W. Kessen (Ed.), *Mussen handbook of child* (4th ed.): *Vol. 1. History, theory and methods* (pp. 357–414). New York: Wiley.

Brook, J. S., Whiteman, M., Brook, D. W., & Gordon, A. S. (1981). Paternal determinants of male adolescent marijuana use. *Developmental Psychology, 17,* 841–847.

Brook, J. S., Whiteman, M., Brook, D. W., & Gordon, A. S. (1984). Paternal determinants of female adolescents' marijuana use. *Developmental Psychology, 20,* 1032–1043.

Brook, J. S., Whiteman, M., & Gordon, A. S. (1983). Stages of drug use in adolescence: Personality, peer, and family correlates. *Developmental Psychology, 19,* 269–277.

Brook, J. S., Whiteman, M., Gordon, A. S., & Brook, D. W. (1984). Identification with paternal attributes and its relationship to the son's personality and drug use. *Developmental Psychology, 20,* 1111–1119.

Brook, J. S., Whiteman, M., Gordon, A. S., & Brook, D. W. (1985). Father's influence on his daughter's marijuana use viewed in a mother and peer context. *Advances in Alcohol and Substance Abuse, 4,* 1–7.

Brook, J. S., Whiteman, M., & Finch, S. (1993). Role of mutual attachment in drug use: A longitudinal study. *Journal of the American Academy of Child and Adolescent Psychiatry, 32,* 982–989.

Bruhn, A. R., & Davidow, S. (1983). Earliest memories and the dynamics of delinquency. *Journal of Personality Assessment, 47,* 476–482.

Buchanan, C. M., Maccoby, E. E., & Dornbusch, S. M. (1991). Caught between parents: Adolescents' experience in divorced homes. *Child Development, 62,* 1008–1029.

Burns, A. (1992). Mother-headed families: An international perspective and the case of Australia. *Social Policy Report, 6,* 1–22.

Butterworth, G. E. (1991). The ontogeny and phylogeny of joint visual attention. In A. Whiten (Eds.), *Natural theories of mind* (pp. 223–232). Oxford: Basil Blackwell.

Cairns, R. B., Cairns, B. D., Neckerman, H. J., Gest, S. D., & Gariepy, J. (1988). Social networks and aggressive behavior: Peer support or peer rejection? *Developmental Psychology, 24,* 815–823.

Carlson, E. A., & Sroufe, L. A. (1995). Contribution of attachment theory to developmental psychopathology. In D. Cicchetti & S. Toth (Eds.), *Development and psychopathology* (Vol 1, pp. 581–617). New York: Wiley.

Carnegie Task Force on Meeting the Needs of Young Children. (1994). *Starting points: Meeting the needs of our youngest children: The report of the Carnegie Task Force on Meeting the Needs of Young Children.* New York: Carnegie Corporation of New York.

Caspi, A., Darryl, J. B., & Glen, J. E. (1989). Continuities and consequences of international styles across the life course. *Journal of Personality, 57,* 375–406.

Cassidy, J., & Marvin, R. S., with the MacArthur Working Group on Attachment. (1989). *Attachment organization in three and four year olds: Coding guidelines.* Unpublished manual.

Chaiken, J. M., & Chaiken, M. R. (1990). Drugs and predatory crime. In M. Tonry & J. Q. Wilson (Eds.), *Crime and justice: A review of research: Vol. 13. Drugs and crime* (pp. 203–240). Chicago: University of Chicago Press.

Cherlin, A. J., Furstenberg Jr., F. F., Chase-Lansdale, P. L., Kiernan, K. E., Robins, P. K., Morrison, D. R., & Teitler, J. O. (1991). Longitudinal studies of effects of divorce on children in Great Britain and the United States. *Science, 252,* 1386–1389.

Chesnais, J. C. (1985). *The consequences of modern fertility trends in the member states of the Council of Europe* (Population Studies, 16). Strasbourg: Council of Europe.

Cicchetti, D., & Beeghly, M. (1987). Symbolic development in maltreated youngsters: An organizational perspective. In D. Cicchetti & M. Beeghly (Eds.), *Symbolic development in atypical children* (pp. 47–68). San Francisco: Jossey-Bass.

Cloninger, C. R. (1987). A systematic method for clinical description and classification of personality variants: A proposal. *Archives of General Psychiatry, 44,* 573–588.

Cohn, D. A. (1990). Child–mother attachment of six-year-olds and social competence at school. *Child Development, 61,* 152–162.

Crnic, K. A., Greenberg, M. T., & Slough, N. M. (1986). Early stress and social support influence on mothers' and high-risk infants' functioning in late infancy. *Infant Mental Health Journal, 7,* 19–33.

Crockenberg, S., & Litman, C. (1990). Autonomy as competence in 2-year-olds: Maternal correlates of child defiance, compliance, and self assertion. *Developmental Psychology, 26,* 961–971.

Cseh-Szombathy, L. (1990). Modelling the interrelation between macro-society and the family. *International Social Science Journal, 126,* 441–449.

Davidow, S., & Bruhn, A. R. (1990). Earliest memories and the dynamics of delinquency: A replication study. *Journal of Personality Assessment, 54,* 601–616.

Dishion, T. J. (1990). The family ecology of boys' peer relations in middle childhood. *Child Development, 61,* 874–892.

Dodge, K. A. (1991). The structure and function of reactive and proactive aggression. In D. J. Pepler & K. H. Rubin (Eds.), *The development and treatment of childhood aggression* (pp. 201–218). Hillsdale, NJ: Erlbaum.

Duncan, G. J., & Hoffman, S. D. (1985). A reconsideration of the economic consequences of marital disruption. *Demography, 22,* 485–498.

Durkheim, E. (1951). *Suicide* (J. Spaulding & G. Simpson, Trans.). New York: Free Press.

Easterlin, R. A. (1968). *Population, labor force and long swings in economic growth: The American experience.* New York: National Bureau of Economic Research.

Eisenberg, N., & Mussen, P. (1989). *The roots of prosocial behaviour in children.* Cambridge, England: Cambridge University Press.

Elder, Jr., G. H., Conger, R. D., Foster, E. M., & Ardelt, M. (1992). Families under economic pressure. *Journal of Family Issues, 13,* 5–37.

Elliott, D. S. (1994). Serious violent offenders: Onset, developmental course, and termination—The American Society of Criminology 1993 Address. *Criminology, 32,* 1–21.

Elliott, D. S., Huizinga, D., & Menard, S. (1989). *Multiple problem youth: Delinquency, substance use and mental health problems.* New York: Springer-Verlag.

Emery, R. E. (1982). Interparental conflict and the children of discord and divorce. *Psychological Bulletin, 92,* 310–330.

Evans, M. (1990). Unsocial and criminal activities and alcohol. In R. Bluglass & P. Bowden (Eds.), *Principles and practice of forensic psychiatry* (pp. 881–895). Edinburgh: Churchill Livingstone.

Eysenck, H. J., & Gudjonsson, G. H. (1989). *The causes and cures of criminality.* New York: Plenum Press.

Fagan, J. (1990). Intoxication and aggression. In M. Tonry & J. Q. Wilson (Eds.), *Crime and justice: A review of research: Vol. 13. Drugs and crime* (pp. 241–320). Chicago: University of Chicago Press.

Fagot, B. I., & Kavanagh, K. (1990). The prediction of antisocial behavior from avoidant attachment classifications. *Child Development, 61,* 864–873.

Farrington, D. P. (1978). The family backgrounds of aggressive youths. In L. A. Hersov, M. Berger, & D. Shaffer (Eds.), *Aggression and antisocial behaviour in childhood and adolescence* (pp. 73–93). Oxford: Pergamon.

Farrington, D. P. (1986). Communities and crime. In M. Tonry & N. Morris (Eds.), *Crime and justice: An annual review of research* (Vol. 7, pp. 189–250). Chicago: University of Chicago Press.

Farrington, D. P. (1989). Later adult life outcomes of offenders and nonoffenders. In M. Brambring, F. Losel, & H. Skowronek (Eds.), *Children at risk: Assessment, longitudinal research, and intervention* (pp. 220–244). New York: Walter de Gruyter.

Farrington, D. P. (1991). Childhood aggression and adult violence: Early precursors and later-life outcomes. In D. Pepler & K. H. Rubin (Eds.), *The development and treatment of childhood aggression* (pp. 5–29). Hillsdale, NJ: Erlbaum.

Farrington, D. P., & Langan, P. A. (1992). Changes in crime and punishment in England and America in the 1980s. *Justice Quarterly, 9,* 5–46.

Farrington, D. P., Loeber, R., Elliott, D. S., Hawkins, D., Kandel, D. B., Klein, M. W., McCord, J., Rowe, D. C., & Tremblay, R. E. (1990). Advancing knowledge about the onset of delinquency and crime. In B. B. Lahey & A. E. Kazdin (Eds.), *Advances in clinical child psychology* (Vol. 13, pp. 283–342). New York: Plenum Press.

Festy, P. (1985). *Divorce, judicial separation and remarriage* (Population Studies, 17). Strasbourg: Council of Europe.

Field, S. (1990). *Trends in crime and their interpretation: A study of recorded crime in postwar England and Wales* (Home Office Research Study 119). London: Her Majesty's Stationery Office.

Flavell, J. H., Green, F. L., & Flavell, E. R. (1986). Development of knowledge about the appearance–reality distinction. *Monographs of the Society for Research in Child Development, 51*(1, Serial No. 212), 1–68.

Fonagy, P., Leigh, T., Steele, M., Steele, H., Kennedy, R., Mattoon, G., Target, M., & Gerber, A. (1996). The relation of attachment status, psychiatric classification, and response to psychotherapy. *Journal of Consulting and Clinical Psychology, 64,* 22–31.

Fonagy, P., Moran, G. S., & Target, M. (1993). Aggression and the psychological self. *International Journal of Psycho-Analysis, 74,* 471–485.

Fonagy, P., Redfern, S., & Charman, T. (in press). Individual differences in theory of mind acquisition: The role of attachment security. *British Journal of Developmental Psychology.*

Fonagy, P., Steele, H., & Steele, M. (1991). Maternal representations of attachment during pregnancy predict the organization of infant–mother attachment at one year of age. *Child Development, 62,* 891–905.

Fonagy, P., Steele, M., & Steele, H. (1993). The integration of psychoanalytic theory and work on attachment: The issue of intergenerational psychic processes. In D. Stern & M. Ammaniti (Eds.), *Attaccamento e psicoanalis.* Bari, Italy: Laterza.

Fonagy, P., & Target, M. (1995). Understanding the violent patient: The use of the body and the role of the father. *International Journal of Psycho-Analysis 76*, 487–502.

Forehand, R., Lautenschlager, G. J., Faust, J., & Graziano, W. G. (1986). Parent perceptions and parent–child interactions in clinic-referred children: A preliminary investigation of the effects of maternal depressive moods. *Behaviour Research and Therapy, 24*, 73–75.

Fox, N. A., Kimmerly, N. L., & Schafer, W. D. (1991). Attachment to mother/attachment to father: A meta-analysis. *Child Development, 62*, 210–225.

Franz, C. E., McClelland, D. C., Weinberger, J., & Peterson, C. (1994). Parenting antecedents of adult adjustment: A longitudinal study. In C. Perris, W. A. Arrindell, & M. Eisemann (Eds.), *Parenting and psychopathology* (pp. 127–144). Chichester: Wiley.

Freud, A. (1965). *Normality and pathology in childhood*. Harmondsworth: Penguin.

Gacono, C. B., & Meloy, J. R. (1992). The Rorschach and the DSM-III-R antisocial personality: A tribute to Robert Lindner. *Journal of Clinical Psychology, 48*, 393–406.

George, C., Kaplan, N., & Main, M. (1996). *The Adult Attachment Interview*. Unpublished manuscript, Department of Psychology, University of California at Berkeley.

Glenn, N. D., & Hoppe, S. K. (1982). Only children as adults: Psychological well-being. *Journal of Family Issues, 5*, 363–382.

Goldsmith, H. H., & Alansky, J. A. (1987). Maternal and infant termperamental predictors of attachment: A meta-analytic review. *Journal of Consulting and Clinical Psychology, 55*, 805–816.

Gordon, A. (1990). Drugs and criminal behaviour. In R. Bluglass & P. Bowden (Eds.), *Principles and practice of forensic psychiatry* (pp. 897–901). Edinburgh: Churchill Livingstone.

Gottfredson, D. C. (1986). An empirical test of school-based environmental and individual interventions to reduce the risk of delinquent behaviour. *Criminology, 24*, 705–731.

Gottfredson, M. R., & Hirschi, T. (1990). *A general theory of crime*. Stanford, CA: Stanford University Press.

Gottfredson, S. D., & Taylor, R. B. (1988). Community contexts and criminal offenders. In T. Hope & M. Shaw (Eds.), *Communities and crime reduction* (pp. 62–80). London: Her Majesty's Stationery Office.

Gove, W. R. (1985). The effect of age and gender on deviant behaviour: A biopsychosocial perspective. In A. S. Rossi (Ed.), *Gender and the life course* (pp. 115–144). New York: Aldine.

Gray, J. A. (1982). *The neuropsychology of anxiety*. New York: Oxford University Press.

Gray, J. A. (1990). Brain systems that mediate both emotion and cognition. *Cognition and Emotion, 4*, 269–288.

Greenberg, M. T., Kusche, C. A., & Speltz, M. (1991). Emotional regulation, self-control, and psychopathology: The role of relationships in early childhood. In D. Cicchetti & S. L. Toth (Eds.), *Rochester Symposium on Developmental Psychopathology: Vol. 2. Internalizing and externalizing expressions of dysfunction* (pp. 21–36). Hillsdale, NJ: Erlbaum.

Greenberg, M. T., & Speltz, M. L. (1988). Contributions of attachment theory to the understanding of conduct problems during the preschool years. In J. Belsky & T. Nezworski (Eds.), *Clinical implications of attachment* (pp. 177–218). Hillsdale, NJ: Erlbaum.

Greenberg, M. T., Speltz, M. L., & DeKlyen, M. (1993). The role of attachment in the early development of disruptive behaviour problems. *Development and Psychopathology, 5,* 191–213.

Grossmann, K. E., & Grossmann, K. (1991). Attachment quality as an organizer of emotional and behavioral responses in a longitudinal perspective. In C. M. Parkes, J. Stevenson-Hinde, & P. Marris (Eds.), *Attachment across the life cycle* (pp. 93–114). London: Tavistock/Routledge.

Gunn, J., Maden, A., & Swinton, M. (1991). *The number of psychiatric cases amongst sentenced prisoners.* London: Home Office.

Gurr, T. R. (1977a). Contemporary crime in historical perspective: A comparative study of London, Stockholm, and Sydney. *Annals, 434,* 114–136.

Gurr, T. R. (1977b). Crime trends in modern democracies since 1945. *International Annals of Criminology, 16,* 41–85.

Gurr, T. R. (1981). Historical trends in crime: A review of the evidence. In N. Morris & M. Tonry (Eds.), *Crime and justice: An annual review of research* (Vol. 3, pp. 295–353). Chicago: University of Chicago Press.

Hare, R. D., & Cox, D. N. (1987). Clinical and empirical conceptions of psychopathy, and the selection of subjects for research. In R. D. Hare & D. Schalling (Eds.), *Psychopathic behaviour: Approaches to research* (pp. 1–21). Toronto: Wiley.

Harris, P. L., Johnson, C. N., Hutton, D., & Andrews, G., & Cooke, T. (1989). Young children's theory of mind and emotion. *Cognition and Emotion, 3,* 379–400.

Haskey, J. (1983). Remarriage of the divorced in England and Wales: A contemporary phenomenon. *Journal of Biosocial Science, 15,* 253–271.

Heidensohn, F. (1996). *Women and crime* (2nd ed.). London: Macmillan.

Hernandez, D. J. (1986). Childhood in sociodemographic perspective. *Annual Review of Sociology, 12,* 159–180.

Herting, J. R., & Guest, A. M. (1985). Components of satisfaction with local areas in the metropolis. *Sociological Quarterly, 26,* 99–115.

Hetherington, E. M. (1988). Parents, children, and siblings: Six years after divorce. In R. A. Hinde & J. Stevenson-Hinde (Eds.), *Relationships within families* (pp. 311–331). Oxford: Clarendon Press.

Hirschi, T. (1969). *Causes of delinquency.* Berkeley: University of California Press.

Hoffman, M. L. (1984). Empathy, its limitations and its role in a comprehensive moral theory. In J. Gewirtz & W. Kurtines (Eds.), *Morality, moral development and moral behaviour* (pp. 283–302). New York: Wiley.

Hoffmann-Nowotny, H. J. (1987). The future of the family. In *European population conference* (pp. 113–200). Helsinki: Central Statistical Office of Finland.

Hope, T., & Hough, M. (1988). Area, crime and incivilities: A profile from the British Crime Survey. In T. Hope & M. Shaw (Eds.), *Communities and crime reduction* (pp. 30–47). London: Her Majesty's Stationery Office.

Huesmann, L. R., Eron, L. D., Lefkowitz, M. M., & Walder, L. O. (1984). Stability of aggression over time and generations. *Developmental Psychology, 20*, 1120–1134.

Isabella, R. A., & Belsky, J. (1991). Interactional synchrony and the origins of infant–mother attachment: A replication study. *Child Development, 62*, 373–384.

Johnston, L. D. (1991). Toward a theory of drug epidemics. In L. Donohew, H. E. Sypher, & W. J. Bukoski (Eds.), *Persuasive communication and drug abuse prevention*. Hillsdale, NJ: Erlbaum.

Kagan, J. (1981). *The second year: The emergence of self awareness*. Cambridge, MA: Harvard University Press.

Kagan, J. (1989). *Unstable ideas*. New York: Basic Books.

Kagan, J. (1984). *The nature of the child*. New York: Basic Books.

Kandel, D. B., & Andrews, K. (1987). Processes of adolescent socialization by parents and peers. *International Journal of the Addictions, 22*, 319–342.

Keilman, N. (1987). Recent trends in family and household composition in Europe. *European Journal of Population, 3*, 297–325.

Kiernan, K. E. (1988). The British family: Contemporary trends and issues. *Journal of Family Issues, 9*, 298–316.

Kiernan, K. E., & Estaugh, V. (1993). *Cohabitation: Extra-marital childbearing and social policy*. London: Family Policy Studies Centre.

Kline, M., Johnston, J. R., & Tschann, J. M. (1991). The long shadow of marital conflict: A model of children's postdivorce adjustment. *Journal of Marriage and the Family, 53*, 297–309.

Kornhauser, R. (1978). *Social sources of delinquency*. Chicago: University of Chicago Press.

Lahey, B. B., McBurnett, K., Loeber, R., & Hart, E. L. (1994). Psychobiology. In G. P. Sholevar (Ed.), *Conduct disorders in children and adolescents: Assessments and interventions* (pp. 27–44). Washington, DC: American Psychiatric Press.

Lamb, M. (1987). Predictive implications of individual differences in attachment. *Journal of Consulting and Clinical Psychology, 55*, 817–824.

Levinson, A., & Fonagy, P. (submitted). Criminality and attachment: The relationship between interpersonal awareness and offending in a prison population.

Lewis, M., Feiring, C., McGuffog, C., & Jaskir, J. (1984). Predicting psychopathology in six-year-olds from early social relations. *Child Development, 55*, 123–136.

Loeber, R., & Dishion, T. (1983). Early predictors of male delinquency: A review. *Psychological Bulletin, 93*, 68–99.

Loeber, R., & Dishion, T. J. (1984). Boys who fight at home and school: Family conditions influencing cross-setting consistency. *Journal of Consulting and Clinical Psychology, 52*, 759–768.

Loeber, R., & Hay, D. F. (1994). Developmental approaches to aggression and conduct problems. In M. Rutter & D. H. Hay (Eds.), *Development through life: A handbook for clinicians.* Oxford: Blackwell Scientific.

Loeber, R., Keenan, K., Green, S. M., Lahey, B. B., & Thomas, C. (1993). Evidence for developmentally based diagnoses of oppositional defiant disorder and conduct disorder. *Journal of Abnormal Child Psychology, 21,* 377–410.

Loeber, R., & Stouthamer-Loeber, M. (1986). Family factors as correlates and predictors of juvenile conduct problems and delinquency. In M. Tonry & N. Morris (Eds.), *Crime and justice: An annual review of research* (Vol. 7, pp. 129–149). Chicago: University of Chicago Press.

Loeber, R., & Stouthamer-Loeber, M. (1987). Prediction. In H. C. Quay (Ed.), *Handbook of juvenile delinquency* (pp. 325–382). New York: Wiley.

Lyons-Ruth, K., Zoll, D., Connell, D., & Grunebaum, H. V. (1989). Familiy deviance and family disruption in childhood: Associations with maternal behavior and infant maltreatment during the first years of life. *Development and Psychopathology, 1,* 219–236.

Magnusson, D. (1987). Adult delinquency in the light of conduct and physiology at an early age: A longitudinal study. In D. Magnusson & A. Ohman (Eds.), *Psychopathology* (pp. 221–234). Orlando, FL: Academic Press.

Magnusson, D., Stattin, H., & Duner, A. (1983). Aggression and criminality in longitudinal perspective. In K. T. Van Dusen & S. A. Mednick (Eds.), *Antecedents of aggression and antisocial behavior.* Boston: Kluwer-Nijhoff.

Main, M. (1991). Metacognitive knowledge, metacognitive monitoring, and singular (coherent) vs. (incoherent) models of attachment: Findings and directions for future research. In C. M. Parkes, J. Stevenson-Hinde, & P. Marris (Eds.), *Attachment across the life cycle* (pp. 127–159). New York: Routledge.

Main, M., & Cassidy, J. (1985). *Assessments of child–parent attachment at six years of age.* Unpublished manual.

Main, M., & Hesse, E. (1990). Adult lack of resolution of attachment-related trauma related to infant disorganized/disoriented behaviour in the Ainsworth Strange Situation: Linking parental states of mind to infant bebaviour in a stressful situation. In M. T. Greenberg, D. Cicchetti, & M. Cummings (Eds.), *Attachment in the preschool years: Theory, research and intervention* (pp. 339–426). Chicago: University of Chicago Press.

Main, M., & Hesse, E. (1992). Disorganized/disoriented infant behavior in the Strange Situation, lapses in the monitoring of reasoning and discourse during the parent's Adult Attachment Interview, and dissociative states. In M. Ammaniti & D. Stern (Eds.), *Attachment and psychoanalysis.* Rome: Gius, Latereza and Figli.

Main, M., Kaplan, N., & Cassidy, J. (1985). Security in infancy, childhood and adulthood: A move to the level of representation. In I. Bretherton & E. Waters (Eds.), Growing points of attachment theory and research. *Monographs of the Society for Research in Child Development, 50*(1–2, Serial No. 209), 66–104.

Martin, J. (1981). A longitudinal study of the consequences of early mother–infant interaction: A microanalytic approach. *Monographs of the Society for Research in Child Development, 46*(3, Serial No. 59), 1–58.

McCord, J. (1980). Patterns of deviance. In S. B. Sells, R. Crandall, M. Roff, J. S. Strauss, & W. Pollin (Eds.), *Human functioning in longitudinal perspective* (pp. 157–165). Baltimore: Williams & Wilkins.

McMahon, R. J., & Forehand, R. (1988). Conduct disorders. In E. J. Mash & L. G. Terdal (Eds.), *Behavioral assessment of childhood disorders* (2nd ed., pp. 105–153). New York: Guilford Press.

Meloy, J. R. (1988a). Violent homicidal behavior in primitive mental states. *Journal of the American Academy of Psychoanalysis, 16,* 381–394.

Meloy, J. R. (1988b). *The psychopathic mind: Origins, dynamics, and treatment.* Northvale, NJ: Jason Aronson.

Meloy, J. R. (1992). *Violent attachments.* Northvale, NJ: Jason Aronson.

Miller, P. A., Eisenberg, N., Fabes, R. A., Shell, R., & Gular, S. (1989). Mothers' emotional arousal as a moderator in the socialization of children's empathy. *New Directions for Child Development, 44,* 65–83.

Moffitt, T. E. (1993). The neuropsychology of conduct disorder. *Development and Psychopathology, 5,* 135–151.

Monkkonen, E. H. (1981). A disorderly people? Urban order in the nineteenth and twentieth centuries. *Journal of American History, 68,* 536–559.

Mortimore, P., Sammons, P., Stoll, L., Lewis, D., & Ecob, R. (1988). *School matters: The junior years.* Wells, Somerset: Open Books.

Moses, L. J., & Flavell, J. H. (1990). Inferring false beliefs from actions and reactions. *Child Development, 61,* 929–945.

Mott, F. L., & Haurin, R. J. (1982). Being an only child: Effects on educational progression and career orientation. *Journal of Family Issues, 3,* 575–593.

Murray, C. A. (1983). The physical environment and community control of crime. In J. Q. Wilson (Ed.), *Crime and public policy* (pp. 107–122). San Francisco, CA: Institute for Contemporary Studies.

Nelson, L. A. (1987). The recognition of facial expressions in the first two years of life: Mechanisms of development. *Child Development, 58,* 889–909.

Norem-Hebeisen, A., Johnson, D. W., Anderson, D., & Johnson, R. (1984). Predictors and concomitants of changes in drug use patterns among teenagers. *Journal of Social Psychology, 124,* 43–50.

Olweus, D. (1979). Stability of aggressive reaction patterns in males: A review. *Psychological Bulletin, 86,* 852–875.

Olweus, D. (1984). Development of stable aggressive reaction patterns in males. In R. J. Blanchard & D. C. Blanchard (Eds.), *Advances in the study of aggression* (pp. 103–137). New York: Academic Press.

Orsagh, T., & Witte, A. D. (1981). Economic status and crime: Implications for offender rehabilitation. *Journal of Criminal Law and Criminology, 72,* 1055–1071.

Patterson, G. R. (1982). *A social learning approach to family intervention: III. Coercive family process.* Eugene, OR: Castalia.

Patterson, G. R. (1986). Performance models for antisocial boys. *American Psychologist, 41,* 432–444.

Patterson, G. R., DeBarsyshe, B. D., & Ramsey, E. (1989). A developmental perspective on antisocial behavior. *American Psychologist, 44,* 329–335.

Patterson, G. R., & Stouthamer-Loeber, M. (1984). The correlation of family management practices and delinquency. *Child Development, 55,* 1299–1307.

Perner, J., Leekam, S. R., & Wimmer, H. (1987). Three-year-olds' difficulty with false belief. *British Journal of Developmental Psychology, 5,* 125–137.

Peterson, P. L., Hawkins, J. D., Abbott, R. D., & Catalano, R. F. (1994). Disentangling the effects of parental drinking, family management, and parental alcohol norms on current drinking by black and white adolescents. *Journal of Research on Adolescence, 4,* 203–227.

Pettit, G. S., & Bates, J. E. (1989). Family interaction patterns and children's behavior problems from infancy to 4 years. *Developmental Psychology, 25,* 413–420.

Popenoe, D. (1987). Beyond the nuclear family: A statistical portrait of the changing family in Sweden. *Journal of Marriage and the Family, 49,* 173–183.

Poulin-Dubois, D., & Shultz, T. R. (1988). The development of the understanding of human behavior: From agency to intentionality. In J. Astington, P. Harris, & D. Olson (Eds.), *Developing theories of mind* (pp. 109–125). New York: Cambridge University Press.

Quay, H. C. (1988). The behavioral reward and inhibition system in childhood behavior disorder. In L. M. Bloomingdale (Eds.), *Attention deficit disorder* (pp. 176–186). Oxford: Pergamon.

Quinton, D., Pickles, A., Maughan, B., & Rutter, M. (1993). Partners, peers and pathways: Assortative pairing and continuities in conduct disorder. *Development and Psychopathology, 5,* 763–783.

Reid, J. B., & Patterson, G. R. (1989). The development of antisocial behavior patterns in childhood and adolescence. *European Journal of Personality, 3,* 107–119.

Reiss, A. J., Jr., & Roth, J. A. (Eds.). (1993). *Understanding and preventing violence.* Washington, DC: National Academy Press.

Reiss, D., Hetherington, E. M., Plomin, R., Howe, G. W., Simmens, S. J., Henderson, S. H., O'Connor, T. J., Bussell, D. A., Anderson, E. R., & Law, T. (1995). Genetic questions for environmental studies: Differential parenting and psychopathology in adolescence. *Archives of General Psychiatry, 52,* 925–936.

Renken, B., Egeland, B., Marvinney, D., Mangelsdorf, S., & Sroufe, L. A. (1989). Early childhood antecedents of aggression and passive-withdrawal in early elementary school. *Journal of Personality, 57,* 257–281.

Rest, J. R. (1983). Morality. In J. H. Flavell & E. M. Markman (Eds.), *Handbook of child psychology: Vol. 3. Cognitive development* (pp. 556–629). New York: Wiley.

Revitch, E., & Schlesinger, L. (1978). Murder: Evaluation, classification, and prediction. In I. Kutash, S. Kutash, & L. Schlesinger (Eds.), *Violence: Perspectives on murder and aggression* (pp. 138–164). San Francisco: Jossey-Bass.

Revitch, E., & Schlesinger, L. (1981). *Psychopathology of homicide.* Springfield, IL: Charles C Thomas.

Richters, J. E., & Walters, E. (1991). Attachment and socialization: The positive side of social influence. In M. Lewis & S. Feinman (Eds.), *Social influences and socialization in infancy* (pp. 185–213). New York: Plenum Press.

Robins, L. N. (1991). Conduct disorder. *Journal of Child Psychiatry and Psychology, 32,* 193–212.

Robins, L. N., & Regier, D. A. (Eds.). (1991). *Psychiatric disorders in America: The epidemiologic catchment area study.* New York: Free Press.

Robinson, E. A. (1985). Coercion theory revisited: Toward a new theoretical perspective on the etiology of conduct disorders. *Clinical Psychology Review, 5,* 577–626.

Roll, J. (1992). *Lone parent families in the European Community.* London: European Family and Social Policy Unit.

Rowe, D. C. (1990). Inherited dispositions toward learning delinquent and criminal behavior: New evidence. In L. Ellis & H. Hoffman (Eds.), *Crime in biological, social, and moral contexts* (pp. 121–133). New York: Praeger.

Rowe, D. C., & Osgood, D. W. (1990). A latent trait approach to unifying criminal careers. *Criminology, 28,* 237–370.

Rowe, D. C., Woulbroun, E. J., & Gulley, B. L. (1994). Peers and friends as nonshared environmental influences. In E. M. Hetherington, D. Reiss, & R. Plomin (Eds.), *Separate social worlds of siblings: The impact of nonshared environment on development.* Hillsdale, NJ: Erlbaum.

Ruotolo, A. (1968). Dynamics of sudden murder. *American Journal of Psychoanalysis, 28,* 162–176.

Rutter, M. (1985a). Family and school influences on behavioral development. *Journal of Child Psychology and Psychiatry, 26,* 349–368.

Rutter, M. (1985b). Resilience in the face of adversity: Protective factors and resistance to psychiatric disorder. *British Journal of Psychiatry, 147,* 598–611.

Rutter, M. (1987). Psychosocial resilience and protective mechanisms. *American Journal of Orthopsychiatry, 57,* 316–331.

Rutter, M. (Ed.). (1988). *Studies of psychosocial risk.* New York: Cambridge University Press.

Rutter, M., Maughan, B., Mortimore, P., Ouston, J., & Smith, A. (1979). *15,000 hours: Secondary schools and their effects on children.* London: Open Books.

Sagi, A., Lamb, M. E., Lewkowicz, K. S., Shoham, R., Dvir, R., & Estes, D. (1985). Security of infant–mother, –father, and –metapelet among kibbutz reared Israeli children. In I. Bretherton & E. Waters (Eds.), Growing points of attachment theory and research. *Monographs of the Society for Research in Child Development, 50*(1–2, Serial No. 209), 257–275.

Sampson, R. J. (1987). Crime in cities: The effects of formal and informal social control. In A. J. Reiss Jr. & M. Tonry (Eds.), *Crime And justice: An annual review of research: Vol. 8. Communities and crime* (pp. 101–136). Chicago: University of Chicago Press.

Sampson, R. J., & Laub, J. H. (1990). Crime and deviance over the life course:

The salience of adult social bonds. *American Sociological Review, 55,* 609–627.

Sampson, R. J., & Laub, J. H. (1993). *Crime in the making: Pathways and turning points through life.* Cambridge, MA: Harvard University Press.

Sampson, R. J., & Wooldredge, J. D. (1987). Linking the micro- and macro-level dimensions of lifestyle: Routine activity and opportunity models of predatory victimization. *Journal of Quantitative Criminology, 3,* 371–393.

Sanson, A., Oberklaid, F., Pedlow, R., & Prior, M. (1991). Risk indicators: Assessment of infancy predictors of preschool behavioral maladjustment. *Journal of Child Psychology and Psychiatry, 32,* 609–626.

Sardon, J. P. (1990). *Cohort fertility in member states of the Council of Europe.* (Population Studies, 21). Strasbourg: Council of Europe.

Schmid, J. (1984). *The background of recent fertility trends in the member states of the Council of Europe* (Population Studies, 15). Strasbourg: Council of Europe.

Schuerman, L., & Kobrin, S. (1987). Community careers in crime. In A. J. Reiss Jr. & M. Tonry (Eds.), *Crime and justice: An annual review of research: Vol. 8. Communities and crime* (pp. 67–100). Chicago: University of Chicago Press.

Shantz, C. U. (1983). Social cognition. In J. H. Flavell & E. M. Markman (Eds.), *Handbook of child psychology: Vol. 3. Cognitive developments* (pp. 495–555). New York: Wiley.

Shaw, D. S., & Bell, R. Q. (1993). Developmental theories of parental contributors to antisocial behavior. *Journal of Abnormal Child Psychology, 21,* 493–518.

Shaw, D. S., & Vondra, J. I. (1993). Chronic family adversity and infant attachment security. *Journal of Child Psychology and Psychiatry, 34,* 1205–1215.

Silbereisen, R. K., Robins, L., & Rutter, M. (1995). Secular trends in substance use: Concepts and data on the impact of social change on alcohol and drug abuse. In M. Rutter & D. J. Smith (Eds.), *Psychosocial disorders in young people: Time trends and their causes* (pp. 490–543). Chichester: Wiley.

Smith, D. J. (1995a). Youth crime and conduct disorders: Trends, patterns and causal explanations. In M. Rutter & D. J. Smith (Eds.), *Psychosocial disorders in young people: Time trends and their causes* (pp. 389–489). Chichester: Wiley.

Smith, D. J. (1995b). Living conditions in the twentieth century. In M. Rutter & D. J. Smith (Eds.), *Psychosocial disorders in young people: Time trends and their causes* (pp. 194–295). Chichester: Wiley.

Smith, D. J., & Tomlinson, S. (1989). *The school effect: A study of multi-racial comprehensives.* London: Policy Studies Institute.

Smith, I. (1990). Alcohol and crime: The problem in Australia. In R. Bluglass & P. Bowden (Eds.), *Principles and practice of forensic psychiatry* (pp. 947–951). Edinburgh: Churchill Livingstone.

Sorce, J., Emde, R., Campos, J., & Klinnert, M. (1985). Maternal emotional signalling: Its effect on the visual cliff behavior of 1 year olds. *Developmental Psychology, 21,* 195–200.

Speltz, M. L., Greenberg, M. T., & DeKlyen, M. (1990). Attachment in preschoolers with disruptive behavior: A comparison of clinic-referred and nonproblem children. *Development and Psychopathology, 2,* 31–46.

Spieker, S. J., & Booth, C. L. (1988). Maternal antecedents of attachment quality. In J. Belsky & T. Nezworski (Eds.), *Clinical implications of attachment theory* (pp. 95–135). Hillsdale, NJ: Erlbaum.

Spitzer, R. L., Williams, J. B. W., Gibbon, M., & First, M. B. (1990). *User's guide for the Structured Clinical Interview for DSM-III-R*. Washington, DC: American Psychiatric Press.

Sroufe, L. A., Carlson, E., & Shulman, R. (1993). Individuals in relationships: Development from infancy through adolescence. In D. C. Funder, R. D. Parke, C. Tomlinson-Keasey, & K. Widaman (Eds.), *Studying lives through time: Personality and development* (pp. 315–342). Washington, DC: American Psychological Association.

Steele, H., Steele, M., & Fonagy, P. (1996). Associations among attachment classifications of mothers, fathers, and their infants. *Child Development, 67*, 541–555.

Strayhorn, J. M., & Weidman, C. S. (1991). Follow-up one year after parent–child interaction training: Effects on behavior of preschool children. *Journal of the American Academy of Child and Adolescent Psychiatry, 30*, 138–143.

Sutherland, E. H., & Cressey, D. R. (1978). *Principles of criminology*. Philadelphia: Lippincott.

Taylor, P. J. (1986). Psychiatric disorder in London's life sentenced prisoners. *British Journal of Criminology, 26*, 63–78.

Thornberry, T. P. (1994). *Violent families and youth violence* (Fact Sheet No. 21). Washington, DC: U.S. Department of Justice, Office of Juvenile Justice and Delinquency Prevention.

Tolan, P., & Guerra, N. (1994). *What works in reducing adolescent violence: An empirical review of the field*. Report submitted to the Center for the Study and Prevention of Violence, University of Illinois at Chicago.

Tomasello, M., Kruger, A., & Ratner, H. H. (1993). Cultural learning. *Behavioral and Brain Sciences, 16*, 495–552.

Tonry, M., Ohlin, L. E., Farrington, D. P., Adams, K., Earls, F., Rowe, D. C., Sampson, R. J., & Tremblay, R. E. (1991). *Human development and criminal behavior: New ways of advancing knowledge*. New York: Springer-Verlag.

Turiel, E. (1983). Domains and categories in social–cognitive development. In W. F. Overton (Ed.), *The relationship between social and cognitive development* (pp. 53–89). Hillsdale, NJ: Erlbaum.

Turner, P. (1991). Relations between attachment, gender, and behavior with peers in the preschool. *Child Development, 62*, 1475–1488.

Urban, J., Carlson, E., Egeland, B., & Sroufe, L. A. (1991). Patterns of individual adaptation across childhood. *Development and Psychopathology, 3*, 445–460.

Voydanoff, P., & Majka, L. C. (1988). *Families and economic distress*. Newbury Park, CA: Sage.

Wallerstein, J. S. (1991). The long-term effects of divorce on children: A review. *Journal of the American Academy of Child and Adolescent Psychiatry, 30*, 349–360.

Weber, C. A., Meloy, J. R., & Gacono, C. B. (1992). A Rorschach study of attachment and anxiety in inpatient conduct-disordered and dysthymic adolescents. *Journal of Personality Assessment, 58*, 16–26.

Weiss, J., Lamberti, J., & Blackman, N. (1960). The sudden murderer II: A comparative analysis. *Archives of General Psychiatry, 2,* 669–678.

Weiss, R. S. (1984). The impact of marital dissolution on income and consumption in single-parent households. *Journal of Marriage and the Family, 46,* 115–127.

Weitzman, L. J. (1985). *The divorce revolution.* New York: Free Press.

Wellman, H. M., & Banerjee, M. (1991). Mind and emotion: children's understanding of the emotional consequences of beliefs and desires. *British Journal of Developmental Psychology, 9,* 191–214.

Wellman, H. M., & Bartsch, K. (1988). Young children's reasoning about beliefs. *Cognition, 30,* 239–277.

Werner, E. E., & Smith, R. S. (1982). *Vulnerable but invincible: A longitudinal study of resilient children and youth.* New York: McGraw-Hill.

Wertham, F. (1966). *A sign for Cain.* New York: Macmillan.

White, J. L., Moffitt, T. E., Earls, F., Robins, L., & Silva, P. A. (1990). How early can we tell? *Criminology, 28,* 507–533.

White, L. K., & Booth, A. (1985). The quality and stability of remarriages: The role of stepchildren. *American Sociological Review, 50,* 689–698.

Wiklund, N., & Lidberg, L. (1990). Alcohol as a causal criminogenic factor: The Scandinavian experience. In R. Bluglass & P. Bowden (Eds.), *Principles and practice of forensic psychiatry* (pp. 941–945). Edinburgh: Churchill Livingstone.

Wilson, J. Q., & Herrnstein, R. (1985). *Crime and human nature.* New York: Simon & Schuster.

Wilson, J. Q., & Kelling, G. (1982, March). Broken windows. *The Atlantic Monthly,* pp. 29–38.

Yoshikawa, H. (1994). Prevention as cumulative protection: Effects of early family support and education on chronic delinquency and its risks. *Psychological Bulletin, 115,* 28–54.

Zahn-Waxler, C., Cole, P., & Barrett, K. C. (1991). Guilt and empathy: Sex differences and implications for the development of depression. In J. Garber & K. Dodge (Eds.), *The development of emotion regulation and dysregulation* (pp. 243–272). Cambridge, England: Cambridge University Press.

Zahn-Waxler, C., Cummings, E. M., McKnew, D., & Radke-Yarrow, M. (1984). Altruism, aggression and social interactions in young children with a manic–depressive parent. *Child Development, 55,* 112–122.

Zahn-Waxler, C., Kochanska, G., Krupnick, J., & McKnew, D. (1990). Patterns of guilt in children of depressed and well mothers. *Developmental Psychology, 26,* 51–59.

Zoccolillo, M., Pickles, A., Quinton, D., & Rutter, M. (1992). The outcome of childhood conduct disorder: Implications for defining adult personality disorder and conduct disorder. *Psychological Medicine, 22,* 971–986.

SECTION III

IN THE CLINIC

9

Toddlers' Internalization of Maternal Attributions as a Factor in Quality of Attachment

ALICIA F. LIEBERMAN

This chapter represents an effort to expand the areas of maternal and infant functioning that are currently being studied to document the parameters of intergenerational transmission of patterns of attachment. Specifically, maternal attributions are discussed as a vehicle for the transmission of important components of the mother's working models of attachment. The argument is made that these attributions are internalized by the infant and become an integral component of the child's working models of attachment and of the self in relation to attachment. Maternal attributions are at the interface between objective, observable, measurable reality and psychological, subjective reality. In this sense, maternal attributions are colored by maternal fantasies (i.e., unconscious wishes and fears) about who the child is and who he or she might become. In describing the role of maternal attributions in the child's emotional development, this chapter attempts to restore fantasy as a legitimate area of inquiry into the attachment process.

Much of our current understanding of babies is anchored on the notion that what happens to them becomes an integral part of who they are. This is particularly evident when we consider the ways babies are treated and the relationships they have. Through their exchanges with attachment figures and other significant people in their lives, infants learn what they can expect from others and in this process they form lasting, viscerally held convictions about their own worth and lovability and their place in the world. This internalization of social reality plays a crucial role in shaping the infant's emotional development, laying the earliest foundations of personality and contributing in major ways to a general predisposition toward mental health versus psychopathology.

No theorist has been as persuasive or as adamant about tracing the reality-based origins of the child's inner life as has John Bowlby (1969/1982, 1973, 1980). Bowlby was trained as a psychoanalyst at a time when children's fantasy life was considered the predominant factor in the genesis of neurosis, and when many child analysts did not meet regularly with the parents of their little patients because the trials and tribulations of everyday life were considered of little import to the progress of the child's analysis. In this theoretical and clinical zeitgeist, Bowlby's insistence on the importance of real-life events and his relentless demonstrations that children's fears, anger, depression, and behavioral problems could be traced to actual parental threats, excessive punitiveness, distortions of reality, inconsistent care, and separation or loss were greeted with skepticism and even derision by many of his colleagues. Even today, when there is a growing rapprochement between certain sectors of psychoanalysis and attachment theory, and when renowned psychoanalysts such as Robert Wallerstein (1973) are calling for a psychoanalytic view of reality, there is still considerable debate about the role of real-life events in personality formation and in the genesis of mental health disorders.

The influences of the mother and the mother–child relationship have been at the forefront in this debate between fantasy and reality because the mother figure comprises the infant's first and most encompassing environment, the environment most intimately connected to early experiences of well-being or distress. As a result, the mother has a mystique unmatched by any other figure in the emotional landscape of humans. She is both archetypal and instinctual, mythical and prosaic, the idealized object of adoration and longing as well as the unforgivable culprit for all that goes wrong. She creates reality and engenders fantasy simply by fulfilling her role. Only a figure as closely associated with physical and psychological survival at the individual and group levels could evoke the tumultuous range of emotions associated with her in public and private life (Neumann, 1955).

Given the difficulties of achieving proper scientific detachment in studying such an affectively charged figure, the great contribution of attachment theory has been to provide a conceptual framework that allows for empirically based investigations of the mother's behavior and its influence on the child–mother relationship and on the infant's development. The use of observable behavior, launched by attachment theorists as an indicator of inner experiences, has bridged a historical gap between clinicians and researchers. It is now possible to investigate important emotional processes in a methodologically sound manner, relying on the knowledge derived from decades of clinical work to ask important questions and to venture researchable hypotheses about possible answers. We can begin to ascertain how what the mother feels and does is perceived and responded to by the child, and in this way we can learn how external reality contributes to create internal reality.

This contribution of attachment theory is most clearly evident in the work of Mary Ainsworth, who set the standard for attachment research when she integrated the use of detailed, clinically driven, longitudinal home observations of mother–infant interaction in the first year of life with the use of the laboratory-based Strange Situation procedure (Ainsworth, Blehar, Waters, & Wall, 1978). Through Ainsworth's seminal studies and others that followed (about a thousand in the last 15 years, by some estimates) we have learned the following:

1. Individual differences in the quality of the baby's attachment can be reliably categorized on the basis of security or anxiousness about the mother's availability.
2. There are fairly predictable links between quality of attachment and the history of the mother–child relationship in the first year.
3. Individual differences in quality of attachment are chronologically stable under stable family conditions but they may shift when family circumstances lead to change in maternal availability.
4. Quality of attachment in infancy is a reasonably good predictor of social–emotional functioning through at least adolescence.
5. The quality of care the mother is able to provide is greatly influenced by the quality of marital or other family support available to her in raising her child.

These conclusions are derived on the basis of careful measurement of maternal and child behavior. The core finding, replicated in different contexts and with different specific measures, is that maternal sensitivity and contingency of response are fairly accurate predictors of the child's security of attachment, whereas her unavailability is associated with different kinds of anxiety in the child. Specifically, mothers who dislike physical contact and are covertly rejecting of the child tend to have infants classified as avoidant in the Strange Situation, mothers who are inconsistently available tend to have infants classified as resistant, and mothers with different forms of psychopathology or unresolved mourning tend to have disorganized babies who lack a coherent strategy to cope with separation and reunion with the mother.

The next question, of course, is: what are the inner structures generating these observable behaviors? Specifically, how are the experiences of attachment, and of the self in relation to attachment, organized at the level of symbolic representation? Mary Main and her students launched the search for an answer through the development of the Adult Attachment Interview, during which mothers were asked to describe in detail their memories and feelings about their relationship with their parents, including experiences of nurturance and comfort as well as those of rejection, separation, and loss. The results uncovered marked structural similarities between the maternal representations of adults as inferred from their answers to the interview and the behavioral manifestations of infants' quality of attachment as observed in the Strange Situation. Whereas babies are classified as secure, avoidant, resistant, or disorganized, mothers are classified as autonomous, dismissive, preoccupied, or unresolved with regard to issues of attachment (Main, Kaplan, & Cassidy, 1985).

How do these structured similarities across development come about? Following Bowlby, Mary Main proposed that the individual differences in the Adult Attachment Interview reflect differences in maternal internal working models of attachment, which are formed and consolidated in the course of development and, once established, provide reliable rules for organizing information relevant to attachment and making this information available or blocking access to it. Those rules are passed on to the next generation because the mother's internal working model of attachment is used not only to organize her own experience, but it also is used as a filter that guides her responses to her own child's affect and behavior. Judy Cassidy (1994) has suggested that the insecure patterns of attachment—namely, the avoidant and resistant patterns in infancy, and the dismissive and preoccupied patterns in adulthood—represent maladaptive strategies regulating negative affect through defenses which minimize affect in the case of avoidant and dismissive patterns, and maximize affect in the case of resistant and preoccupied types. In contrast, the secure pattern involves flexible access to negative affect and the ability to regulate it adaptively through integration with positive affect.

If internal working models of attachment serve to provide or block access to affective experiences and to regulate negative affect, it makes sense to predict the intergenerational transmission of patterns of attachment from mother to child. Mothers would essentially be modeling to their children how to cope with negative affect, teaching them what is acceptable or forbidden to feel and to express. Indeed, there is emerging evidence of a link between maternal representations and child quality of attachment (Fonagy, Steele, & Steele, 1991; Zeanah et al., 1993; see also van IJzendoorn & Bakermans-Kranenberg, Chapter 5, this volume). These studies report that not only do autonomous mothers tend to have secure children and anxiously attached mothers tend to have anxiously attached children, but also, more specifically, dismissing mothers are likely to have avoidant babies, and preoccupied mothers are likely to have resistant babies. If replicated, these studies would indicate that the basic structure of early defenses shows a remarkable similarity in mothers and their young infants, at least as assessed by theoretically compatible research instruments.

CLINICAL CONTRIBUTIONS TO THE UNDERSTANDING OF INTERGENERATIONAL TRANSMISSION

The intergenerational continuities that are emerging through this research confirm clinical reports that overly intense maternal ambivalence is associated with disturbances in the child's attachment and in the social and emotional development of the infant. Selma Fraiberg captured this phenomenon most vividly when she coined the now-famous expression "ghosts in the nursery," which refers to the infant's engulfment in the mother's unresolved psychological conflicts (Fraiberg, Adelson, & Shapiro, 1975). Based on this insight, Fraiberg and her colleagues developed infant–parent psychotherapy as a clinical method of intervention designed to address the manifestations of the mother's ambivalence in her attitudes and interactions with her baby. The goal of infant–parent psychotherapy is to trace the origins of this ambivalence by eliciting the mother's emotional experience of her own attachment figures. In this process, the mother learns to identify those negative responses to the baby that are displacements in the present of the anger, fear, and other painful affects she experienced in her interactions with attachment figures. When the mother achieves an emotional differentiation between her feelings toward her baby and her unresolved feelings toward attachment figures from her childhood, the baby can in effect be freed from the malevolent "ghosts" of the mother's past (Fraiberg, 1980). The effectiveness of this approach in reversing disorders of attachment was demonstrated in a randomized trial in which infants and mothers receiving infant–parent psychotherapy in the infant's second year of life were found to have significantly more adaptive scores than did an untreated comparison group in measures derived from attachment theory, including goal-corrected partnership, maternal empathy, and child anger, avoidance, and resistance toward the mother (Lieberman, Weston, & Pawl, 1991).

The clinical process of infant–parent psychotherapy is of great value in tracing the intergenerational transmission of disorders of attachment (Lieberman, 1985, 1991; Lieberman & Pawl, 1988, 1990, 1993). The narrative records of infant–parent psychotherapy sessions consist of detailed and, whenever possible, verbatim accounts of what mother and baby said and did during each session. The therapist uses these clinical notes to reflect on the psychological processes that emerge and to devise a specific, individually tailored approach to intervention. In addition to this clinical function, the notes also provide access to detailed descriptions of maternal attitudes, feelings, memories, and associations, her wishes and fears, her behavior toward her infant, and her infant's behavior toward her. In this sense, clinical notes are comparable in their hypothesis-generating value to the detailed transcripts of home observations that comprised the basis of Mary Ainsworth's seminal research on the development of attachment in the first year of life (Ainsworth et al., 1978).

From this rich observational and narrative material, maternal attributions toward the baby have emerged as a particularly useful area of inquiry for understanding the process of intergenerational transmission of conflicts about attachment. In our clinical population mothers often perceive their babies along dimensions that are dictated by their own psychological difficulties rather than by normative developmental concerns. In other words, they attribute to the baby characteristics and motives that are rooted in their own internal conflicts and do not reflect the baby's motivations and needs. The pressure to comply with these maternal attributions is gradually internalized by the baby, who often comes to behave in ways that are strikingly concordant with the mother's attributions. These observations suggest that maternal attributions represent a valuable route for studying the intergenerational transmission of disorders of attachment from mother to child.

MATERNAL ATTRIBUTIONS AS EXPRESSIONS OF WORKING MODELS

Maternal attributions could be described as fixed beliefs that the mother has about her child's existential core, beliefs that she perceives as objective, accurate perceptions of the child's essence but might in fact reflect the mother's fantasies, including her fears, conflicts, and wishes about the child and the child's function in her life. Of course, parents routinely make attributions to their children, and many of those attributions are essential for the child's healthy development. Dix and Grusec (1985) outlined four essential features of the social context for normative parental attributions. First, parents make inferences about the developmentally determined motives and limitations characteristic of specific ages. Second, attributions need to keep pace with the rate of change inherent in the child's development. Third, the external pressures affecting a child are incorporated into the parental attribution process. Fourth, attributions reflect the parents' need to see themselves as competent in raising their children and to take pleasure in the child as a reflection of themselves.

This conceptualization of parental attributions incorporates the information-processing features that are characteristic of attribution theory. It stresses that parents' responses to their children are determined by an ongoing assessment of the causes of their children's behavior, including the role of the children's characteristic traits and the impact of situational factors as causative factors. This conceptual framework emphasizes the flexibility of the parental attributional process. Parental attributions are described as changing according to the child's age, personal characteristics, and life circumstances. There is also an emphasis on the role of pleasure and positive self-esteem that parents derive from their children. The model depicts the normative attributional process of ordinary, reasonably well-adjusted, "good enough" parents whose positive feelings substantially outweigh their ambivalence toward their children.

In a clinical population of parents and infants with severe disorders of attachment, parental attributions are characterized by the absence of precisely those features identified by Dix and Grusec (1985). Babies become the recipients of pervasively negative or developmentally inappropriate parental perceptions. Rather than flexibly attuned to the characteristics of the child's age, personality characteristics, and situational factors, parental attributions are rigid, constricting, and not amenable to change. Instead of reflecting maternal self-esteem and pleasure in the child's positive characteristics, such attributions reflect the mother's fears, anger, or other suppressed or unacknowledged parts of herself.

Negative attributions can be more or less rigid and more or less attuned with reality in the sense that their content may be relatively consistent with the child's own characteristics and developmental stage, or they may be frankly bizarre and even delusional. Negative attributions may also be rather isolated or permeate the mother's entire perception of the child. One mother, for example, perceived her 3-month-old daughter as so cunning that, according to the mother, she jumped from her crib adjacent to the parental bed to breastfeed while the mother was asleep, and then jumped back to her crib. This was the mother's explanation for not having as much milk in the mornings as she expected. This rather bizarre attribution could be very worrisome depending on the context, but in fact it remained isolated from other perceptions of the child and had a rather harmless origin: the mother's hope that her daughter could take care of herself even when the mother was not consciously available to her, for example, when she was asleep. Negative maternal attributions can begin before the child's birth. One pregnant woman, who was preoccupied with her voracious appetite for food and with her anger when her eating was interrupted, described her unborn baby as "demanding" and "devouring of every bit of energy" the mother had. When her daughter was 2 days old, the mother commented, "She is pretty, but she is very greedy." In keeping with her fantasies during pregnancy, this mother misinterpreted her baby daughter's healthy appetite as a sign of voraciousness. If the baby cried while the mother was eating, this woman attributed the baby's crying to her greediness and her desire to deprive the mother of food. When recounting her own experiences with food as a young child, this mother reexperienced the anger and fear associated with not having enough food. As the oldest of five children, she was the last in line at the table and she remembered routinely finding that the best morsels were gone by the time the platters of food reached her.

As this example indicates, maternal attributions are usefully conceptualized as products or reflections of the mother's internal working models of the infant and of herself in relation to attachment. These attributions embody the ways in which the mother experiences herself and her infant, and they carry the imprint of the mother's early experiences of self in relationship to her own attachment figures. The study of maternal attributions yields specific information about these experiences and their transmission to the infant. Whereas current conceptualizations of working models of attachment describe predominant defensive styles that are abstracted from the mother's narrative (i.e., dismissive, preoccupied, disorganized, autonomous), maternal attributions offer an unedited view of fantasies and concrete perceptions that guide the mother's actual ministrations toward the child and directly shape the infant's emerging working model of the self in relation to attachment.

Maternal attributions shape which baby behaviors the mother can become attuned to and which behaviors are ignored or misinterpreted. Daniel Stern (1985) coined the expression "selective attunement" to describe how mothers share in the subjective experiences of their infants and influence these experiences in ways that correspond to the mother's own agendas. By attuning to some subjective states of their babies and not to others, mothers inject their own fantasies, desires, fears, and prohibitions into the baby's sense of what they are and are not permitted to feel. Christopher Bollas (1987), in his influential book *The Shadow of the Object,* framed this process using a psychoanalytic perspective but an equally compelling image. He described the mother as a "transformational object," that is, a person who through her actions changes the baby's sense of self. When we think of the multiple concrete actions of the mother that transform the baby's subjective experience—from feeding and diapering to soothing a crying baby or engaging a restless baby in play—and when we think of the microscopic, moment-to-moment interpretations of the baby's behavior that mothers make before they intervene (Stern, 1985, p. 206, calculates that on the average there is one maternal attunement per minute), we can grasp the extent to which the mother's interpretations of the baby and her resulting ministrations get woven into the very texture of how the baby experiences himself. In the case of the mother who saw her 2-day-old daughter as "greedy," this attribution of greediness had a rather straightforward expression. The mother let the baby cry for long periods of time (30 to 40 minutes) if the crying occurred while the mother was eating. She first finished her meal, however long it took, and only then did she tend to her baby. By then the child was often so overwrought and disorganized that she could not be calmed down and choked on the milk the mother tried to feed her. This was interpreted by the mother as a confirmation of her perception that her daughter was greedy, overly demanding, and had an "unrealistic" expectation that her needs should be met before her mother's.

Observations of the mother and daughter revealed that this mother's attributions, and the behaviors through which she expressed them, were creating in her child the same anxiety about the availability of food and the same frantic need to eat immediately that the mother suffered from. At a very young age, this baby was learning that hunger can be so intense and prolonged that it cannot be satisfied even when food is finally available. The mother's resentment and feelings of being exploited, which manifested themselves in tense and jerky movements and an angry facial expression, compounded the daughter's experience of hunger as a painful visceral sensation that was accompanied by an equally painful alienation from her mother. This baby was learning that the person she depended on could become the source of privation and suffering rather than of comfort and protection. In this dyad, the mother was indeed a transformational object, but one who transformed average discomfort and bearable hunger pangs into intense agony rather than well-being as the baby wailed for the milk that first choked her and only later could succeed in filling her up. As a result, the baby was developing an eating disorder that shared many features of her mother's eating disorder.

THE INFANT'S INTERNALIZATION OF MATERNAL ATTRIBUTIONS

Experiences like those described above are encoded at the most visceral, nonverbal levels of the child's sense of self long before the baby is able to form a stable mental representation of the mother. These experiences become sensorimotor memories that build the foundations of an existential sense of self through the creation and storage in memory of states of being. As Bollas (1987) describes it, the mother is "known less as a discrete object with particular qualities than as a process linked to the infant's being and the alteration of his being" (p. 4). Unless negative maternal attributions can be transformed through the mother's inner development, these sensorimotor memories become integrated with similar experiences that occur at a later age and are semantically encoded by the child, giving rise to symbolic representations of the self and the mother. Gradually, the maternal attributions shape the child's sense of who he is. When this occurs, children come to see themselves and to behave in the ways their mothers see them and expect them to behave. The early sensorimotor memories coalesce with semantic memories to form an image of who the mother is and who the child is in relation to her.

Sometimes the same negative maternal attribution is visited and revisited on the child throughout his formative years and even into adulthood, as in the case of the mother who said of her 40-year-old son, "He was a con artist from the day he was born." Other times the negative attribution takes different expressions as the child's developmental acquisitions elicit different conflicts in the mother. One mother, for example, seeing a squashed bug on her sleeping baby daughter's forehead, said, "This means that her dead father took possession of her." Two years later, the same mother believed that her daughter, now a toddler, was oversexualized ("just like her father") because she briefly touched her vagina. The attribution of possession by the dead father remained stable, but the specific expression of this maternal identification of the daughter with the father changed with the child's developmental stage.

The integration of sensorimotor memories with semantic memories first becomes apparent in the second and third years of life, when the child begins to use symbolic representation as a way of encoding his or her perceptions of the world, including sense of self and of others. This is a ripe age for eliciting negative maternal attributions because the toddler's increasing autonomy enables him or her to become an increasingly active partner in the mother's conflicts. Even allowing for pronounced individual differences, infants' relatively undifferentiated emotional functioning during the first year of life makes them more likely to serve as "blank screens" for their parents' attributions. Toddlers, on the other hand, tend to fuel their parents' negative attributions through their intense curiosity in exploring the world and themselves, learning through trial and error what is permitted and what is forbidden, persisting in trying to attain what they want, and responding with noncompliance, negativism, and aggression to parental efforts to stop or redirect unwanted pursuits. Even reasonably loving and well-functioning parents are known to respond with exasperation to the power struggles that inevitably ensue in raising a toddler. Parents with clinical levels of ambivalence toward their toddlers find themselves in a particularly difficult position, and often attribute their children's unruly behavior to their being a "monster," "tyrant," or "devil," labels recurrently used by parents of toddlers in our clinical work.

Paradoxically, the toddler's quest for autonomy coexists with an intense desire to please attachment figures. In the second year of life, toddlers become increasingly aware of adult standards and strive to live up to them, becoming anxious and distressed when unable to do so (Kagan, 1981). The wish to please is so powerful a motive in the toddler years that the predominant anxiety of this age is the fear of losing the mother's love. Taken together, the wish to please and the complementary anxiety regarding losing the mother's love constitute a powerful incentive for the development of a moral conscience and a sense of social belonging in the child (see also Fonagy et al., Chapter 8, this volume).

The developmental task of integrating autonomy and the wish to please applies also to the child's self-definition. When the mother's predominant attributions are positive ("You are a wonderful, lovable child and I am proud of you"), the child internalizes those attributions, believing what the mother says and complying with it to please her. Unfortunately, the same process of internalization through compliance takes place when the mother's attributions are negative. The child complies with the mother's perceptions of his or her being a tyrant, a devil, or a monster by selectively engaging in behaviors that confirm the parental attributions, such as disobedience, recklessness, and acts of aggression.

Psychoanalytic theory offers the concept of projective identification as a way of understanding this process of attribution and compliance with the attribution on the part of its recipient (Klein, 1948). Ogden (1982) described projective identification as a three-part process. In the first phase, involving projection, one person attributes or projects an unwanted part of him- or herself on to another person. In the second phase, the projector pressures the recipient of the projection to behave in ways that are consistent with it—in other words, to justify the projection. In the third phase, the recipient of the projection yields to the pressure and behaves in ways that are consistent with the projection. Although this process was described to clarify aspects of the analyst–analysand relationship in psychotherapy, it also applies to our understanding of the mother–toddler relationship in our clinical population (Lieberman, 1992).

What are the similarities and differences between attributions and projections? A thorough analysis of this question is beyond the scope of this chapter, but one important similarity is that both concepts partake of an information-processing approach. In the case of attributions, the person making the attributions is assumed to use developmental, situational, and individual traits as the data from which the attributions are inferred. In the case of projections, the data for the inference are assumed to come from the projector's effort to resolve internal conflicts about the self by disowning a particular trait and attributing it to another person. Using the terms of attachment theory, one might argue that projections are no more than the attributions to another person of unconscious or suppressed components of the internal working models of the self. Regardless of the specific terms used, the pressure on the recipient to comply with the attribution is present in all three theoretical scenarios. Three clinical examples serve to illustrate this phenomenon.

Sapphire, 2 years old, was perceived by her mother as follows: "She was always very sensual from the time she was born. But now she really became a Love Goddess, she is so cute and so seductive." This mother's attributions had such an organizing effect on the way she related to her daughter that the message on her telephone answering machine was, "Hi, this is the household of Nancy and of Sapphire, the Love Goddess." Sapphire was bombarded by maternal requests for kisses and hugs and by exposure to her mother's oversexualized lifestyle. She found herself celebrated and cherished when she lived up to maternal attributions, an irresistible lure to become more and more the way her mother wanted her to be. Sapphire insisted on running naked around the house and often lay on the floor with her legs open, touching her vagina while smiling at the therapist. When walking on the street, she would point at the crotches of the men passing by while saying "penis" in a loud voice. Interestingly, at 3½ years of age, Sapphire still wore diapers to bed although she was dry through the night. When the therapist asked her why, Sapphire replied, "If I don't wear diapers, my mom will forget I'm still a little girl." This child found a safe place to take a respite from her mother's pressure for precocious sexualization—she incorporated her mother's attributions but also kept for herself an area where she could remain a little girl.

At 18 months old, Rita had a mother whose depression immobilized her. She could hardly go out of the house, found no pleasure in daily life, and moved and talked in a lethargic way. Rita was the only source of pleasure for her. In one session after another, she looked at her daughter tenderly and said, "She is so funny. She makes me laugh. She is a real clown." Rita complied with this maternal attribution. In one session she put on a funny hat and pranced in front of her mother, wearing a phony, overly bright and fixed smile. She repeated again and again gestures that made her mother laugh, while she herself laughed in an artificial manner. The put-on nature of this precocious effort to live up to her mother's attributions was evident in Rita's often somber, sad expression when her mother was not paying attention to her.

Timmy, 30 months old, was a veritable "terror." He seemed bent on a path of destructiveness. He bit his baby brother, ran away from his mother while crossing the street, refused to comply with his mother's requests, and constantly engaged in activities that were dangerous to himself, to others, and to objects in the household. He was accident prone and had broken many things, including some of his favorite toys. When he was aggressive to his baby brother, his mother would tell him he was a "murderer," and she confided to the therapist that he might become a serial killer. Her speech to him was filled with labels that denigrated him. She told him he was "bad," "impossible," "a pest to live with," and openly said in front of him that she did not like him. The distress and anger these attributions generated in Timmy were clearly expressed in an overly intense separation anxiety as well as in random acts of physical and verbal aggression toward his mother, including a well-entrenched habit of calling her "bitch."

These examples illustrate how maternal attributions affect the child's working model of attachment and of the self. The study of maternal attributions is very useful in uncovering the themes, rather than the morphological structure, of patterns of attachment. Themes and structure are both important in understanding internal working models, and specific themes affect behavioral structure, leading to a better understanding of the dynamics of the interaction between mother and child. In this sense, the study of maternal attributions opens new perspectives in our understanding of what transpires in the texture of mother–child attachment, complementing the picture offered by studying maternal sensitivity and the representation of attachment in working models of the self. Whereas maternal internal working models have proven more powerful than has maternal sensitivity in predicting infant security of attachment, there is only partial knowledge of how attachment representations are transmitted (the transmission gap; van IJzendoorn, 1995; see also van IJzendoorn & Bakermans-Kranenberg, Chapter 5, this volume). The study of maternal attributions and their internalization by the child could contribute in valuable ways to the narrowing of that transmission gap.

REFERENCES

Ainsworth, M. D. S., Blehar, M. C., Waters, E., & Wall, S. (1978). *Patterns of attachment: A psychological study of the Strange Situation.* Hillsdale, NJ: Erlbaum.

Bollas, C. (1987). *The shadow of the object.* New York: Columbia University Press.

Bowlby, J. (1973). *Attachment and loss: Vol. 2. Separation: Anxiety and anger.* New York: Basic Books.

Bowlby, J. (1980). *Attachment and loss: Vol. 3. Sadness and depression.* New York: Basic Books.

Bowlby, J. (1982). *Attachment and loss: Vol. 1. Attachment.* New York: Basic Books. (Original work published 1969)

Cassidy, J. (1994). Emotion regulation: Influences of attachment relationships. In N. Fox (Ed.), The development of emotion regulation: Biological and behavioral considerations. *Monographs of the Society for Research in Child Development, 59*(1–2, Serial No. 240), 228–249.

Dix, T. H., & Grusec, J. E. (1985). Parent attribution in the socialization of children. In I. E. Sigel (Ed.), *Parental belief systems: Psychological consequences for children.* Hillsdale, NJ: Erlbaum.

Fonagy, P., Steele, H., & Steele, M. (1991). Maternal representations of attachment during pregnancy predict the organization of infant–mother attachment at one year of age. *Child Development, 62,* 891–905.

Fraiberg, S., Adelson, E., & Shapiro, V. (1975). Ghosts in the nursery: A psychoanalytic approach to the problem of impaired infant–mother relationships. *Journal of the American Academy of Child Psychiatry, 14*(3), 1387–1422.

Fraiberg, S. (Ed.). (1980). *Clinical studies in infant mental health.* New York: Basic Books.

Kagan, J. (1981). *The second year.* Cambridge, MA: Harvard University Press.

Klein, M. (1948). *Contributions to psychoanalysis, 1921–1945.* London: Hogarth Press.

Lieberman, A. F. (1985). Infant mental health: A model for service delivery. *Journal of Clinical Child Psychology, 14,* 196–201.

Lieberman, A. F. (1991). Attachment theory and infant–parent psychotherapy: Some conceptual, clinical and research considerations. In D. Cicchetti & S. Toth (Eds.), *Rochester Symposium on Developmental Psychopathology: Vol. 3. Models and integrations* (pp. 261–288). Hillsdale, NJ: Erlbaum.

Lieberman, A. F. (1992). Infant–parent psychotherapy with toddlers. *Development and Psychopathology, 4,* 559–574.

Lieberman, A. F., & Pawl, J. H. (1988). Clinical applications of attachment theory. In J. Belsky & T. Nezworski (Eds.), *Clinical implications of attachment* (pp. 327–351). Hillsdale, NJ: Erlbaum.

Lieberman, A. F., & Pawl, J. H. (1990). Disorders of attachment and secure base behavior in the second year of life: Conceptual issues and clinical intervention. In M. T. Greenberg, D. Cicchetti, & E. M. Cummings (Eds.), *Attachment in the preschool years* (pp. 375–398). Chicago: University of Chicago Press.

Lieberman, A. F., & Pawl, J. H. (1993). Infant–parent psychotherapy. In C. Zeanah (Ed.), *Handbook of infant mental health* (pp. 427–442). New York: Guilford Press.

Lieberman, A. F., Weston, D., & Pawl, J. H. (1991). Preventive intervention and outcome with anxiously attached dyads. *Child Development, 62,* 199–209.

Main, M., Kaplan, N., & Cassidy, J. (1985). Security in infancy, childhood, and adulthood: A move to the level of representation. In I. Bretherton & E. Waters (Eds.), Growing points of attachment theory and research. *Monographs of the Society for Research in Child Development, 50*(1–2, Serial No. 209), 66–104.

Neumann, E. (1955). *The Great Mother: An analysis of the archetype.* Princeton: Princeton University Press.

Ogden, T. H. (1982). *Projective identification and psychotherapeutic technique.* New York: Academic Press.

Stern, D. (1985). *The interpersonal world of the infant.* New York: Basic Books.

van IJzendoorn, M. H. (1995). Adult attachment representation, parental responsiveness, and infant attachment: A meta-analysis on the predictive validity of the Adult Attachment Interview. *Psychological Bulletin, 117,* 387–403.

Wallerstein, R. S. (1973). Psychoanalytic perspectives on the problem of reality. *Journal of the American Psychoanalytic Association, 21,* 5–33.

Zeanah, C., Benoit, D., Batton, M., Regan, C., Hirshberg, L. M., & Lipsitt, L. P. (1993). Representations of attachment in mothers and their one year-old infants. *Journal of the American Academy of Child and Adolescent Psychiatry, 32,* 278–286.

10

Intergenerational Transmission of Relationship Psychopathology: A Mother–Infant Case Study

CHARLES H. ZEANAH
ELIZABETH FINLEY-BELGRAD
DIANE BENOIT

The idea that individuals enter relationships with certain propensities for interpreting experiences and behavior traces its contemporary history to Freud's (1920) description of the compulsion to repeat. A specific version of the repetition compulsion has been central to clinical work with infants and their families; namely, that adults recreate early relationship experiences in subsequent relationships. Fraiberg's (1989) clinical work suggested that such relationship reenactments might be unconsciously passed on to the subsequent generation in what she described as "terrible and exacting detail" (p. 165). Following Bowlby's conceptual framework (Bowlby, 1969/1982, 1973, 1980), attachment research has provided empirical support for these assertions by operationalizing patterns of behaviors in parents and infants that are presumed to reflect similarities in representational processes. Intergenerational transmission of patterns of attachment has been demonstrated via concordances between attachment patterns from Strange Situation classifications of infants (Ainsworth, Blehar, Waters, & Wall, 1978) and Adult Attachment Interview classifications of parents (George, Kaplan, & Main, 1984) in numerous samples by different investigators in several different cultures around the world (van IJzendoorn, 1995; see also van IJzendoorn & Bakermans-Kranenburg, Chapter 5, this volume).

In this chapter we examine a single case of intergenerational transmission of attachment relationship psychopathology, focusing on an adolescent mother and her two oldest children. The purpose of this examination is to move beyond broad indices of concordance and to consider the similarities and divergences in how one young mother related both to her own mother and to her children (see Lieberman, Chapter 9, this volume). The case we present is uniquely suited for such an examination because records are available from an initial clinical treatment that began just before the young mother's delivery of her first child, from participation in a longitudinal research project which began in the latter part of her second pregnancy and continued until her son was 2 years old, and from a clinical treatment which began when he was 2 years old and continued for another 2½ years after that.

The intergenerational pattern that we will describe is one of angry rejection by the parent, frustration and bewilderment in the child, intolerance of dependence in self and other, and mutual derogation and teasing. In particular, we will focus on derogation, a term introduced by Main and Goldwyn (1994) to describe an unusual pattern of dismissal in the Adult Attachment Interview. According to Main and Goldwyn (1994), derogation is that form of dismissal in which attachment experiences, and especially attachment figures, are actively and contemptuously devalued. The *Oxford English Dictionary* defines derogation as: "to take away or detract from, diminish, disparage; to take away something from a thing so as to lessen or impair it." At the behavioral level, this is manifest by a teasing/taunting interaction, whereas at the level of discourse this is manifest by a devaluing rejection.

Anna Freud (1936) described identification with the aggressor as a defense in which a child who is threatened by aggression responds by becoming aggressive to cope with extreme fear and helplessness. In the case we discuss a young mother whose response to her mother's demeaning criticism of her was to become dismissing of her mother's power over her and of her own neediness, as well as to bully and tease her own children. Thus, derogation may be considered a form of identification with the aggressor in which feelings of intense vulnerability, created by interactions with a demeaning, threatening, and more powerful other, are defensively transformed into contemptuous disregard *for* the other, which then mirrors the original contemptuous disregard *from* the other. Sroufe and Fleeson (1986) emphasized that both sides of infant–caregiver relationship patterns are internalized by young children, thereby facilitating intergenerational transmission.

In addition to considering the intergenerational transmission of the derogating/teasing relationship pattern, the case we present also lends itself to a discussion of the process of changing the pattern. Although attachment research has emphasized concordances in representations of attachment in infants and parents, clinicians must struggle with how to change generational patterns. Features within the derogating/teasing pattern possibly related to the capacity for change will be important to note. Also, we will try to highlight key features of the therapeutic relationship which were crucial to improvement.

FIRST CLINICAL ENCOUNTER

Aleisha was 15 years old and 7 months pregnant when she was referred to an outpatient psychiatry clinic for evaluation of depression and suicidal ideation. She was referred by a social worker who was based at an obstetrical hospital but who spent time at a school-based program for adolescent mothers. In the evaluation, Aleisha reported that she had been "OK" until she found out that she was pregnant 4½ months before. Since that time, she had been intermittently preoccupied by thoughts of suicide and on two occasions she had attempted to kill herself. In both cases she said that she had wanted to die and to kill the baby also. In fact, she said that she still wanted to die because her mother was so enraged about her pregnancy. She reported several instances of abusive treatment by her mother, including at least one previous investigation by child protective services that had not resulted in any charges.

Dr. A, the resident child psychiatrist who conducted the evaluation, dictated in her report at the time:

> "Aleisha feels that her only problem is her relationship with her mother, that her mother doesn't care about her, never did care about her, and never will care about her, and that if it wasn't for her mother, she wouldn't be depressed and wouldn't want to kill her baby or herself. In fact, Aleisha is convinced that her mother wishes she were dead."

In the next session Aleisha and her mother, Ms. D, were seen together. Ms. D gave Dr. A little reason to doubt Aleisha's fear. Ms. D dismissed any concerns about Aleisha, saying that she could not be worried about Aleisha since worrying would be "a sin in God's Kingdom." Further, she said that they had never had a "real" mother–daughter relationship. When asked how she felt about Aleisha's expressions of suicidality, she replied chillingly, "She'd better do it right, or I might do it myself." She acknowledged that she was extremely angry about Aleisha's pregnancy, and she threatened to kill the baby's father if she ever saw him. Interestingly, she acknowledged that she was angry in part because Aleisha's pregnancy reminded her of her own pregnancy with Aleisha's oldest brother when she had been 16 years old.

This led to a discussion of her own history. Ms. D had grown up with a mother who was difficult, hostile, rejecting, and abusive and a father who had been largely absent. She said that she had been the "black sheep" of the family, and that her mother was enraged when she learned that Ms. D was pregnant at age 16. She recalled a scene in which her mother, who was extremely obese, tried to choke her and to abort the baby by jumping on Ms. D's abdomen. At the age of 19, Ms. D left home and had not seen her mother until she moved back in with her 2 years previously. Ms. D and her husband had separated when Aleisha was 3 months old, and Ms. D had had a number of relationships with men since then. After a number of stressful events, Ms. D began to abuse alcohol, marijuana, and cocaine. After she moved back in with her mother, she joined a church, was "saved, revived, sins were repented," and she stopped using drugs and alcohol. At the time of the evaluation, she said that she went to church several times a week and that she considered herself to be a very religious person. Having obtained this history, Dr. A believed that despite all of the obvious reasons for concern, there were some reasons for hope. Aleisha and her mother were both obviously in pain, and they both said that they wanted help. Despite saying that she was not worried about Aleisha, Ms. D did appear to show some genuine concern and seemed to accept some responsibility for Aleisha's distress. Dr. A recommended focused family psychotherapy for Aleisha and Ms. D, and because her rotation at the hospital would be ending in 3 months, she recommended that after the baby was born, Aleisha and the baby be referred to a teen–tot clinic at the hospital. This was a pediatric clinic that featured an array of supportive services for adolescent mothers and infants.

Initial Treatment

In the few sessions held before the baby's birth, Aleisha and Ms. D showed remarkable progress and improvement. Aleisha no longer felt suicidal. She and her mother found that they enjoyed shopping together, and they spoke excitedly about the expected baby. They both agreed that they were grateful for their "new beginning." This, of course, made Dr. A nervous. She wondered how long they could maintain their fragile peace, and she noted signs of trouble in the midst of their chipperness. Aleisha was quite passive in their sessions, and as her mother became more controlling, she seemed to withdraw further. The D's also missed a few sessions, but there were no significant complaints and all was generally well. Aleisha met with the pediatrician in charge of the teen–tot clinic and made arrangements to attend with her baby after birth.

Aleisha delivered a baby girl, Ellen, about a week after her due date. Aleisha adjusted reasonably well in the initial postpartum weeks, and she and her mother attended sessions fairly regularly with Dr. A. For the next 6 weeks, sessions with Aleisha, Ellen, and Ms. D went smoothly. Aleisha vacillated a bit in her confidence about her caregiving and about Ellen's attachment to her, but all of this appeared to be within the expectable range. Her suicidal ideation had disappeared after the initial contact and had not reappeared. Having arranged a successful transfer to the teen–tot clinic, Dr. A terminated with the family. Aleisha and her mother appeared to have negotiated the early postpartum adjustment well, and they agreed to continued intervention through the new program.

Resumption of Treatment

Six weeks later Ms. D called Dr. A requesting an appointment for Aleisha immediately. She said that Aleisha had become quite depressed and much less interested in Ellen than before. An appointment was scheduled for the three of them the following day. Dr. A learned at that appointment that since she had seen them last, the family had moved to a new neighborhood which Aleisha did not like. She and Ms. D had been fighting about the father of the baby, with whom Aleisha wanted to remain involved. When Dr. A pointed out that Aleisha seemed to have dealt with her anger toward her mother by withdrawing from the baby, Aleisha burst into tears and said that she was very angry, but she hadn't realized that she was "making Ellen pay for it." Withdrawal when angry was a pattern already apparent for Aleisha with her mother; this session suggested a transfer of the pattern to her relationship with Ellen. Another appointment was scheduled, but the family did not keep it.

After several false starts, Dr. A persuaded the Ds to resume treatment. Over the next few weeks, Aleisha missed several appointments but she began to complain bitterly about Ms. D, whom she said yelled at her constantly. She declared her intentions to find an apartment and to move out on her own. She said that she had not been truthful about how things had been going with her mother all along; in fact, they had been terrible. A 17-year-old friend who was living on her own with a baby had invited Aleisha to come and live with her. Dr. A responded to this news by attempting to have Aleisha consider the numerous problems she would likely encounter if she left her mother's and to consider alternatives in the form of other supportive programs.

Adult Attachment Interview

Dr. A administered the Adult Attachment Interview (AAI) to Aleisha to help her understand Aleisha's perspective on her early childhood experiences. This structured interview covers an adult's reports of childhood relationship experiences and the individual's current perspective on those experiences (see van IJzendoorn & Bakermans-Kranenburg, Chapter 5, this volume). A number of features were striking. Aleisha described a troubled childhood in which her mother had treated her harshly, and at times abusively. She saw less of her father than she would have liked, and her mother made frequent moves. As a result, Aleisha described having no one to turn to for comfort or solace. When her parents were together they often argued or became violent, and they both apparently drank excessively at times. Aleisha's paternal grandmother died when she was 6 or 8 years old. This grandmother appeared to have been the most positive parental figure in Aleisha's childhood, and Aleisha responded to her death by refusing to believe that she was really dead. It was clear that she had not resolved the loss at the time of the interview.

The interview also made clear that Aleisha strongly idealized her father, describing him in glowing terms, but she provided no specific memories of his availability to her. In fact, his absence was especially notable given her apparent need for protection from her mother's punitiveness. Aleisha seemed to be trying in her descriptions to lessen the effect of her mother's power over her, in part by not allowing herself or the interviewer to know that she had been hurt. She described her relationship with her mother in the following way: "I didn't like her. Ain't nothing else." Later, when asked directly, Aleisha said that her relationship with her parents had had no effects on her development. She also described her mother on several occasions as a nobody, contemptuously disavowing the importance of her mother and their relationship. This pattern, in conjunction with the other dismissing features of the responses, were illustrative of derogation.

At other times in the AAI, Aleisha acknowledged that her mother had hurt her, although she fought to hide this hurt from her mother. The message from Aleisha, which is clear throughout the interview, might be described as, "She didn't hurt me, or even if she did, I wasn't going to let her know it." This was more than dismissing the effects her harsh and punitive upbringing had had on her; there was also an implicit power struggle going on in which Aleisha could fight her mother's domination only through a stubborn, passive resistance. Nevertheless, demonstrating a brief flash of insight, she did suggest as an afterthought that some of her own anger and impatience with children might be due to her mother's incessant anger and criticism of her. Aleisha also reported numerous examples of Ms. D's derogation of her throughout her childhood. For example, Aleisha recalled an incident in which her mother rebuked her for saying that she had already completed her homework in school. Her mother didn't believe her: "I'll kick your behind if you don't bring your homework home every day," she said. Aleisha's brother tried to defend her by pointing out that it was possible that Aleisha had been given time in study hall to complete her homework. Aleisha recalled that her mother's response to this was, "So what, she ain't nothing special!" From the standpoint of Aleisha's experience, this was the core message of her relationship with her mother.

Finally, despite the generally dismissing quality of her descriptions, there was also an undercurrent of unmet neediness and confusion about what had elicited her mother 's responses to her. Aleisha gave a number of examples of how she did not seek comfort from her mother during childhood. When she became upset, she said, she tended to go off by herself or hug her dolls. Toward the end of the interview she was asked about her current relationship with her mother. She said that it had not changed at all; then she added, "I still don't, you know, talk to my mother as much as I want to."

Working Model of the Child Interview

Around this same time, Dr. A also interviewed Aleisha with the Working Model of the Child Interview (Zeanah & Benoit, 1995) to obtain a more formal assessment of her perceptions of Ellen and her relationship with her. In this interview, conducted when Ellen was 5 months old, Aleisha conveyed confusion and ambivalence about the baby, who seemed already to reenact aspects of Aleisha's relationship with her own mother. Aleisha described repeatedly her bewilderment about Ellen's crying, which she felt was Ellen's most difficult behavior.

DR. A: Can you give me a typical example of what happens at the time that she cries?

ALEISHA: I don't know, she just starts crying. She won't be hungry, she won't be wet, she'll just cry.

DR. A: I see. What do you feel like doing at those times?

ALEISHA: I be saying, "What's the matter with you?" I be asking her, and she'll stop, and she'll look at me, and she'll cry again. It's like she's saying, "Don't you know what's the matter with me?" I'm like, "No!"

Dr. A recognized in this scenario that the baby reenacted Aleisha's own bewildered pain in her relationship with Ms. D ("Don't you know what's the matter with me?"). Furthermore, Ellen's crying, which Aleisha experienced as criticism, reenacted the "indicting other," whom Aleisha was at a loss as to how to please. This was the first obvious illustration of the next level of generational repetition of some aspects of the relationship pattern. Aleisha also made it clear that Ellen was a source of comfort for her at times.

DR. A: You said "lovable."
ALEISHA: Oh, well, when we both feeling down, we always hug each other.
DR. A: Do you have a specific memory that you could tell me more about?
ALEISHA: Uh-huh, that's when we moved over there. My mother had yelled at me and she was, she was yelling at the baby 'cause the baby kept crying. And so when I, I, when I got the baby, she stopped crying, and we went into the room, and we just, we just sat there hugging each other. I'll hold, stand her up and she'll hug me, and I'll hug her back.

Dr. A believed that the interviews had confirmed her working impression of an intergenerational pattern of angry rejection of a needy child by a caregiver, bewilderment on the child's part about what had elicited the rejection, and mutual derogation by parent and child. She also noted the poignant link between Aleisha, the scared child hugging her dolls for comfort, and Aleisha, the scared mother hugging her baby for comfort. There was obvious reason for concern about this pattern as an indication of role reversal, but also some evidence of Aleisha's reaching out for others.

Following these interviews Dr. A developed a list of possible services for Aleisha, but the family missed a number of visits. The teen–tot clinic began to note Aleisha's sometimes rough handling of Ellen. Within a month, things had deteriorated significantly. Ms. D finally returned for an appointment. There, accompanied by Ellen but not Aleisha, she told Dr. A that she was very angry with Aleisha. She had whipped Aleisha the week before, prompting Aleisha to call the police. When the police arrived, Ms. D had screamed to them that she would beat Aleisha to death if they let her come into the house. Ms. D said that she called Child Protective Services (CPS), and they advised her to call an attorney about having Aleisha removed from her home. She said that she would never forgive Aleisha for having called the police, and that she had no intention of ever working anything out with her. This was, she held, Aleisha's third big mistake (the first being a fire she set when she was 6 years old in which the family lost their belongings, and the second being her pregnancy with Ellen). "It's a closed case," she announced firmly. She refused to sign permission for Aleisha to attend any of the programs identified by Dr. A.

Dr. A told her that she had concerns about everyone's anger, threats, and vulnerabilities, and that she wanted to call CPS herself before anyone got hurt. As a result of this call, CPS became involved, and Aleisha was transferred to a shelter in a neighboring town. Ellen remained with Ms. D while Aleisha was away. Dr. A had only a few phone contacts with Aleisha from a couple of different shelters and transitional housing facilities. Aleisha requested appointments more than once but did not keep them. Dr. A did not hear from Aleisha again after the first month she left home, and Dr. A completed her training and moved out of the area 8 months later.

ANOTHER TREATMENT ATTEMPT

Aleisha was lost to follow-up for a period of time, but after several months she returned to the teen–tot clinic with Ellen, now approaching 2 years old. Aleisha was also pregnant for a second time. After she delivered her second child, Antoine, she was referred for treatment to an experienced therapist who worked in the teen–tot clinic.

This therapist established a good start with Aleisha through a combination of home and clinic visits, but Aleisha decided to visit her father, who lived in a large city several hours away. Although she had not seen or talked to him in years and didn't know exactly where he lived, she set out to find him, taking Ellen and Antoine with her. When Aleisha returned from her visit several weeks later, she discontinued the treatment on the advice of her Social Services case worker, who suggested that Aleisha had too many services and that she, the case worker, would provide all needed interventions to Aleisha herself.

RESEARCH CONTACTS

In the meantime, during the third trimester of her pregnancy with Antoine, Aleisha was recruited to participate in a research project at the original hospital where she had received her initial psychiatric treatment. The study involved a series of laboratory and home visits during pregnancy and at infant ages 4, 10, 15, 20, and 24 months. The research team also had occasional informal contacts with Aleisha and her children between scheduled times of assessment to maintain contact with her, and they remained concerned about Aleisha and her children throughout the study. Aleisha's self-reports of distress were extremely high, with scores on the Beck Depression Inventory (Beck, Ward, Mendelson, Mock, & Erbaugh, 1961) frequently in the severely depressed range. She moved frequently and reported ongoing conflict with her extended family. She was scrutinized by CPS during the study and was investigated formally at least twice. Summaries of the home and laboratory visits follow.

Pregnancy Laboratory Visits

Aleisha and Ellen were seen together for a structured interactional assessment involving free play, clean-up, teaching tasks, and separation and reunion episodes (Crowell & Feldman, 1988) when Ellen was 25 months old. The most striking part of their interaction occurred in the reunion episode following a 3-minute separation. Ellen was distressed by her mother's leaving the playroom, and she cried softly by the door. When Aleisha returned, Ellen stopped crying immediately, and her mother picked her up briefly, inquiring, "Whatsa' matter?" Aleisha then put Ellen down and took a seat at a table where the two of them had worked on tasks earlier. Aleisha tried to connect a pair of earphones to a hand-held radio and paid no attention to Ellen, who stood beside the table clutching a small blanket and looking at her mother. Almost imperceptively, Ellen put the corner of the blanket into her mouth, and Aleisha responded immediately, "Take it outcha mouth." Ellen then smiled and began to bite the blanket repeatedly while looking directly at her mother for some acknowledgment. Aleisha said nothing, but she laughed aloud each time Ellen bit the blanket. Ellen then collapsed playfully to the floor and her mother laughed again. Ellen began to roll slowly back and forth on the floor, and her mother said only, "Why you wanna do that?" This theme of teasing would be repeated in virtually every interaction between Aleisha and her children that was observed.

In the AAI administered a week later as part of the investigation, much of the information about Aleisha's childhood that she had reported in the initial AAI (completed 2 years previously) was repeated. The same features of abusive treatment by her mother, followed by bewilderment and finally dismissing the effects of such harsh treatment, were all apparent again. When asked to describe her childhood relationship with her mother, Aleisha said, "There wasn't no relationship. I was just a daughter that when the boys [her brothers] do something, I get the blame for it. It was like, it was like, we didn't have no kind of relationship."

4-Month Home Visit

A home visit, scheduled to encompass a feeding but otherwise intended to be naturalistic observation, was videotaped when Antoine was 4 months old. During much of Antoine's feeding Aleisha was absorbed in watching a television soap opera; in one poignant image, she placed Antoine's pacifier in her mouth and kept it there for several minutes as she held a bottle for Antoine.

After the feeding, a teasing interaction with Ellen ensued. The "game" began with Ellen reaching for Antoine, and Aleisha responded by pushing her away. Ellen giggled excitedly as she repeatedly approached her mother, and Aleisha pushed her away again and again. Although this was clearly play, it was rough, and Ellen's squeal sounded at times a bit shrill and anxious. Finally, after several minutes the game ended when Aleisha raised her voice and sharply rebuked Ellen, who then walked away tearfully.

10-Month Home Visit

At the next videotaped home visit Ellen was away at daycare and Antoine and his mother were home alone. Loud music played through stereo speakers throughout the hour-long visit. Antoine was in a walker, and he was left alone with the music playing loudly for much of the visit. Several times, however, his mother entered the room without his realizing it (he could not hear her because of the music). Once, she snuck up behind him and grabbed his head from behind. He startled, and she looked at him and smiled. Several other times when she entered the room without his realizing it, Aleisha surprised Antoine. Often, she did this by roughly kicking his walker, sending him sliding across the floor. Throughout this visit, Aleisha's teasing behaviors were rough, and also frightening. Antoine spent prolonged minutes nearly motionless in the walker, with a blank expression on his face as the music played on.

15-Month Home and Laboratory Visits

In the videotape of the next home visit, Aleisha was watching another young child for a neighbor in addition to watching Ellen and Antoine. Aleisha and Antoine were lying on a mattress and box springs in the bedroom, while Ellen and the other child played around the edge of the mattress. The most notable interaction concerned Antoine's pleading for gum, which he saw his mother chewing. She denied having any gum, and she laughed at him as he cried in frustration. Variations on this pattern continued, with her "showing" him that she had none by hiding the gum and opening her mouth, until finally Antoine rolled away slowly from her on the mattress, and began to writhe in frustration. She swatted at him with a pillow, and then placed it over him as he cried. Aleisha laughed as he cried even louder, and he began to rake his fingers across his face in rapid succession. At this point, Aleisha turned away from him. He approached her again, reaching up towards her mouth, and she nibbled his fingers. As he cried out again in frustration, she took the gum out of her mouth and put it into his, turned away from him again, and then began to watch television. This was a clear example of Antoine being taught not to trust his own perceptions and cognitions, which Bowlby (1973) described as creating incoherent models in young children if the incongruences were severe and persistent enough.

Aleisha and Antoine also visited the laboratory for a Strange Situation procedure 1 week later. In the first reunion Antoine was fairly avoidant, but the second reunion was quite unusual. Antoine was a bit distressed during the second separation, but when his mother returned, he took two steps toward the door and then stopped. He looked as if he might try to walk out the door, but his mother closed it behind her and walked past him silently. After she reached the other side of the playroom, she asked, "Were you crying?" By this time, Antoine was quite preoccupied with a toy, and he sat with his back to his mother, not looking at her nor vocalizing at all. After about a minute, he turned to face her, but instead of approaching her, he began to roll slowly around on the floor with a dazed look on his face. In the final 30 seconds of the reunion, she put a cookie monster puppet on her hand, approached him on the floor where he laid, and began to "get" him with the puppet as he laughed in response.

20-Month Laboratory Visit

Antoine was seen in a semistructured social interaction procedure at 20 months. He played first with an examiner and a standard set of toys as his mother completed questionnaires in a corner of the playroom, and then he played with his mother after the examiner left the room. Differences in his play with the two adults were notable. With the examiner, he was an enthusiastic and sociable participant as they played with various toys together. He talked to her, demonstrated good joint attention, and noticed her reactions. He sat close to her (unusually close for a boy his age in our experience), and he even rested his hand on her leg as he played with a pop-up box at one point. The examiner later reported that she had felt during the session as if Antoine were appealing to her to care for him through his sociable but emotionally hungry behavior.

After the examiner left the room, Antoine and his mother began to play with the same set of toys. After only a few seconds, Antoine tried to put the top on a plastic bucket, but Aleisha blocked his effort with a toy bear, perhaps trying to introduce a new play material. Antoine reacted immediately, crying out and pushing against the bear his mother held. She reached for the top that he held, and he angrily pulled it away from her, exclaiming, "Mine!" She then covered the top of the bucket with her hand, and he slammed the top down on her. She said, as she positioned her arms in an exaggerated defensive posture, "You're abusin' me—what's wrong with you?" They continued to struggle over the bucket for several minutes. At times, Aleisha feigned injury as Antoine pushed her hands away and cried out in frustration. As they left the laboratory at the end of the 10-minute session, Aleisha said sardonically to Antoine, "Now it's time to leave your lap of luxury." The interactions during this visit illustrated clearly the relationship specificity of the derogating/teasing pattern from Antoine's point of view. At this age, the conflicted and aggressive interactions had not spread to interactions with others, such as the examiner in this session or to his daycare providers.

24-Month Laboratory Visit

Antoine and Aleisha were seen together when he was 24 months old in the same structured interactional assessment procedure that Aleisha and Ellen had participated in 2 years earlier. The entire procedure was more conflicted with Antoine that it had been with Ellen. Even the free play episode was punctuated by conflict. Antoine also was unable to use his mother for support in solving tasks because their interaction repeatedly degenerated into bickering and teasing. Further, the pattern of rolling away from his mother with a dazed expression that had been evident in the Strange Situation at 15 months was apparent again.

Summary of Research Contacts

Although Antoine and his mother were not the most worrisome dyad in the investigation, they generated considerable anguish among the investigators. Aleisha's angry and depressed moods were palpable, and the painful pattern of teasing and derogation was apparent. All of this concern had led the team to ongoing discussions about intervention, but Aleisha had received a number of largely unsuccessful attempts at intervention throughout the time she was involved in the research. The investigators decided to make a final attempt to engage her in treatment at the conclusion of the research project. In a debriefing wrap-up session at the completion of the study, Aleisha accepted a referral of Antoine for home-based evaluation and treatment.

RECENT TREATMENT

The team met with Dr. C, a resident child psychiatrist, who had expressed a willingness to provide in-home treatment to Aleisha and to Antoine. Given Aleisha's history of difficulty in sustaining treatment, the basic establishment and maintenance of a therapeutic relationship was defined as the initial goal. Following this, the plan was to discover with Aleisha the links between her own childhood relationship experiences and her experiences as a mother.

Initial Session

When Dr. C first met Aleisha, she and her two older children had been living on the third floor of a three-family house in an "inner city" area. Aleisha's maternal grandmother lived on the first floor and her aunt and her large family lived on the second floor.

Dr. C's initial session with Aleisha was memorable. In her own words:

> "After locating the house, I pulled my car over, securely locked it and headed up the front steps. I pushed wide the partially open front door and advanced into the darkened entry way which housed an overflowing garbage can. I carefully climbed the two darkened flights of stairs, ever ready to flee from running rodents I anticipated though never saw. As I ascended, I was greeted by the light of a window on the third floor landing. I found the handleless door and knocked. I heard a muffled, 'Come!' from inside. I pushed the door open. I entered a darkened apartment. A few paces took me into the living room where two women sat on either end of the battered couch. I asked, 'Aleisha?' and one of the women looked up and said, 'Yeah.'
>
> "Aleisha sat slumped at one end of the couch wearing dark clothes. I could barely discern her features in the darkness but for the light of the large television across the room blaring a rap video. I introduced myself and extended my hand which she took limply. She motioned for me to sit in a deep, overstuffed chair to the side of the couch. She never introduced her companion, who never spoke.
>
> "Between the two women on the couch was a soundly sleeping boy who appeared to be about two years old, and I assumed that this must be Antoine. I asked her about her understanding of my being there. She explained that she understood that I was there to talk with her. She immediately began complaining about Antoine

awakening her early in the morning and her needing to lock him out of her room.

"Soon, Aleisha woke Antoine by roughly shaking him. She explained to me this was so he would go to bed at a reasonable hour that night. When he sat up, she stuck a cookie in his mouth which he grabbed and removed. She then took a cookie and began eating it herself. She said he liked to watch videos and put the remote control in his hands. Taking his hand, she pushed the buttons while telling him how important it was to know how to change channels.

"Antoine was clean, though he had a perpetually runny nose. He sat on the couch for the duration of my visit without any toys or significant activities with which to busy himself. Aleisha got up once to go to the door in response to a knock. When she returned, Antoine had picked up the television control. Aleisha pushed him roughly and said, 'Are you mad at me?' He did not respond. She pushed him again, and he responded by hitting back at her. A few minutes later, Antoine was sitting very still and had almost fallen back to sleep. Aleisha hit him lightly, saying, 'Wake up!' He hit back at her several times. She looked over at me and explained that 'he's just falling back to sleep.' Soon after that I got up to go. When I said good-bye, Antoine spontaneously began to cry" (Finley-Belgrad, 1994, p. 7).

First Early Turning Point

Aleisha and Dr. C met weekly, often in her still-darkened apartment with rap video playing. Usually, the children were present and she was able to talk about her frustrations with their constant neediness and her own feelings of neediness and emptiness. At times, family or friends would be there when Dr. C arrived for the appointments. At other times, someone barged into the house or the room, interrupting the sessions. At these times, Aleisha behaved as though powerless to alter this pattern, which would emerge as a major theme in the treatment. As they continued to meet, Dr. C felt rapidly integrated into Aleisha's extended family with everyone knowing that she was "Aleisha's doctor" and making social contact with her. Their relationship was established, but was it going anywhere?

After several initial visits, Aleisha was not at her apartment at the appointed time. She was not there the next time, nor the next. Dr. C continued to call at the usual appointment time. She waited for some time each visit, then left a written note for Aleisha, but not a single visit occurred. Finally, after a gap of 6 weeks, Aleisha was there and the visits resumed. Dr. C tried to discuss the missed appointments with Aleisha, but at the time she had little to say about it. Only during the termination of treatment would Dr. C learn what Aleisha had thought about those missed appointments.

As Dr. C consistently kept weekly appointments, Aleisha became more engaged and able to talk about what it was like for her to have the stresses of being financially dependent on public assistance (Aid for Dependent Children) and having an active 2-year-old boy and 4-year-old girl. She was able to talk about her frustrations and about Antoine's challenging behavior, which she experienced as "aggressiveness." They began to discuss normal developmental expectations.

Second Early Turning Point

A breakthrough occurred, and Dr. C gained some insight into her relationship with Aleisha after about 7 months. Aleisha, over several sessions, began mentioning and then became increasingly disturbed about her new CPS worker. Her social worker, whom she had met only briefly on a few occasions, was talking about removing her two children from her home.

Aleisha had first become involved with the department several years previously around a question of sexual abuse of her daughter by a boyfriend, but nothing had been substantiated. Contact had continued without significant activity. Aleisha had a parent aid two days a week through CPS. It was unclear why the possibility of removing her children had arisen—both to Aleisha and to Dr. C. Initially, Aleisha had been hesitant to involve Dr. C with CPS. She experienced the department as a threatening, antagonistic bureaucracy which had not been helpful at all. In contrast, she had begun to trust Dr. C and to feel that she could be helpful. She seemed almost afraid, as she discussed it with Dr. C, that their relationship might be tainted in some way by association with the bureaucracy of CPS. Dr. C thought that she also might be afraid that she might disappoint her by being "like the others" or by being powerless to help.

Nevertheless, Dr. C gently but repeatedly suggested that it might be helpful to their work together for her to be present at meetings with the CPS worker. Dr. C attended the next meeting with Aleisha and her CPS worker. To her great surprise, Dr. C was astonished at how confrontational, abrasive, and directive the worker was with Aleisha. Without having spent any time with her or the children, and without having attempted to find out what was going on now between Aleisha and the children, the worker was accusatory and making unfounded assumptions based on material in a departmental file on Aleisha. In the process, she provoked Aleisha into an angry, withholding, and uncooperative stance. Dr. C tried to intervene to interrupt this destructive process, but to little avail. The worker continued to berate Aleisha. Dr. C was incensed by the worker's conduct, and she later wrote a letter describing her observations and objections to the worker, but the precipitous plans for removing the children continued, unaffected. Dr. C then wrote a letter to the court, and this led to swift action. At the judge's insistence, the worker was removed from the case and the plan for removal was dropped. The newly assigned worker ultimately became an important ally of Aleisha's. Clearly, this concrete advocacy was another turning point in Dr. C's relationship with Aleisha because it interrupted what must have seemed to Aleisha another version of the devaluing derogation that she had experienced with her mother. Several other times during the treatment, Dr. C would again help Aleisha challenge authority figures constructively. Each time, Aleisha seemed to be strengthened as a partner in the process.

Themes in the Middle Phases

The middle phase of treatment focused on three additional significant areas for Aleisha beyond advocacy with various social systems. First, Aleisha demonstrated growing appreciation of her children's experience and an increasing ability to view experiences through their eyes. Second, she struggled to clarify and then to accept her relationships with her father and then with her mother. Third, Aleisha began to acknowledge and to attempt to resolve a destructive relationship with her boyfriend.

In a typical session early in the middle phase of treatment, Dr. C arrived and was let in to a cluttered living room with papers and clothes strewn about. Aleisha was not in sight, but Antoine and Ellen were running around the room, and four young adults were watching television silently. Aleisha came out of her bedroom and flung a pair of pants in the direction of Antoine. Dr. C suggested that she and Aleisha go somewhere quiet to talk. First, Aleisha said gruffly to no one in particular, "All of you leave." When no one responded she led Dr. C into the children's bedroom and again announced to the room, "Everyone stay out!" Aleisha began to talk to Dr. C. All of a sudden, Ellen came running into the room crying, followed by Antoine, who looked startled. Ellen reported that one of the women in the other room had punched her arm. Aleisha stormed out into the living room, yelling at the four adults that no one had the right to hit her child. While she was gone, Ellen climbed up in Dr. C's lap and cried softly. As Aleisha came back into the room, Dr. C said to Ellen, realizing that she was talking to everyone, "It's very scary when people yell and hit each other. Sometimes it's hard to feel safe." About this time, the young son of one of the women in the other room wandered into the bedroom, and Aleisha shoved him roughly as if to avenge Ellen's hurt. As Dr. C discussed this with her, however, Aleisha acknowledged how hard things must be for this boy and how much he must have felt hurt, as she associated to her own painful experiences. Slowly, she was beginning to appreciate the perspective of the other in her interactions with Ellen and Antoine also.

Soon afterward, Aleisha decided again to visit with her father, who lived several hours away. She did not discuss the visit at length with Dr. C, but it seemed that afterward she viewed him less idealistically than she had previously. She began to acknowledge his shortcomings and no longer looked to him as a realistic resource for her and the children. On the other hand, Dr. C noted also that she was neither angrily preoccupied nor assailed by his letting her down. Instead, she seemed a bit disappointed but also resigned to his having a fairly peripheral role in her life. A couple of weeks later, in a rare moment of quiet in Aleisha's living room, Dr. C pointed out to Aleisha a curious paradox. On the one hand, it was often hard for them to have any privacy at all, because someone was always barging in and interrupting them. On the other hand, there were significant parts of herself that Aleisha kept completely private from everyone. Aleisha seemed surprised, pleased, and hesitant all at once as she said, "You noticed that, huh?" Dr. C replied quietly, "Yeah." At that moment, as if to underscore the lack of privacy, the kids burst through the door, home from school. Nevertheless, Dr. C had communicated her understanding that Aleisha needed and deserved her privacy, but also how much Aleisha hid from others and perhaps at times from herself.

After this session Aleisha began talking with Dr. C about her fear of "becoming" her mother. This involved many long discussions about Aleisha's childhood abuse, and her anger with her mother about not being more available and not protecting her. An important breakthrough occurred when she told Dr. C about a television talk show she had seen in which a number of adults had discussed their personal histories of sexual abuse as children. Aleisha was struck by a woman who had been raped 25 years before, but she was still talking about it with obvious pain. The night following the program, Aleisha had a traumatic dream about her own abuse. Dr. C asked Aleisha why she thought the people had discussed their abuse on the program. She said, "I think that they want to get it off their chest—reduce their burden." Dr. C asked if Aleisha ever thought about getting it off of her chest. Aleisha replied, "If I told my family, they would hate me. They wouldn't believe me. My mother wouldn't believe me. If she'd been a mother, it never would have happened." Dr. C pointed out her sadness about not being understood or believed. Aleisha responded, "Yeah. This one man on the show, he talked about just sitting around silent all the time. I know what that's like. I do that. Sometimes, my boyfriend touches me, and I just don't like it. I tell him I don't feel like it, but I can't tell him why." Aleisha said that if the painful memories ever troubled her when she was with her children, she forced herself to divert her attention away from them.

Following this session, Aleisha did talk to her mother about her own sexual abuse at the hands of one of the mother's boyfriends and about the rape at age 12. Aleisha seemed greatly relieved afterward that her mother not only believed her, but also had responded supportively. Dr. C noted a definite change in Aleisha's attitude about her mother that had grown slowly over the previous year and was increasingly apparent after this conversation. Aleisha made reference to her mother having done the best she could have during Aleisha's childhood, and later she acknowledged with insight and compassion that her mother's life had been hard. In addition, Dr. C noted that Aleisha now set firmer limits with her mother and with the rest of the extended family. This new peace made it possible for her mother to become more involved with Aleisha when she had her third child, Constance, a short time later. Notably, Aleisha decided to name Constance after Ms. D. Dr. C believed that Aleisha had become better able to allow her mother to be a part of her life without expecting too much from her. She seemed to have begun the important process of making peace with her mother's shortcomings for the first time in her life.

Although not the father of either Ellen or Antoine, Ronald became an important part of Aleisha's life several months after Dr. C met her. Dr. C had met Ronald on a few occasions and had been impressed by what she had heard about him from Aleisha. He was a responsible worker who held a full-time job, was fond of the children and spent time with each of them, and he took up for Aleisha in her ongoing squabbles with her extended family. Nevertheless, a dark side to Ronald and Aleisha's relationship would develop and then Dr. C would hear considerably more. Aleisha began to describe fights with Ronald. At first, these were verbal arguments, but they became more physical and Dr. C became more concerned. One day when Dr. C came for her weekly appointment she found the front door to Aleisha's apartment missing. Aleisha was sitting in the living room holding Constance, who was dozing. Dr. C asked what had happened. Aleisha was obviously shaken as she replied, "Ronald." She said that she had started to call Dr. C during the fight but that she had been afraid that Ronald would be sent to jail.

After this session, Aleisha and Ronald reconciled and agreed to meet with Dr. C as a couple. In the first couple session, they described a nonviolent argument the previous day in which Ronald had complained that Aleisha did not dress femininely enough. Aleisha wanted to make her own choices about dress. This introduced a theme that would continue about Ronald's efforts to control her. The final outcome of the couple sessions was that Aleisha and Ronald decided not to stay together, although he remained involved with the children. Dr. C was struck by

Aleisha's reaction to the breakup. When Ronald moved out, Antoine became quite distraught and he cried frequently if Ronald was even mentioned. He told his mother that he hated Ronald, but Aleisha responded to him compassionately nonetheless. She told Dr. C that she thought that Antoine's reaction was understandable, given that Ronald was the only father that he had ever known. Dr. C thought about how far Aleisha had come in being able to step out of her own struggles to consider Antoine's feelings and perspectives.

Termination Phase

The reason for the termination date was that Dr. C was pregnant and planning to take time off from clinical work. She discussed this with Aleisha on many occasions and noted that Aleisha expressed more regret than anger about the impending loss. Aleisha also indicated that Dr. C's taking time off for her children made sense to her. Dr. C felt that the termination was probably premature from the standpoint of Aleisha's needs, but she hoped that Aleisha's identification with her as a mother would sustain her nonetheless.

The final phase of treatment actually began soon after her breakup with Ronald, when Aleisha moved out of the apartment in which she had been surrounded by her extended family and relocated in another part of town. Dr. C thought, as she helped Aleisha pack and listened again to the rationale for the move, that it was a constructive effort by Aleisha to assert her independence. Aleisha recognized that she would continue to need to rely on her family for help in the future but that she did not need to be in their midst constantly to be involved with them. Further, she realized that she had allowed herself to be used as a doormat in many ways. She also acknowledged missing Ronald, but notably, she seemed more concerned about how Antoine and Ellen were handling it.

A new crisis ensued not long after the move. Aleisha was pregnant for the fourth time, and she was feeling fatigued and stressed by the demands of her children. At one of her prenatal visits she complained to a social worker, who called Dr. C to let her know about Aleisha's distress. Apparently, a visiting nurse called CPS because Aleisha said something about wanting to be "rid of" the kids. Dr. C knew from previous experiences that this was the kind of thing that Aleisha said when she was worn out, and she was not worried about the children's safety. She tried to communicate this to CPS, but for reasons that were never clear, the children were removed. As Dr. C advocated vigorously for the children's return, a new allegation emerged that Ronald had physically abused Ellen. It was never clear to Aleisha or to Dr. C who made this allegation and nothing was ever substantiated, but it resulted in the children spending 6 weeks in foster care before being returned to Aleisha. Aleisha used this time productively to strengthen her resolve, to declare her devotion to Ellen, Antoine, and Constance, and to fight to have them returned to her. In being apart from them and under threat, she realized in a new way how much they meant to her. She also laid claim to her children psychologically more deeply than she ever had before. At the same time, she had the leisure to focus on her pregnancy and to work through some of her ambivalent feelings about the anticipated baby.

Aleisha also reviewed with Dr. C their entire relationship together: what it had meant to her and what she had learned from it. Dr. C helped Aleisha list the concrete indicators of progress. Aleisha had signed up for and begun working diligently on her high school equivalence examination. She was a member of the Parents' Committee at Antoine's Head Start program. She was living on her own but had established good working relationships with a number of different programs. Most importantly, however, she felt better about herself, especially about herself as a mother. She was more sensitive and competent in her interactions with Antoine and with Ellen, and better able to appreciate their perspectives. She was also able to advocate for her children's educational and emotional needs. She also directly expressed to Dr. C how much she had meant to her.

In one of their final sessions, Dr. C arrived as Aleisha was wrapping up with a parent aid who had taken her on an errand. The aid, whom Dr. C had seen on a few other occasions, was laughing about how much Aleisha had been "jabbering." "I just couldn't shut her up!" she said teasingly. Aleisha replied, "Yeah, but I wasn't always that way. When I met Dr. C, I blew off our meetings for six weeks, but I still couldn't get rid of the girl. That's when I knew she really cared about me. Now, I don't know what I'm going to do without her."

DISCUSSION

Aleisha's story is one in which an intergenerational pattern of angry rejection, derogation, and disavowal of neediness was interrupted through a therapeutic relationship. We will first describe the pattern itself and then discuss the crucial features related to change.

The most striking manifestation of the intergenerational pattern we describe is derogation. Although there is an overriding devaluing coolness about attachment relationships as described by individuals classified as derogating, Main and Goldwyn (1994) also indicate that the derogating individual may be perceptive and passionate, and may even convey a continuing capacity for attachment. Clearly, the conflicted relationship between Aleisha and her mother and between Aleisha and Antoine were passionate and the passion underlying the conflicts may well have contributed to Aleisha's treatability. There were a number of examples of Aleisha's derogating descriptions of her mother as a "nobody" in the AAIs she completed, as well as in her therapy sessions with Dr. C. Interestingly, Aleisha's hurt from her relationship with her mother was always apparent to Dr. C, who understood Aleisha's derogation as a defense against her mother's shaming of her. Aleisha also reported many examples of her mother derogating her, and several others were witnessed by Dr. A in the original treatment. Most important of these was the incident in which Aleisha's mother referred to her as "nothing special."

In retrospect, we speculate that Aleisha's suicidal ideation was a manifestation of transgenerational identification with the aggressor. Aleisha's wish to die and to kill her baby was an identification with her mother's homicidal rage at her, which reenacted Ms. D's mother's homicidal rage at Ms. D when she became pregnant. Death wishes may represent the ultimate form of derogation. There was also interpersonal derogation apparent in Aleisha's interactions with her children, especially with Antoine. Although teasing was apparent with Antoine as early as the 10-month home visit, the openly derogating dismissal of him became apparent at the 15-month home visit in the hidden gum interchange, as she repeatedly shoved him away from her as he approached her. At 20 months, and again at 24 months, the full interactive pattern was evident. Aleisha first provoked Antoine through teasing and then by retaliating against him by swatting at him. Antoine responded by aggressively lashing out at Aleisha, seeming to overinterpret her every move as an attack. This is the essence of derogation: lashing out aggressively at others to lessen or weaken them. What is curious about this pattern in the case of Antoine and Aleisha, of course, is that Antoine was not even 2 years old when his mother began to act as if he were threatening to her (see Lieberman, Chapter 9, this volume, for treatment of maternal attributions), as when she protested that he was abusing her and feigned a defensive posture in their play interaction at 20 months. Aleisha's teasing of Antoine, which often initiated their conflicted interactions, served the function of provoking Antoine into aggressive and attacking behavior, which then justified both her perception of him as threatening and her derogation of him to weaken him and therefore to protect herself from the "threat" that he posed to her.

Galdston (1984), who linked teasing interactions to violence within families, has pointed out that the process has four identifiable stages: (1) the excitement of desire is stimulated by word or sight; (2) the incitement to action is elicited by one partner who offers his or her body as "bait" to be acted upon by the other; (3) the recipient is provoked to respond, in essence, "You asked for it," and (4) retaliation ensues. This pattern of teasing was evident in the interactions between Aleisha and Antoine, as well as in both interactional and representational levels of Aleisha's relationship with her mother. We suggest that teasing in the context of this relationship pattern simultaneously expresses contempt for the other as a manifestation of derogation, and it also provokes the other into aggressive behavior. By the latter part of Antoine's second year of life, Aleisha's aggression increasingly provoked counteraggressive responses from Antoine as a part of maintaining the interaction. Treatment intervened before Antoine had begun to initiate the interactive pattern himself, although our experience is that as children enter the third and especially the fourth years they are increasingly likely to initiate the aggressive interactions themselves. Such patterns might be described by the participants as "only playing," but the play is overly rough and developmentally inappropriate for the child, as demonstrated repeatedly in interactions between Antoine and Aleisha.

The defensive function of derogation is that a more conscious aggressive and dominating sense of self defends against a less conscious, helpless and vulnerable sense of self (Zeanah, 1993). In their study of play patterns among preschoolers, Troy and Sroufe (1987) found that only children with avoidant attachment classifications interacted with their peers as both victims and victimizers. It is likely that both victim and victimizer self-representations are present within the same dismissing/avoidant state of mind and that contextual factors play a role in which state of mind is most evident at a particular time. We suggest that this particular coexistence of contradictory self-representations characterizes the derogating/teasing relationship pattern, an example of what Bowlby (1973) described as multiple models of attachment.

The co-occurrence of a dominant, aggressive, and exploitative self-representation and a weak, helpless, and vulnerable self-representation in the same individual also was illustrated by Harmon, Wagonfeld, and Emde (1982). They described long-term outpatient psychotherapy of a school-aged child who had been diagnosed as having an anaclitic depression in his infancy. Two transference characters this boy created were a powerful, contemptuous, aggressive, and dominant character, known as "Cool Cat," and a weak, incompetent, and submissive character, known as "George" (which was the boy's given name). The boy and his behavior toward the therapist alternated between these two characters for some time during the treatment until Cool Cat eventually acknowledged his loneliness and soon thereafter disappeared from the sessions. George, like Aleisha, illustrates the self-representations which underlie the derogating/teasing pattern of relating.

Having identified the intergenerational pattern of derogation/teasing, the clinician must then decide how to intervene to interrupt it. The first principle of intervention in such cases is to anticipate that the derogation likely represents a reenactment of the parent's own childhood experiences and to search for links between past and present. Second, it is important to help the parent recognize not only the behavioral pattern of derogation and teasing, but also the affective and subjective experiences that accompany it. Once this has been accomplished it may be possible to help the parent appreciate the links between the here-and-now pattern with the baby and the old pattern from their own childhood. For the intergenerational pattern in this case to be interrupted, several other conditions were probably also necessary. First, Aleisha herself maintained an ability to reach out to others and to mobilize them, which kept large numbers of intervenors involved with her. The first apparent break in the intergenerational pattern was Aleisha's remaining aware (albeit it incompletely and inconsistently) of her own neediness. Although she maintained a gruff outward stance with others and often turned her attention away from her own distress and from others as potential sources of support, she never completely banished her own longing for closeness, and she made others aware of this at times. Clearly, it took some extraordinary therapeutic efforts to have her recognize these feelings in herself more fully, and especially to reveal this side of herself to others, but it seemed to have been implicitly palpable all along. This was a great strength, as it motivated many others who were interested in helping her to remain involved. Being aware of one's neediness and having the capacity to accept such neediness is also not what we would ordinarily expect from someone with a dismissing/avoidant state of mind with respect to attachment. Nevertheless, it is important to recall that infants and preschoolers classified as avoidant with their mothers have been shown to exhibit dependent behavior with their mothers at home (Ainsworth et al., 1978) and with their teachers at school (Sroufe, 1983). This suggests that disavowal of one's neediness may be variably evident in individuals with this relationship pattern.

Second, from a developmental perspective, Aleisha at 19 years old was no longer as emotionally involved with nor as instrumentally dependent upon her mother as she had been when Dr. A had met her as a 15-year-old. She made important strides, with the help of Dr. C, in deidealizing her mother and her father, an important task of adolescence. Interestingly, as she began to relinquish the internal image of the longed-for (perfectly gratifying) mother, she also became better able to maintain an adaptive amount of physical and psychological distance from her mother. When her daily interaction with her mother had diminished substantially, Aleisha was in a better position to address her internal representation of her mother. Most importantly, she came to imbue her mother with much less power, thereby obviating the need to derogate her and enabling her to view her mother in a more balanced manner.

Third, characteristics of Dr. C and of the treatment approach were also important. Fraiberg (1989) eloquently described the advantages of home-based interventions for infant–parent psychotherapy. Home visits to Aleisha communicated a powerful message about Dr. C's reaching out, and they meant that Dr. C assumed the burden of being on "foreign turf," which is no doubt how Aleisha had felt in a number of treatment settings herself. Dr. C also communicated her availability to Aleisha at an emotional level, leading eventually to Aleisha's relationship changes.

The establishment of a therapeutic alliance seemed to be facilitated by a number of factors. These included Dr. C's commitment and dependability, her interest in Aleisha as an individual, her helping Aleisha articulate her feelings about helpers, and her advocating for Aleisha with the social service system (which Aleisha had experienced only as an insensitive and impersonal bureaucracy). All of these factors must have gratified Aleisha's yearning to feel special, as she could not with her mother. Attachment theory has not always emphasized sufficiently the crucial importance of the child's feeling noticed and valued as a distinct individual by the attachment figure. The feeling of specialness that Dr. C conveyed to Aleisha, primarily through the nonspecific aspects of the psychotherapy, were probably crucial. In attachment terms, what Dr. C gave to Aleisha was an unwavering belief in Aleisha's value and an acceptance of her neediness. This, of course, enhanced Aleisha's belief in herself and facilitated in her a reasonable tolerance for her own imperfection. When she could accept vulnerability in herself, she had less need for defensive distortions such as derogation.

Dr. C's responding to Aleisha's derogation by the CPS worker also was especially crucial in retrospect. At the time, it could not have been clear to Dr. C that by siding with Aleisha and advocating constructively for her, Dr. C was introducing in a powerful way the possibility that change for Aleisha was possible and that her old feelings of being treated unfairly had some validity. It has long been a central premise of infant–parent psychotherapy that when a parent's own feelings of hurt and deprivation are identified, articulated, and linked to painful events, the parent may then be freer to respond more sensitively to his or her child (Fraiberg, 1989; Lieberman & Pawl, 1993). In conveying this understanding and acceptance of Aleisha, Dr. C gave the emotional support that countered the lessening, weakening, and impairing effects of derogation.

Having established the alliance, it was possible for change to occur both externally and internally for Aleisha with regard to her important relationships. The key issues were facing her father's fallibility more realistically, discussing her childhood sexual abuse with her mother, developing an appreciation for her mother's struggles, setting concrete limits on interaction with her extended family, and ending the violent relationship with Ronald. These changes made possible other changes related to revising models of her self as a woman, herself as a parent, and her children. These changes required accepting dependence within herself, seeing the world through the eyes of her children, and identifying with Dr. C as a mother. In a sense, each of these changes required giving up the contemptuous dismissal of herself, of her children, of motherhood, and of attachment relationships that had characterized the previous derogating/teasing pattern of relating.

This case illustrates one constellation of an intergenerational pattern of relationship psychopathology and its alteration through intensive infant–parent psychotherapy. It is worth noting in this regard that at least one investigation has demonstrated the positive benefits to the developing mother–infant relationship of this form of therapy (Lieberman, Weston, & Pawl, 1991). Clearly, more such investigations are needed to address the larger questions of how to change of intergenerationally transmitted patterns of disturbed and disordered attachments.

ACKNOWLEDGMENTS

The authors appreciate the helpful comments of Drs. Neil Boris, Michael Scheeringa, and Leslie Atkinson about an earlier version of this chapter.

REFERENCES

Ainsworth, M. D., Blehar, M. C., Waters, E., & Wall, S. (1978). *Patterns of attachment.* Hillsdale, NJ: Erlbaum.

Beck, A. T., Ward, C. H., Mendelson, M., Mock, J., & Erbaugh, J. (1961). *Archives of General Psychiatry, 4,* 561–569.

Bowlby, J. (1973). *Attachment: Vol. 2. Separation: Anxiety and danger.* New York: Basic Books.

Bowlby, J. (1980). *Attachment and loss: Vol. 3. Loss: Sadness and depression.* New York: Basic Books.

Bowlby, J. (1982). *Attachment and loss: Vol. 1. Attachment.* New York: Basic Books. (Original work published 1969)

Crowell, J. A., & Feldman, S. S. (1988). Mothers' internal working models of relationships and children's behavioral and developmental status: A study of mother–child interaction. *Child Development, 59,* 1273–1285.

Finley-Belgrad, E. (1994). Tales from training. *The Signal, 2,* 6–9.

Fraiberg, S. (1989). *Assessment and therapy of disturbances in infancy.* Northvale, NJ: Jason Aronson.

Freud, A. (1936). *The ego and the mechanisms of defense*. New York: International Universities Press.

Freud, S. (1920). Beyond the pleasure principle. In *The complete works of Sigmund Freud* (Vol. 18, pp. 7–64). London: Hogarth Press.

Galdston, R. (1984). Teasing as an inducer to violence. In J. Call, E. Galenson, & R. L. Tyson (Eds.), *Frontiers of infant psychiatry* (pp. 307–312). New York: Basic Books.

George, C., Kaplan, N., & Main, M. (1984). *The Adult Attachment Interview*. Unpublished manuscript, University of California at Berkeley.

Harmon, R. J., Wagonfeld, S., & Emde, R. N. (1982). Anaclitic depression: A follow-up from infancy to puberty. *Psychoanalytic Study of the Child, 37*, 67–94.

Lieberman, A. F., & Pawl, J. (1993). Infant–parent psychotherapy. In C. H. Zeanah (Ed.), *Handbook of infant mental health* (pp. 427–442). New York: Basic Books.

Lieberman, A. F., Weston, D. R., & Pawl, J. H. (1991). Preventive intervention and outcome with anxiously attached dyads. *Child Development, 62*, 199–209.

Main, M., & Goldwyn, R. (1994). *Adult Attachment Interview classification system: Version 6.0*. Unpublished manuscript, University of California at Berkeley.

Sroufe, L. A. (1983). Infant–caregiver attachment and patterns of adaptation in preschool: The roots of maladaptation and competence. In M. Perlmutter (Ed.), *Minnesota Symposia in Child Psychology* (Vol. 16, pp. 41–81). Hillsdale, NJ: Erlbaum.

Sroufe, L. A., & Fleeson, J. (1986). Attachment and the construction of relationships. In R. A. Hinde & J. Stevenson-Hinde (Eds.), *Relationships and development* (pp. 27–47). Hillsdale, NJ: Erlbaum.

Troy, M., & Sroufe, L. A. (1987). Victimization among preschoolers: Role of attachment relationship history. *Journal of the American Academy of Child and Adolescent Psychiatry, 26*, 166–172.

van IJzendoorn, M. (1995). Associations between adult attachment representations and parent–child attachment, parental responsiveness and clinical status: A meta-analysis on the predictive validity of the Adult Attachment Interview. *Psychological Bulletin, 117*, 387–403.

Zeanah, C. H. (1993). Subjectivity in infant–parent relationships: Contributions from attachment research. In S. C. Feinstein & R. C. Marohn (Eds.), *Adolescent psychiatry* (Vol. 19, pp. 121–136). Chicago: University of Chicago Press.

Zeanah, C. H., & Benoit, D. (1995). Clinical applications of a parent perception interview. In K. Minde (Ed.), *Infant psychiatry: Child and adolescent psychiatric clinics of North America* (Vol. 4, pp. 539–554). Philadelphia: W. B. Saunders.

Index